Ocular Surface Disease

Springer
*New York
Berlin
Heidelberg
Barcelona
Hong Kong
London
Milan
Paris
Singapore
Tokyo*

Ocular Surface Disease
Medical and Surgical Management

Edward J. Holland, MD

Clinical Professor of Ophthalmology
University of Cincinnati
Director of Cornea Services
Cincinnati Eye Institute
Cincinnati, Ohio

◆

Mark J. Mannis, MD, FACS

Professor and Vice-Chair
Director of Cornea, External Disease
and Refractive Surgery
Department of Ophthalmology
University of California, Davis
Sacramento, California

Illustrations by Nelva B. Richardson

With 201 Illustrations

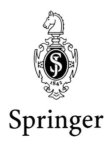

Springer

Edward J. Holland, MD
Director of Cornea Services
Cincinnati Eye Institute
and
Clinical Professor
University of Cincinnati
10494 Montgomery Road
Cincinnati, OH 45242
USA

Mark J. Mannis, MD, FACS
Professor and Vice Chairman
Director of Cornea, External Disease
 and Refractive Surgery
Department of Ophthalmology
University of California, Davis
4860 "Y" Street, Suite 2400
Sacramento, CA 95817
USA

Library of Congress Cataloging-in-Publication Data
Ocular surface disease: medical and surgical management / editors, Edward J. Holland,
 Mark J. Mannis.
    p. ; cm.
  Includes bibliographic references and index.
  ISBN 0-387-95161-X (h/c : alk. paper)
   1. Anterior segment (Eye)—Diseases.   2. Adnexa oculi—Diseases.   I. Holland, Edward J.
II. Mannis, Mark J.
   [DNLM: 1. Corneal Diseases—therapy.   2. Cornea—anatomy & histology.
3. Cornea—physiology.   WW 220 O21 2001]
RE334 .O26 2001
617.7'19—dc21   2001031419

Printed on acid-free paper.

Production managed by Lesley Poliner; manufacturing supervised by Jerome Basma.
Typeset by Matrix Publishing Services, Inc., York, PA.
Printed and bound by Maple-Vail Book Manufacturing Group, York, PA.
Printed in the United States of America.

9 8 7 6 5 4 3 2 1

ISBN 0-387-95161-X   SPIN 10785181

Springer-Verlag   New York Berlin Heidelberg
A member of BertelsmannSpringer Science+Business Media GmbH

◆

To our fellows
Whose hard work, long hours, and dedication to patient care
have allowed us the opportunity to help
the most challenging of ophthalmic patients.

◆

Preface

The evolution in our understanding of the anatomy and physiology of the ocular surface and the accompanying revolution in the management of ocular surface disease has been a process spanning at least three decades. Despite enormous advances in corneal transplantation, the advent of immunosuppressive therapy, and advances in contact lens physiology, ocular surface disease has remained a constant and often a confounding problem. Diseases of the ocular surface range from mild dry eye—one of the most common diagnoses in clinical practice—to the less common, but devastating and blinding, abnormalities that result from chemical and thermal injuries. Clinical advances notwithstanding, this broad range of diseases has remained a medical and surgical challenge.

Clarification of the role of the cellular components of the ocular surface and of the relation of these components to tear function, cell adhesion, and surface renewal has renewed interest in more effective and successful intervention in this group of problems. At this writing, even as we appreciate the demonstrated role of new classes of cells that renew the ocular surface, we are just beginning to learn about the chemical signals that drive the process of physiologic surface restoration. We stand at the verge of a wealth of new scientific and clinically useful information that will serve patients who, until now, had limited resources.

In this text, we have endeavored to provide a succinct but thorough overview of this emerging field. The anatomy and physiology of the ocular surface is detailed. Diseases of the ocular surface are described with special attention given to the disorders affecting ocular surface stem cells. A significant portion of the book is devoted to the medical and surgical management of these disorders.

Our goal was to produce a textbook that organizes what we currently know about the emerging field of ocular surface disease and transplantation, and to stimulate new ideas for the future. Recent advances have improved outcomes for patients with blinding corneal surface diseases. Many of these patients have regained useful vision, which was thought to be impossible as recently as 10 to 20 years ago. Other patients, however, remain refractory to current therapies. It is for these patients that we continue to strive for future breakthroughs, and it is our sincere hope that this textbook will assist clinicians, and ultimately our patients, in accomplishing better therapeutic outcomes.

EDWARD J. HOLLAND, MD
MARK J. MANNIS, MD
2001

Acknowledgments

Many individuals have contributed to this effort. First, we wish to thank our contributing authors, many of whom are the pioneers in the field of ocular surface disease. We asked the authors for a very rapid turnaround of their work. Despite busy schedules, all responded with timely and outstanding work.

We would especially like to thank Christy Rains, Executive Secretary in Cincinnati, who has overseen the entire project. Christy has masterfully kept track of all the text, illustrations, and timetables. Without her, the project would not have been possible. Likewise, we would like to thank Rita Snyder, who coordinated the effort in Sacramento.

Our appreciation is also extended to Merry Post, as well as to Nelva Richardson, a talented medical illustrator, who were forced into very tight work schedules and responded outstandingly. We would also like to thank Judy Mannis, who designed the book cover and who, more importantly, provided great support and acted as peacekeeper between the authors.

Finally, a very special thanks to Gary Schwartz, MD, who made significant scientific and editorial contributions to this project.

EDWARD J. HOLLAND, MD
MARK J. MANNIS, MD
2001

Contents

Contributors

CHRISTOPHER R. CROASDALE, MD
Davis Duehr Dean
Assistant Clinical Professor Ophthalmology
Department of Ophthalmology and Visual Sciences
University of Wisconsin, Madison
Madison, WI, 53792 USA

JASON K. DARLINGTON, MD
School of Medicine
University of California, Davis
4860 "Y" Street, Suite 2400
Sacramento, CA 95817, USA

SHERAZ M. DAYA, MD, FACP, FACS, FRCS (ED)
Director & Consultant
Corneo-Plastic Unit
Corneoplastic Unit, Queen Victoria Hospital NHS
  Trust
Holyte Road
East Grinstead, W. Sussex RH193DZ, UK

ALI R. DJALILIAN, MD
Senior Staff Fellow
National Eye Institute
10 Center Drive, Bldg 10
Bethesda, MD 20892, USA

HARMINDER S. DUA, MBBS, FRCS, MD, PhD
Chair and Professor of Ophthalmology
University of Nottingham
B Floor, South Block
University Hospital, Queens Medical Centre
Nottingham NG7 2UH, UK

GARY N. FOULKS, MD, FACS
Professor & Chairman of Department of
  Ophthalmology
University of Pittsburgh, School of Medicine,
203 Lothrop Street
Pittsburgh, PA 15213, USA

FREDERICK W. FRAUNFELDER, MD
Assistant Professor of Ophthalmology
Oregon Health Sciences University
Casey Eye Institute
3375 SW Terwilliger Blvd.
Portland, OR 97201, USA

JOSÉ A.P. GOMES, MD
Cicatricial Ocular Diseases Study Group
  Coordinator
External Diseases and Cornea Service
Federal University of São Paulo (UNIFESP/EPM)
São Paulo/SP, Brazil

EDWARD J. HOLLAND, MD
Director of Cornea Services
Cincinnati Eye Institute
Clinical Professor
University of Cincinnati
10494 Montgomery Road
Cincinnati, OH 45242, USA

R. RIVKAH ISSEROFF, MD
Professor of Dermatology,
Director of Tissue & Bioengineering Lab
University of California, Davis
Dermatology Department
One Shields Avenue, TB192
Davis, CA 95616, USA

B. ALYSE KHOSLA-GUPTA, MD
Duke University
Ophthalmology Department
9008 Lansdale Drive
Raleigh, NC 27617, USA

TERRY KIM, MD
Assistant Professor of Ophthalmology
Cornea and Refractive Surgery
Duke University Eye Center
Box 3802-Erwin Road
Durham, NC 27710, USA

FREDERICH E. KRUSE, MD
Professor of Ophthalmology
University of Heidelberg
Heidelberg, Germany

MARIAN S. MACSAI, MD
Chief Division of Ophthalmology, Evanston
    Northwestern Healthcare
Professor and Vice Chair Ophthalmology,
    Northwestern University
2050 Pfingsten Road, Suite 220
Evanston, IL 60025, USA

JACKIE V. MALLING, RN, CEBT
Technical Director
Minnesota Lions Eye Bank
420 Delaware St, SE MMC 493
Minneapolis, MN 55455, USA

MARK J. MANNIS, MD, FACS
Professor & Vice-Chair Department of Ophthalmology
Director of Cornea, External Disease & Refractive
    Surgery
University of California, Davis
4860 "Y" Street, Suite 2400
Sacramento, CA 95817, USA

Michael L. Nordlund, MD, PhD
University of Cincinnati &
Cincinnati Eye Institute
10494 Montgomery Road
Cincinnati, OH 45242, USA

Robert B. Nussenblatt, MD
Scientific Director
National Eye Institute
10 Center Drive, Bldg 10
Bethesda, MD 20892, USA

Stephen C. Pflugfelder, MD
Professor of Ophthalmology
Cullen Eye Institute, Baylor College of Medicine
6565 Fannin, NC 205
Houston, TX 77030, USA

Larry F. Rich, MS, MD
Professor of Ophthalmology
Director of Cornea Service & Refractive Surgery
Casey Eye Institute
Oregon Health Sciences University
3375 SW Terwilliger Blvd.
Portland, OR 97201, USA

IVAN R. SCHWAB, MD
Professor of Ophthalmology
Corneal, External Disease & Uveitis
University of California, Davis, Medical Center
4860 "Y" Street, Suite 2400
Sacramento, CA 95817, USA

GARY S. SCHWARTZ, MD
Clinical Assistant Professor
University of Minnesota
8650 Hudson Blvd., Suite 110
Lake Elmo, MN 55042, USA

ABRAHAM SOLOMON, MD
Cornea Fellow, Department of Ophthalmology
University of Miami, School of Medicine
900 NW 17th Street
Miami, FL 33136, USA

JOEL SUGAR, MD
Professor of Ophthalmology
Vice Chairman, Department of Ophthalmology
Director of Cornea Services
University of Illinois at Chicago
1855 W. Taylor
Chicago, IL 60612, USA

DONALD T.H. TAN, FRCS
Deputy Director, Singapore National Eye Centre
Associate Professor, National University of Singapore
11 Third Hospital Avenue
Singapore 168751, Singapore

Joseph Tauber, MD
Clinical Professor of Ophthalmology
Kansas University School of Medicine
Hunkeler Eye Centers
4321 Washington, Suite 6000
Kansas City, MO 64111, USA

Scheffer C. G. Tseng, MD, PhD
Charlotte Breyer Rodgers Chair Professor
Bascom Palmer Eye Institute
University of Miami School of Medicine
1638 NW 10th Avenue
Miami, FL 33136, USA

Kazuo Tsubota, MD
Professor of Ophthalmology
Tokyo Dental College
Ichikawa General Hospital
5-11-13 Sugano
Ichikawa, Chiba
272-8513 Japan

Part I

Introduction

1
Anatomy and Physiology of the Ocular Surface

Kazuo Tsubota, Scheffer C.G. Tseng, and Michael L. Nordlund

Introduction

The anatomical ocular surface is composed of the mucosa that lines the globe and palpebral surfaces, the corneoscleral limbus, the corneal epithelium, and the tear film. The anatomical ocular surface, however, is dependent on adjacent structures such as the anterior lamellae of the lids, the lashes and the lacrimal system for normal function. The role of the ocular surface is to maintain optical clarity of the cornea by regulating the hydration of the cornea and conjunctiva and to protect the globe from mechanical, toxic, and infectious trauma. Additionally, the ocular surface provides for free movement of the globe to assist in visual tracking. Several anatomical and physiologic specializations have evolved in the ocular surface and its adnexal tissues to facilitate their unique functions. In the event of a breakdown in the defense mechanisms, the ocular surface and adnexal tissues have developed unique repair responses that heal the injury with minimal effect on optical clarity. With chronic or severe damage, however, the ocular surface responds aggressively to ensure survival of the eye. Such vigorous responses can result in permanent distortion of the ocular surface anatomy and degradation of the optical clarity of the cornea. The normal structure and function of these tissues are described in this chapter.

Lid Anatomy and Function

The eyelids are unique structures that provide a movable mucosal lining that covers the entire ocular surface. Thus, the eyelids constitute the first line of defense of the ocular surface against dehydration and trauma. If anatomical or functional abnormalities of the lid are found, the first therapy in alleviating an associated ocular surface condition is to attempt to restore normal lid physiology.

Structurally, the eyelid is composed of seven layers (Figure 1.1).[1] Proceeding from the superficial surface, the layers are keratinized skin, eyelid protractors (orbicularis oculi muscles), orbital septum, orbital fat, eyelid retractors (levator muscle and aponeurosis and Müller's muscle), tarsus and conjunctiva. The region of the lids in apposition to the globe is primarily responsible for maintaining a healthy ocular surface and is the region most commonly involved in ocular surface pathology. Structurally, this portion of the lid begins where the orbital septum fuses with the levator aponeurosis a few millimeters superior to the tarsus in the upper lid. Thus, there is no orbital fat in the "functional" lid. The structure and function of the remaining six layers of the lid are described below.

Eyelid Skin

The skin on the eyelid, like most skin, is composed of a keratinized stratified squamous epithelium overlying a basement membrane and subcutaneous connective tissue.[2] It extends from the orbital rims to the mucocutaneous junction on the lid margin. The mucocutaneous junction is located immediately posterior to the tarsus and the meibomian gland orifices and demarcates the transition of the skin to mucosa. Eyelid skin is unique in that it contains no subcutaneous fat. The skin is firmly attached to underlying orbicularis muscle and connective tissue. This specialization makes the skin on the eyelid the thinnest skin on the body and allows it to accordion fold with minimal resistance during opening. An additional specialization of eyelid skin is the near absence of follicles in the pretarsal, preorbicularis and preseptal skin, and the presence of cilia near the lid margin. The 100 upper lid lashes and the 50 lower lid lashes exit just anterior to the tarsal plate and project anteriorly.[1] The upper lashes arch superiorly and the lower lashes arch inferiorly, which assists in catching and preventing small debris from depositing on the ocular surface.

Histology of the skin of the eyelid reveals an epidermis composed of keratinized stratified squamous ep-

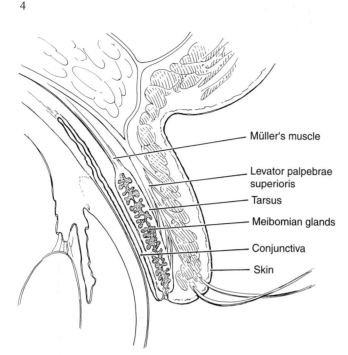

Figure 1.1. The lid and its components and their relation to the ocular surface. The anatomical ocular surface is bordered by the mucocutaneous junction of the lid margins and the caruncle. The palpebral conjunctiva lining the posterior surface of the lids constitutes a large percentage of the ocular surface. The adjacent anterior lamella of the eyelid provides a mechanical barrier to protect the ocular surface and contains the structures required to open and close the eyelid. Normal function of the eyelid is essential for maintenance of a stable tear film and a healthy ocular surface. Additionally, because of the immediate proximity of the anterior eyelid structures to the ocular surface, pathology of any of these structures can indirectly compromise the health of the ocular surface. This intimate relationship between the eyelid and the anatomical ocular surface constitutes the functional ocular surface.

ithelium that rests on a dense basement membrane (Figure 1.2).[2,3] Keratinocytes constitute the primary cellular component of the epidermis. These cells form four identifiable layers. The basal layer is a single row of proliferative keratinocytes. Daughter cells are displaced superficially and adopt a flatter polygonal shape and constitute the stratum spinosum or squamous layer. As these cells are further displaced toward the surface, they produce additional keratin, which aggregates into intracellular keratohyalin granules. The abundance of these granules defines the next layer of cells, called the stratum granulosum or granular layer. The external layer is the stratum corneum or horny layer, and is composed of granular keratinocytes that have adopted a flat morphology and lost their nuclei. Keratinization is a specialization of skin that restricts water loss and absorption and provides additional protection against mechanical insults.

The epidermis also contains two types of dendritic cells. Melanocytes produce the pigment melanin, which

is internalized by the keratinocytes and is responsible for the color of the skin. Langerhans cells are the second dendritic cell type and are antigen-presenting cells that assist in the initiation of the immune responses of the skin. The epithelium is attached to the basement membrane of the skin, which is predominantly composed of type IV collagen. The basement membrane is important for the integrity and adherence of the epithelium, and is a target of pathology in several dermatologic conditions, such as pemphigus. Deep to the basement membrane is subcutaneous connective tissue. In the eyelid, this layer is unique in that it contains no fat. As mentioned, this specialization makes the eyelid skin the thinnest on the body.[1]

The similarity of the skin of the eyelid to the skin of the body makes it susceptible to dermatologic conditions and many systemic diseases that are known to affect skin elsewhere on the body. Systemic diseases such as systemic lupus erythematosis, scleroderma and amyloidosis all can affect the skin of the eyelids.[4–6] Desquamating dermatologic conditions, such as epidermolysis bullosa and toxic epidermal necrolysis, have all been de-

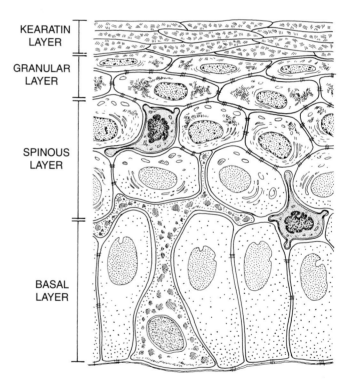

Figure 1.2. Epidermis and its cellular components. The differentiation of keratinocytes from proliferative basal cells into squamous cells, then granular cells, and finally into terminally differentiated cells of the stratum corneum, is diagrammed. The keratin layer prevents dehydration of the epidermis and provides an additional mechanical barrier to environmental insults. Also shown are the dendritic cells of the skin. Melanocytes are responsible for production of pigment, and the Langerhans cells are the antigen-presenting cells of the skin.

scribed to involve the lids.[7,8] Allergic conditions such as contact dermatitis are commonly observed in the ophthalmologist's office.[9] Skin tumors such as nevi, melanoma, basal cell carcinoma, squamous cell carcinoma and sebaceous cell carcinoma occur in the eyelids as well.[10] The number of skin diseases that can affect the lids is extensive and beyond the scope of this book.

Normal eyelid skin and lashes are essential for maintaining a healthy ocular surface. Dermatologic and systemic conditions that affect the skin, subcutaneous connective tissue or follicles can result in scarring and lid retraction and trichiasis. These conditions, in turn, can cause mechanical trauma to the ocular surface and can lead to exposure.

Eyelid Protractors

The orbicularis oculi muscles are responsible for proper closure of the lid during sleep and blinking. Additionally, the orbicularis muscle contributes to normal lid tension and the pumping of tears into the lacrimal sac. The muscle is oriented in a concentric fashion around the palpebral fissure and is anchored to the medial and lateral canthal tendons and the upper and lower tarsal plates. The orbicularis muscle functions in a sphincter-like fashion and induces closure of the lids with contraction. The muscle is divided into pretarsal, preseptal and orbital components. The pretarsal portion is primarily responsible for unconscious blinking, and the preseptal and orbital portions are primarily involved during voluntary closure.[1,3] The muscle is innervated by the seventh cranial nerve.

Dysfunction of the orbicularis oculi muscle may be manifest as lagophthalmos, as lower lid ectropion or laxity with mild or no lagophthalmos, or as a decreased blink rate or incomplete blink. Each of these conditions results in chronic ocular surface exposure. The many etiologies of orbicularis dysfunction can be classified by the site of pathology. Primary myopathies affect the orbicularis muscle. Disorders such as myasthenia gravis interrupt normal transmission across the neuromuscular junction. The seventh nerve innervates the orbicularis and is commonly compromised by compressive lesions, iatrogenic trauma, or inflammatory conditions like Bell's palsy. Central nervous system disorders can primarily affect the seventh nerve fascicles or nucleus, or result in decreased mentation resulting in poor blink rate or incomplete blink. Finally, excessive activity of the orbicularis is a different type of dysfunction and is found in benign essential blepharospasm and hemifacial spasm.

Eyelid Retractors

The levator palpebrae muscle and Müller's muscle are responsible for elevating the upper lids. The levator is the primary retractor and is under voluntary control via the third cranial nerve. The muscle arises from the an-

nulus of Zinn, courses anteriorly and 14–20 mm before inserting on the tarsus transitions to a connective tissue aponeurosis. The aponeurosis then condenses with other connective tissue to form Whitnall's ligament before continuing anteriorly where it divides into anterior and posterior lamellae. The anterior lamellae course throughout the orbicularis to insert on subcutaneous septa forming the lid crease. The posterior fibers insert on the anterior aspect of the tarsus approximately 2 mm above its inferior margin. The levator muscle is assisted by Müller's muscle, which is responsible for 1–2 mm of elevation of the upper lid. Müller's muscle originates from the underbelly of the levator, inserts on the superior border of the tarsus, and is regulated by the sympathetic nervous system. The lower lid retractors are less defined, but are comprised of slips of muscle extending from the inferior rectus muscle.

Dysfunction of the upper lid retractors can result from neurogenic, myogenic, aponeurotic, mechanical and traumatic mechanisms and is manifest as ptosis and dermatochalasis. Typically, these conditions do not adversely affect the ocular surface.[1] They are, however, common in the aging population and frequently require surgical correction because they are cosmetically disturbing, or interfere with the superior visual field. Surgical overcorrection of these conditions is a common etiology of lagophthalmos, and exposure keratopathy and can contribute to ocular surface pathology.[11] In contrast, disinsertion of the lower lid retractors releases the inferior tarsus, allowing it to invert. Disinsertion of the lower lid retractors is a common cause of lower lid entropion.[12,13] Surgical correction of entropion is required to prevent exposure keratopathy and mechanical trauma to the ocular surface through contact with inverted lashes and keratinized skin.

Tarsus

The tarsal plates are condensations of connective tissue that function as the skeleton of the upper and lower lid.[14] The vertical height of the tarsal plates is 10 mm and 4 mm for the upper and lower plates, respectively. Both run nearly the entire width of the lid and insert into the periosteum of the orbit medially and laterally. The plates serve as attachment sites for the levator, the orbicularis, and the orbital septum. The structural rigidity of the tarsal plates also provides resistance against inversion of the lid margins. Finally, the tarsal plates contain the meibomian glands that secrete lipid into the tear film. The lipid layer of the tear film has tremendous importance and functions as a surfactant to promote uniform distribution of the tear film and to retard evaporation of the aqueous tear film.[15,16] The meibomian glands are commonly affected in chronic inflammatory conditions such as blepharitis, acne rosacea, and ocular cicatricial pemphigoid. Chronic inflammation of the meibomian glands can lead to distichiasis and contribute to ocular surface pathology.

Conjunctival Anatomy and Function

The conjunctiva is an ectodermally derived mucosal epithelium that extends from the mucocutaneous junction of the eyelid margins to the corneoscleral limbus.[17] The surface area of the conjunctiva is greater than that of the palpebral and bulbar surfaces, and the excess forms multiple folds. The folds are most pronounced in the fornices, and function to allow movement of the globe. Medially, there is no fornix and the folding of the conjunctiva creates the plica semilunaris. At the corneoscleral limbus, the conjunctiva forms radial folds called the palisades of Vogt. Occasionally, debris can be trapped in the crypts of these folds.

The histologic structure of the conjunctiva is that of a stratified columnar or cuboidal nonkeratinized epithelium (Figure 1.3).[17] Columnar morphology is more commonly seen on the tarsal conjunctiva, and cuboidal epithelium is typically found on the palpebral and bulbar conjunctiva. The thickness of the epithelium varies regionally from 2–3 cell layers in the tarsal and forniceal conjunctiva to 6–9 layers in the bulbar conjunctiva. The epithelium also contains goblet cells. Goblet cells are large cells that constitute 5–10% of the cells in the conjunctival epithelium and produce mucin, a carbohydrate rich substance. The importance of mucin will be addressed in the discussion of the tear film. Goblet cells are found in greatest numbers on the inferonasal bulbar

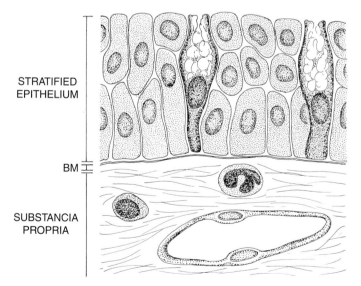

Figure 1.3. A schematic drawing of conjunctival epithelium showing the difference between stratified columnar and stratified cuboidal morphologies. Goblet cells are an important component of the conjunctival epithelium, and in combination with the epitheliocytes are responsible for mucin production and secretion.

conjunctiva and in the tarsal conjunctiva.[17,18] Recent studies have demonstrated the preferential location of conjunctival epithelial stem cells and proliferating goblet cells in the fornix; some stem cells are present in the bulbar and limbal conjunctiva.[19] The location of the stem cells in the fornix provides formidable protection of these cells from environmental hazards, and may explain why conjunctival epithelium is typically capable of regeneration following severe injuries. Further characterization of these cells is needed.

Ultrastructurally, the membranes of adjacent epithelial cells contain invaginations and outpouchings that create intercellular pockets where antibodies and inflammatory cells can accumulate.[17] The superficial location of these components of the immune system enables the conjunctiva to respond quickly to infections and trauma, but also makes it particularly sensitive to allergic and other immunologic pathology. The apical surface of the epitheliocytes has microvilli and secretes glycoproteins that form a thick glycocalyx.[20,21] The glycocalyx is highly negatively charged, and thus confers a hydrophilic state to the conjunctival surface. Functionally, the glycocalyx promotes even distribution of the tear film and decreases the adhesion of bacteria.

Underlying the epithelium is the basement membrane, which is primarily composed of type IV collagen.[22] Below the basement membrane is the substantia propria, a fibrovascular connective tissue that provides structural support and contains vasculature and immune cells. The substantia propria can be further divided into two layers. The superficial layer is loosely attached to the epithelium via connection to the basement membrane and contains lymphocytes and other immune cells.[17] The deeper layer is adherent to the episclera and contains vasculature from the anterior ciliary arteries and sensory nervous innervation from the ophthalmic division of the trigeminal nerve.

Dysfunction of the conjunctiva can be manifest as different conditions. In nutritional deficiency, or with chronic low grade inflammation, the conjunctiva responds with increased mucous secretion. With resolution of the inflammatory stimulus, the conjunctiva will revert to its normal state. With chronic inflammation, the conjunctiva undergoes a process of squamous metaplasia.[23,24] Squamous metaplasia is characterized by the development keratinization and loss of goblet cells with decreased mucous production. Loss of goblet cells results in an unstable tear film, and keratinization results in mechanical injury to the ocular surface. Mechanical injury and an unstable tear film result in inflammation that induces further damage to the conjunctiva and goblet cells. As a result, squamous metaplasia progresses and a vicious cycle ensues in which attempts to heal and protect a distorted conjunctival anatomy provide additional stimuli for the progression of the anatomical distortion. In treating ocular surface disease, it is impera-

The figure has labels: STRATIFIED EPITHELIUM, BM, SUBSTANCIA PROPRIA

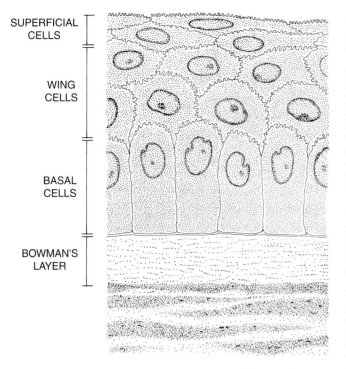

SUPERFICIAL CELLS

WING CELLS

BASAL CELLS

BOWMAN'S LAYER

Figure 1.4. A schematic drawing of corneal epithelium showing the differentiation of proliferative basal cells into wing cells, and finally into superficial cells. The absence of keratin makes the cornea particularly susceptible to dehydration. Maintenance of a stable tear film is the evolutionary solution to prevent dehydration. Also shown are the basement membrane, and Bowman's layer. The corneal epithelium contains no goblet cells.

tive to break this cycle to prevent permanent damage to the ocular surface. With progression of the cycle, or with severe injury or inflammation, the conjunctiva will be irreversibly damaged and scarring will occur. Scarring results in foreshortening or loss of the fornices, symblepharon, altered blink, ocular motility restriction, lagophthalmos and chronic exposure. Additionally, severe injuries often directly destroy the goblet cell population, resulting in an unstable tear film. The combination of an unstable tear film, chronic exposure and mechanical trauma associated with scarring and squamous metaplasia will ultimately result in irreversible keratinization, conjunctival overgrowth of the cornea, and corneal scarring.

Corneal Anatomy and Function

The cornea is the portal through which visual information from the environment enters the eye. As such, it is a highly specialized optical tissue that must maintain transparency to visible light, regularly refract visible light and resist adverse external forces such as dehydration, microbial invasion and trauma. It is the primary tissue that the ocular surface has evolved to protect. Structurally, the cornea is an avascular tissue consisting

of five layers: the epithelium, Bowman's layer, the stroma, Descemet's membrane and the corneal endothelium (Figure 1.5). Over 90% of the cornea is composed of stroma.[25,26] The stroma is relatively paucicellular and is predominantly composed of extracellular type 1 collagen. The collagen fibrils are uniform is size and spacing, a specialization that allows the transmission of visible light.[27] In a simplified description, the endothelium and Descemet's membrane regulate the hydration status of the stroma, and the epithelium and Bowman's layer provide protection against the environment.

A normal corneal surface is crucial to its function. The corneal epithelium is a nonkeratinized, stratified squamous epithelium approximately 5–7 cells thick.[25] Microscopically, it consists of a monolayer of columnar basal cells which are adherent to a basement membrane. The basement membrane of the corneal epithelium is attached to Bowman's layer—a condensation of type 1 and 3 collagen that is approximately 12 microns thick. Traditionally, it was thought that Bowman's layer was important to maintain normal anatomy and physiology of the corneal epithelium. However, Bowman's layer does not regenerate following injury and many patients continue to have normal corneal epithelium following ablation of the layer in photorefractive surgery.[28,29] Thus, its function remains to be elucidated.

As in skin, the basal epithelial cells are mitotic cells and give rise to daughter cells that differentiate as they migrate toward the surface. The immediate descendants of basal cells are wing cells, which derive their name from characteristic wing-like processes. These cells possess numerous gap junctions, intercellular interdigitations, and desmosomes important in nutritional and structural support.[30,31] Wing cells subsequently flatten to 2–6 microns thick and develop a polygonal morphology as they differentiate into the superficial cells of the corneal epithelium. Unlike skin, however, the superficial cells possess little keratin and do not further differentiate into a keratinized layer. The absence of keratinization makes the surface particularly susceptible to dehydration and trauma. As seen in conjunctival epithelium, the superficial cells possess many surface microvilli and secrete abundant glycoprotein that forms a rich glycocalyx.[32,33] These specializations increase the surface area for oxygen diffusion into the avascular cornea and improve the surface hydrophilicity, and, thus, tear film distribution. Superficial cells ultimately undergo apoptosis and are sloughed into the tear film.[34,35]

Limbus and Stem Cell Anatomy and Function

The limbus is the anatomical transition of sclera and conjunctival epithelium into cornea and is believed to be the location of the epithelial stem cells of the cornea.

At the limbus, the stratified columnar conjunctival epithelium moves to the stratified squamous epithelium of the cornea, and the vascular substantia propria of the conjunctival epithelium ends in a rich vascular limbal plexus. The vascular plexus is believed to be important in providing nutrients and oxygen to the mitotically active limbal stem cells. Additionally, the limbus may function to restrict conjunctival cells from the corneal epithelium.

The stem cell population responsible for repopulation of the corneal epithelium remains poorly described. Early studies documented a centripetal movement of corneal epithelial cells from the limbus to the central cornea, suggesting that proliferating precursor cells were present at the limbus.[36] The concept of limbal-based stem cells was further supported by the observation that it was impossible to create permanent corneal epithelial defects in laboratory animals without damaging the limbus.[37] Finally, it had long been realized that circumferential damage of the limbus, or damage of a portion of the limbus, produced a varying extent of conjunctival epithelial ingrowth.[38–40] The observed changes were characterized by vascularization, chronic inflammation, poor epithelial integrity as manifested by an irregular surface, recurrent erosion, or persistent epithelial defect, destruction of basement membrane and fibrous ingrowth. These changes are now known to result from limbal stem cell deficiency and together constitute the hallmark clinical features used to identify stem cell insufficiency.

Identification of limbal stem cells has been difficult. That a mitotic cell population resides at the limbus has been demonstrated.[41] Additionally, it has been shown that these mitotic cells do not express the keratin markers seen in all other corneal epitheliocytes.[42] The absence of this marker of differentiation of corneal epithelium in this mitotic subset of cells is consistent with the classic understanding of pluripotential undifferentiated stem cells proliferating to produce daughter cells that demonstrate progressive differentiation. Additionally, the monoclonal marker 4G10.3 has been demonstrated to stain a subset of mitotic basal limbal cells in the rat.[43,44] In models of thermal or mechanical injury to the rat cornea, 4G10.3-positive cells dramatically increase in number during the reparative phase of the injury. Unfortunately, a marker clearly identifying stem cells has not been identified in humans. The success of replenishing normal human corneal epithelium with transplantation of limbal tissue, or with transplantation of cells harvested from the limbus and expanded in vitro, clearly confirms the presence of stem cells in the human limbus.[45–52] Together, these data strongly suggest a limbal location of the stem cells of the corneal epithelium.

The current model of stem cell differentiation and function is that corneal epithelial stem cells are located in the basal limbus. Stem cells can differentiate down two pathways (Figure 1.5).[53] Along one pathway, differentiating stem cells function to repopulate the corneal epithelium. This process begins with the centripetal horizontal movement of stem cells onto the cornea as they

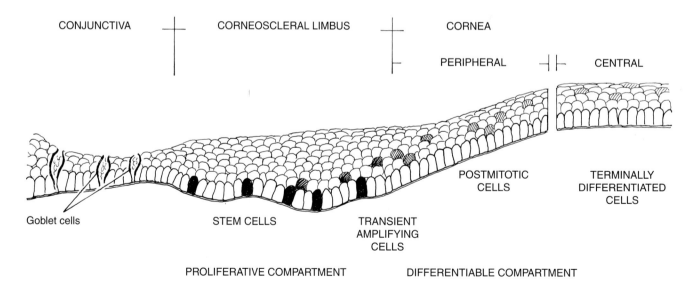

Figure 1.5. The location of corneal epithelial stem cells at the corneoscleral limbus. A fraction of the basal epithelial cells at the limbus are stem cells (SC) for the corneal epithelium. Stem cell differentiation can occur via two pathways. Differentiating stem cells that move centripetally onto the cornea become transient amplifying cells (TAC). These cells, located in the basal layer of the cornea, proliferate and differentiate into the postmitotic cells (PMC) of the suprabasal corneal epithelium. Further differentiation of PMC results in the terminally differentiated cells (TDC) of the superficial corneal epithelium. Alternatively, stem cells can differentiate and migrate superficially. This process is believed to be important in establishing a barrier to separate the conjunctiva and cornea.

differentiate into transient amplifying cells. Transient amplifying cells constitute the basal layer of the cornea and proliferate and differentiate into the postmitotic cells of the suprabasal corneal epithelium. The postmitotic cells are identifiable as wing cells on histologic sections. Further differentiation of the postmitotic cells results in the terminally differentiated cells of the superficial corneal epithelium. The second pathway of stem cell differentiation results from vertical migration of the stem cells as they differentiate. Little is known about the specifics of this process, but it is believed to be important in establishing a barrier to separate the conjunctiva and cornea.

The importance of the stem cells of the corneal epithelium has only been appreciated in the past decade, and this recent understanding has led to the development of surgical procedures to transplant healthy stem cells. Prior to stem cell transplantation, penetrating keratoplasty was commonly performed in patients with limbal stem cell deficiency, and these grafts universally failed.[54,55] It is now clear that healthy stem cells are required to maintain a normal corneal epithelium, and to prevent overgrowth of the cornea by conjunctival epithelium. Conditions that can adversely affect the health of the stem cells include chemical and thermal injuries, cryotherapy or multiple surgeries involving the limbus, chronic contact lens wear, erythema multiforme major (Stevens–Johnson syndrome), or severe microbial infection (Table 1.1). These conditions directly damage the stem cells and constitute one class of causes of stem cell deficiency. A second group of diseases are those in which there is gradual loss of limbal stem cells without an identifiable mechanism of the injury. Examples of these diseases are aniridia, keratitis associated with multiple endocrine deficiencies, neurotrophic keratopathy, and pterygium/pseudopterygium. Table 1.1 classifies conditions of stem cell loss based on etiology. The right-hand column lists the number of patients with each condition. As mentioned, the pathogenesis of stem cell loss

in these conditions is unknown, but the absence of obvious direct injury to the stem cells suggests that humoral, neuronal, vascular, and inflammatory factors may be important regulators of the stem cell environment. Disruption of one or more of the factors may alter the stem cell environment and result in stem cell loss. Consistent with this theory is the demonstration that several growth factors and cytokines may be important in the regulation of stem cell and stromal fibroblast proliferation.[56] Further characterization of stem cells and their environment may provide insight into the pathogenesis of stem cell loss, and therapies to prevent it.

Tear Film Anatomy and Function

A stable tear film is a prerequisite to good vision, and its maintenance is a complicated process (Figure 1.6). The structural roles of the tear film are to provide a smooth uniform refractive surface, to lubricate the ocular surface, and thus to facilitate comfortable movement of the lids while minimizing mechanical trauma. Additionally, however, the tear film is an integral component of ocular surface defense against microbial invasion and environmental trauma, and it provides trophic support to the cells of the ocular surface (Table 1.2).[57–66] The tear film is composed of mucin secreted from conjunctival goblet cells and epithelium, aqueous tears secreted by the lacrimal glands, and lipids secreted by the meibomian glands.[20,21] The three components combine to form a trilaminar structure (Figure 1.7).[67] Mucin forms the layer most proximal to the corneal surface and directly interacts with the conjunctival glycocalyx, providing a hydrophilic layer upon which aqueous tears layer.[21] The hydrophilic nature of the mucin promotes even distribution of the aqueous tears. The aqueous surface is then covered by lipid secreted from meibomian glands.[15] The lipid layer is essential to retard evaporation and prevent early breakup of the tear film. The trilaminar structure

Table 1.1. Corneal diseases with limbal deficiency.

	No. of Patients
Category 1 Aplasia: Total Loss of Stem Cells due to Primary Destruction	**53**
Chemical/thermal injuries	34
Stevens–Johnson syndrome	7
Multiple surgeries or cryotherapies of the limbal region	4
Contact-lens-induced keratopathy	5
Severe microbial keratitis	3
Category 2 Hypofunction: Gradual Loss of Stem Cell Function	**41**
Aniridia (hereditary)	13
Keratitis associated with multiple endocrine deficiencies (hereditary)	2
Neurotrophic keratopathy (neuronal or ischemic)	13
Peripheral inflammatory disorders and chronic limbitis	5
Idiopathic	8
TOTAL	94

Figure 1.6. The complexity of maintaining a stable tear film. Production and secretion of tear components, redistribution of the tears through blinking, and drainage of tears must be precisely regulated. Disruption of any of the components of this complicated regulatory cycle can result in tear film instability and the associated symptoms of injection, irritation, and blurred vision. The challenge to the clinician is to define the dysfunction of the tear film, and to re-establish normal or nearly normal tear film anatomy and function.

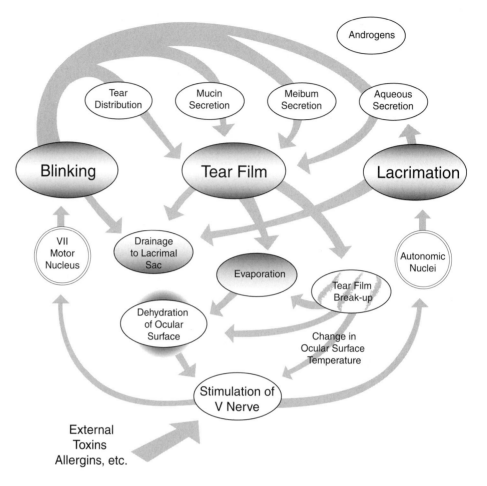

provides stability that allows the eye to remain open from 10–200 seconds without disruption of the tear film in normal individuals.[68–70] Patients with disorders of mucin or of meibomian gland secretion have markedly reduced tear stability, which results in discomfort and blurred vision.[71,72] As discussed, blinking redistributes a fresh tear film on the ocular surface approximately every 5–6 seconds.[73]

New evidence suggests that the conventional trilaminar model of the tear film may not be correct. Laser inferometry has demonstrated that the mucin layer is more evenly distributed throughout the entire thickness of the tear film.[74] Additionally, ultrastructural analysis using in vivo cryofixation has failed to demonstrate a pure aqueous layer.[75] These new data are intriguing and may change our concepts of how the components of the tear film interact.

Tear film insufficiency can occur as a result of deficiency of any one of the three components, and is the hallmark finding in patients with tear film instability. Symptomatically, patients with tear film insufficiency experience foreign-body sensation, redness and blurred vision. The most widely recognized abnormality of the tear film is aqueous tear deficiency that results in keratitis sicca. Age-related decreases in tear production and autoimmune diseases such as Sjögren's syndrome or rheumatoid arthritis are common etiologies of keratitis sicca. The Schirmer test can be performed easily in the office and is typically reduced in these patients. In contrast, patients with mucin deficiency or meibomian gland dysfunction have normal aqueous tear production. These patients can be identified with the simple clinical test of tear breakup time. Typically, patients with meibomian gland disease or mucin deficiency demonstrate a tear breakup time of less than 10 seconds.[76] Patients with meibomian gland disease also have increased tear evaporation and high tear osmolality.[77,78]

Lacrimal System

Ocular tear film stability is dependent on the maintenance of the precise ratio of the three components. Excess or deficiency of any of the components compromises tear film stability. Although little is known about the regulation of meibomian gland and goblet cell function,[79,80] aqueous tear secretion is a precisely regulated and complicated process. The lacrimal gland is a specialized sebaceous gland located superotemporal to the

Table 1.2. Components of tear and serum.

Components	Concentration	
	Tear (Basal)	Serum[a]
PROTEINS		
Total protein	7.37 gm/liter	68–82 gm/liter
Lysozyme	2.39 gm/liter	4.0–15 mg/liter
Lactoferrin	1.51 gm/liter	ND
Albumin	54 mg/liter	35–55 gm/liter
IgA	411 mg/liter	0.9–4.5 gm/liter
IgD	ND	3.0–300 mg/liter
IgE	ND	0.25–0.7 mg/liter
IgG	32 mg/liter	8–18 gm/liter
IgM	ND	0.37–2.8 gm/liter
CuZn-SOD	103 ng/mg protein	ND[c]
GROWTH FACTORS		
EGF	1.66 ng/ml	0.72 ng/ml
TGF-α (males)	247 pg/ml	147 pg/ml
TGF-α (females)	180 pg/ml	(males & females)
TGF-β1	ND	140.3 ng/ml
TGF-β1[b]	2.32 ng/ml	
TGF-β2	55 pg/nl	
VITAMIN		
Vitamin A	16 ng/ml	883 ng/ml
Vitamin C	117 μg/ml	7–20 μg/ml
ANTIOXIDANT		
Tyrosine	45 μM	77 μM
Glutathione	107 μM	ND[c]
CARBOHYDRATE		
Glucose	26 mg/l	0.6–1.2 gm/liter
ELECTROLYTES		
Na^+	145 mEq/l	135–146 mEq/liter
K^+	24.1 mEq/1	3.5–5.0 mEq/liter
Ca^{2+}	1.5 mM	1.1 mM
Cl^-	128 mM	96–108 mM
HCO_3^-	26 mM	21–29 mM
NO_3^-	0.14 mM	0.19 mM
PO_4^{3-}	0.22 mM	1.42 mM
SO_4^{2-}	0.39 mM	0.53 mM

CuZn-SOD = Cu,Zn super-oxide dismutase; EGF = epidermal growth factor; TGF = transforming growth factor; ND = not detected

[a] Each value is the normal concentration in serum

[b] Acid activated tear

[c] These components are present in red blood cells at high concentration

globe. It secretes tears through ducts emptying into the superior temporal fornix in response to parasympathetic stimulation via the seventh cranial nerve. The accessory lacrimal glands of Krause and Wolfring are located in the superior fornix and have no known neuronal innervation. Basal tear secretion from the accessory glands provides tears to the superior fornix and the tears are redistributed to the ocular tear film by blinking. In contrast, the main lacrimal glands are thought to be responsible for reflex tearing. The tearing reflex is triggered by irritation of the ocular surface, which is transmitted via the trigeminal nerve to the trigeminal sensory nucleus, and to the autonomic nuclei.[81,82] Parasympathetic fibers leaving the autonomic nuclei

travel along the facial nerve to the lacrimal gland, where they stimulate tear secretion. Emotional stimuli can also trigger reflex tearing.[82] Reflex tearing results in secretion of a relatively large volume of tears, which is important in flushing and diluting foreign materials such as debris, allergens and toxins from the ocular surface.

Traditionally, reflex tearing had not been thought to be important in the basal secretion of aqueous tears. This hypothesis has been challenged by the finding that tear production is significantly diminished in conditions of decreased corneal sensitivity. For example, decreased tear secretion has been documented during sleep, with general and local anesthesia, and in neurotrophic keratitis.[83–85] This finding suggests that normal corneal sensitivity is necessary for maintenance of normal tear secretion, and thus reflex tearing is an important component of basal tearing. A role for reflex tearing in the minute-to-minute regulation of tear secretion would explain the high prevalence of dry eye seen clinically in conditions with decreased corneal sensitivity.

Regulation of tear secretion may be even more complicated. It has recently been shown that anesthesia of the nasal mucosa results in decreased tear secretion.[86] The significance of this finding remains to be determined, but it may indicate that the structures other than the ocular surface that are innervated by the trigeminal nerve may contribute to the regulation of reflex, and

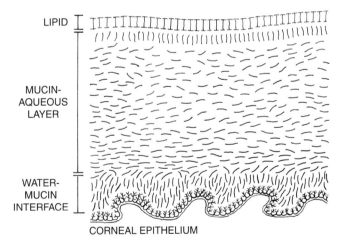

LIPID

MUCIN-AQUEOUS LAYER

WATER-MUCIN INTERFACE

CORNEAL EPITHELIUM

Figure 1.7. A schematic drawing of the tear film and its components. Shown are the production and secretion of mucin by corneal and conjunctival epitheliocytes to produce a mucin-rich glycocalyx. The glycocalyx interacts with mucin secreted by goblet cells. The mucin layer imparts a hydrophilic quality to the cell surface, facilitating even distribution of the overlying aqueous tear layer. Lipids provided by the meibomian glands of the lids constitute the third layer of the tear film and function to retard evaporation of the aqueous layer. A stable tear film is essential for a smooth optical surface, and to prevent dehydration of the cornea.

thus basal tearing. For example, irritation of the eyelashes or the skin on the eyelids may help drive tear secretion.

Blinking

Stability of the ocular tear film requires not only the appropriate mixture of its constituents, but also normal blinking. Blinking redistributes the tear film in a uniform layer, promotes secretion of tears from the accessory tear glands, and pumps excess tears into the lacrimal sac.[89,90] The normal blink rate is approximately 6 hertz.[73] The rate is dramatically increased in normal individuals under conditions of increased evaporation such as windy and dry conditions. Interestingly, the blink rate is reduced with visual activities requiring focused concentration, such as with computer work, driving and reading.[89] Some studies have documented a reduction of 50 percent in these situations.

Control of blinking is regulated by multiple inputs. Blinking can be induced by pain or touch of the ocular surface and transmitted via the fifth cranial nerve, or by light stimuli via the optic nerve.[90] The stimulus is transmitted to the trigeminal sensory nucleus and other supranuclear regions, where it is processed.[91] The efferent stimulus to blink is carried to the pretarsal orbicularis muscle by the zygomatic branch of the seventh nerve. Abnormalities of the fifth cranial nerve, as seen following Herpes simplex or Varicella zoster infections, can prevent conduction of the sensory stimulus to the brain stem and decrease blink rate, or cause incomplete blinking. Similarly, disruption of the condition of the efferent impulse via the seventh cranial nerve as seen in Bell's palsy can alter normal blinking. Finally, any cause of generalized dysfunction of the central nervous system with decreased mentation can disrupt the blink reflex.

While incomplete and infrequent blinking are the primary abnormalities of blinking, excess blinking can occur and cause ocular surface pathology. Blepharospasm is a condition characterized by involuntary overactivity of the orbicularis. The resultant increased blink rate and lid tension may cause microtrauma and mechanical disruption of the ocular surface. Similarly, normal blinking can induce microtrauma in the dry eye as a result of increased friction between the lid and the bulbar conjunctiva. This process is thought to contribute to the pathology of superior limbic keratoconjunctivitis.[92]

The sensory stimulus primarily responsible for the basal regulation of blinking in the absence of noxious stimuli has not been identified. Recent evidence using infrared radiation thermometry, or high-speed and high-resolution thermography, suggest that the change in corneal temperature that occurs with the early breakup of the tear film may be the basic stimulus.[93,94] It has been hypothesized that, in patients with an unstable tear film, temperature changes associated with tear breakup may not be sufficient to induce blinking, and thus blink rates may actually be reduced in severely affected patients.[95] Thus, the pathogenesis of conditions associated with ocular tear film instability may be not only a result of exposure of the ocular surface from early tear breakup, but also a result of exposure from incomplete and infrequent blinking.

Tear Dynamics

The ocular tear film is a transient and dynamic structure. To maintain the health of the ocular surface, the tear film must be continually cleared and replaced. The rate of removal of newly produced tears is called tear clearance, and it is regulated by the rate of production of new tear components, the dynamics of tear redistribution on the ocular surface through the action of blinking, and the rate of drainage of old tears into the nasolacrimal sac. An important implication of this model is that clearance of tears is dependent not only on the pumping of tears into the nasolacrimal sac by blinking, but also on the production of new tears. Thus, patients with dry eyes and poor tear secretion have decreased tear clearance. Tear clearance can be measured by fluorophotometry, and this technology has documented a significant reduction in tear clearance in dry-eye patients.[96,97] An alternative method for evaluating tear clearance in the clinic is to place fluorescein in the eye as a tracer and to use serial Schirmer test strips to determine the time for clearance of the fluorescein. Measurements using this method are consistent with those obtained by fluorophotometry.[98,99] The simplicity and low cost of this method make it a readily available tool for every ophthalmologist. Clinically, testing of tear clearance is useful to accurately diagnose dry eyes, distinguishing Sjögren's-type dry eye from non-Sjögren's type, and distinguishing aqueous tear deficiency from lipid tear deficiency. The significance of a reduction in tear clearance is that inflammatory cytokines in the tear film or preservatives or other chemicals in topical medications are not diluted or cleared as quickly. As a result, these compounds are present in increased concentrations and have prolonged exposure to the ocular surface. This may explain the increased sensitivity of the dry eye to environmental, host and iatrogenic compounds. A better understanding of tear clearance and the dynamics of tear secretion, distribution and evaporation is important in developing better therapies for ocular surface and tear disorders.

Summary

The ocular surface is a complex structure dependent on the successful integration of multiple tissues to maintain its health and normal visual function. As our understanding of this important structure has improved, we have developed new therapies for many blinding and disabling conditions that were previously untreatable. Further understanding of the normal anatomy and physiology of the ocular surface, and the pathogenesis of its dysfunction in disease, is needed to continue our progress in this exciting field.

References

1. Kersten R et al. Orbit, Eyelids and Lacrimal System, in *Basic and Clinical Science Course*, K Hecht et al., editors. 2000, The Foundation of the American Academy of Ophthalmology: San Francisco, p. 122–131.

2. Font R. Eyelids and lacrimal drainage system. *Ophthalmic Pathology*, ed. Spencer WH. Vol. 3. 1986, Philadelphia: WB Saunders. 241–336.

3. Wolfley DE. Eyelids. *Cornea*, ed. J Krachmer, M Mannis, and E Holland. 1997, St. Louis: Mosby.

4. Kearns W, Wood W, Marchese A. Chronic cutaneous lupus involving the eyelid. *Ann Ophthalmol* 1982; 14(11): 1009–10.

5. Krieg T, Meurer M. Systemic scleroderma. Clinical and pathophysiologic aspects. *J Am Acad Dermatol* 1988; 18(3): 457–81.

6. Breathnach SM. Amyloid and amyloidosis. *J Am Acad Dermatol*. 1988; 18(1 Pt 1):1–16. Review.

7. McDonnell PJ, S.O.M.S.D.J.E.R.A. Eye involvement in junctional epidermolysis bullosa. *Arch Ophthalmol* 1989; 107(11):1635–7.

8. Gans LA. Eye lesions of epidermolysis bullosa. Clinical features, management, and prognosis. *Arch Dermatol* 1988; 124(5):762–4.

9. Nethercott JR, Nield G, Holness DL. A review of 79 cases of eyelid dermatitis. *J Am Acad Dermatol* 1989; 21(2 Pt 1):233–30.

10. Loeffler M, Hornblass A. Characteristics and behavior of eyelid carcinoma (basal cell, squamous, cell sebaceous gland, and malignant melanoma). *Ophthalmic Surg* 1990; 21(7):513–8.

11. Lowry JC, Bartley GB. Complications of blepharoplasty. *Surg Ophthalmol* 1994; 38(4):327–50.

12. Bashour M, Harvey J. Causes of involutional ectropion and entropion—age-related tarsal changes are the key. *Ophthal Plast Reconstr Surg* 2000; 16(2):131–41.

13. Schaefer AJ. Variation in the pathophysiology of involutional entropion and its treatment. *Ophthalmic Surg* 1983; 14(8):653–655.

14. Maus M. Basic Eyelid Anatomy. 1 ed. *Principles and Practice of Ophthalmology* ed. D Albert and F Jakobiec. Vol. 3. 1994, Philadelphia: WB Saunders. 1689–1692.

15. Tiffany JM. The role of meibomian secretion in the tears. *Trans Ophthalmol Soc U K* 1985; 104(Pt 4):396–401.

16. Bron AJ, Tiffany JM. The meibomian glands and tear film lipids. Structure, function, and control. *Adv Exp Med Biol* 1998; 438:281–95.

17. Nelson J, Cameron J. The Conjunctiva. 1 ed. *Cornea*, ed. J Krachmer, M Mannis, and E Holland. Vol. 1. 1997, St. Louis: Mosby. 41–47.

18. Ralph RA. Conjunctival goblet cell density in normal subjects and in dry eye syndromes. *Invest Ophthalmol* 1975; 14(4):299–302.

19. Wei ZG et al. Label-retaining cells are preferentially located in fornical epithelium: implications on conjunctival epithelial homeostasis. *Invest Ophthalmol Vis Sci* 1995; 36(1):236–46.

20. Dilly PN, Mackie IA. Surface changes in the anaesthetic conjunctiva in man, with special reference to the production of mucous from a non-goblet-cell source. *Br J Ophthalmol* 1981; 65(12):833–42.

21. Dilly PN. Contribution of the epithelium to the stability of the tear film. *Trans Ophthalmol Soc U K* 1985; 104(Pt 4): 381–9.

22. Foster CS et al. Conjunctival epithelial basement membrane zone immunohistology: normal and inflamed conjunctiva. *Int Ophthalmol Clin* 1994; 34(3):209–14.

23. Nelson JD, Havener VR, Cameron JD. Cellulose acetate impressions of the ocular surface. Dry eye states. *Arch Ophthalmol* 1983; 101(12):1869–72.

24. Tseng SC. Staging of conjunctival squamous metaplasia by impression cytology. *Ophthalmology* 1985; 92(6):728–33.

25. Nishida T. Cornea. 1 ed. *Cornea*, ed. J Krachmer, M Mannis, and E Holland. Vol. 1. 1997, St. Louis: Mosby. 2253.

26. Hogan M, Alvarado J, Weddell J. *Histology of the human eye*. 1971, Philadelphia: WB Saunders.

27. Maurice D. The cornea and sclera. 3 ed. *The Eye*, ed. H Davison. Vol. 1B. 1984, Orlando: Academic Press.

28. Goodman GL et al. Corneal healing following laser refractive keratectomy. *Arch Ophthalmol* 1989; 107(12):1799–803.

29. Marshall J et al. Long-term healing of the central cornea after photorefractive keratectomy using an excimer laser. *Ophthalmology* 1988; 95(10):1411–21.

30. Suzuki K et al. Coordinated reassembly of the basement membrane and junctional proteins during corneal epithelial wound healing. *Invest Ophthalmol Vis Sci* 2000; 41(9): 2495–500.

31. Barry PA et al. The spatial organization of corneal endothelial cytoskeletal proteins and their relationship to the apical junctional complex. *Invest Ophthalmol Vis Sci* 1995; 36(6):1115–24.

32. Nichols B, Dawson CR, Togni B. Surface features of the conjunctiva and cornea. *Invest Ophthalmol Vis Sci* 1983; 24(5):570–6.

33. Andrews PM. Microplicae: characteristic ridge-like folds of the plasmalemma. *J Cell Biol* 1976; 68(3):420–9.

34. Estil S, Primo EJ, Wilson G. Apoptosis in shed human corneal cells. *Invest Ophthalmol Vis Sci* 2000; 41(11):3360–4.

35. Wilson SE. Role of apoptosis in wound healing in the cornea. *Cornea* 2000; 19(3 Suppl):S7–12.

36. Hanna C. Proliferation and migration of epithelial cells during corneal wound repair in the rabbit and the rat. *Am J Ophthalmol* 1966; 61(1):55–63.

37. Srinivasan BD, Eakins KE. The reepithelialization of rabbit cornea following single and multiple denudation. *Exp Eye Res* 1979; 29(6):595–600.

38. Chen JJ, Tseng SC. Corneal epithelial wound healing in partial limbal deficiency. *Invest Ophthalmol Vis Sci* 1990; 31(7):1301–14.

39. Chen JJ, Tseng SC. Abnormal corneal epithelial wound healing in partial-thickness removal of limbal epithelium. *Invest Ophthalmol Vis Sci* 1991; 32(8):2219–33.

40. Huang AJ, Tseng SC. Corneal epithelial wound healing in the absence of limbal epithelium. *Invest Ophthalmol Vis Sci* 1991; 32(1):96–105.

41. Cotsarelis G et al., Existence of slow-cycling limbal epithelial basal cells that can be preferentially stimulated to proliferate: implications on epithelial stem cells. *Cell* 1989; 57(2):201–9.

42. Schermer A, Galvin S, Sun TT. Differentiation-related expression of a major 64K corneal keratin in vivo and in culture suggests limbal location of corneal epithelial stem cells. *J Cell Biol* 1986; 103(1):49–62.

43. Zieske JD, Bukusoglu G, Yankauckas MA. Characterization of a potential marker of corneal epithelial stem cells. *Invest Ophthalmol Vis Sci* 1992; 33(1):143–52.

44. Chung EH, Bukusoglu G, Zieske JD. Localization of corneal epithelial stem cells in the developing rat. *Invest Ophthalmol Vis Sci* 1992; 33(7):2199–206.

45. Copeland RA, Jr, Char DH. Limbal autograft reconstruction after conjunctival squamous cell carcinoma. *Am J Ophthalmol* 1990; 110(4):412–5.

46. Kenyon KR, Tseng SC. Limbal autograft transplantation for ocular surface disorders. *Ophthalmology* 1989; 96(5): 709–22; discussion 722–3.

47. Kenyon KR. Limbal autograft transplantation for chemical and thermal burns. *Dev Ophthalmol* 1989; 18:53–8.

48. Jenkins C et al. Limbal transplantation in the management of chronic contact-lens-associated epitheliopathy. *Eye* 1993; 7(Pt 5):629–33.

49. Tsai RJ, Tseng SC. Human allograft limbal transplantation for corneal surface reconstruction. *Cornea* 1994; 13(5):389–400.

50. Tsubota K et al. Reconstruction of the corneal epithelium by limbal allograft transplantation for severe ocular surface disorders. *Ophthalmology* 1995; 102(10):1486–96.

51. Ronk JF et al. Limbal conjunctival autograft in a subacute alkaline corneal burn. *Cornea* 1994; 13(5):465–8.

52. Tan DT, Ficker LA, Buckley RJ. Limbal transplantation. *Ophthalmology*, 1996; 103(1):29–36.

53. Lehrer MS, Sun RR, Lavker RM. Strategies of epithelial repair: modulation of stem cell and transit amplifying cell proliferation. *J Cell Sci* 1998; 111(Pt 19):2867–75.

54. Gomes JA et al. Recurrent keratopathy after penetrating keratoplasty for aniridia. *Cornea* 1996; 15(5):457–62.

55. Kremer I et al. Results of penetrating keratoplasty in aniridia. *Am J Ophthalmol* 1993; 115(3):317–20.

56. Tseng SC. Regulation and clinical implications of corneal epithelial stem cells. *Mol Biol Rep* 1996; 23(1):47–58.

57. McNamara NA, Fleiszig SM. Human tear film components bind Pseudomonas aeruginosa. *Adv Exp Med Biol* 1998; 438:653–8.

58. Qu XD, Lehrer RI. Secretory phospholipase A2 is the principal bactericide for staphylococci and other gram-positive bacteria in human tears. *Infect Immun* 1998; 66(6): 2791–7.

59. Van Setten G, Schultz G. Transforming growth factor-alpha is a constant component of human tear fluid. *Graefes Arch Clin Exp Ophthalmol* 1994; 232(9):523–6.

60. Ohashi Y et al. Presence of epidermal growth factor in human tears. *Invest Ophthalmol Vis Sci* 1989; 30(8):1879–82.

61. Van Setten GB et al. Epidermal growth factor is a constant component of normal human tear fluid. *Graefes Arch Clin Exp Ophthalmol* 1989; 227(2):184–7.

62. Van Setten GB, Schultz GS, Macauley S. Growth factors in human tear fluid and in lacrimal glands. *Adv Exp Med Biol* 1994; 350:315–9.

63. Watanabe K, Nakagawa S, Nishida T. Stimulatory effects of fibronectin and EGF on migration of corneal epithelial cells. *Invest Ophthalmol Vis Sci* 1987; 28(2):205–11.

64. Nishida T et al. Fibronectin promotes epithelial migration of cultured rabbit cornea in situ. *J Cell Biol* 1983; 97(5 Pt 1):1653–7.

65. Dursun D et al. The effects of experimental tear film removal on corneal surface regularity and barrier function. *Ophthalmology* 2000; 107(9):1754–60.

66. Tervo T et al. Tear hepatocyte growth factor (HGF) availability increases markedly after excimer laser surface ablation. *Exp Eye Res* 1997; 64(4):501–4.

67. Dilly PN. Structure and function of the tear film. *Adv Exp Med Biol* 1994; 350:239–47.

68. Mengher LS, Pandher KS, Bron AJ. Non-invasive tear film breakup time: sensitivity and specificity. *Acta Ophthalmol (Copenh)* 1986; 64(4):441–4.

69. Mengher LS et al. A non-invasive instrument for clinical assessment of the pre-corneal tear film stability. *Curr Eye Res* 1985; 4(1):1–7.

70. Mengher LS et al. Effect of fluorescein instillation on the pre-corneal tear film stability. *Curr Eye Res* 1985; 4(1):9–12.

71. Mathers WD et al. Meibomian gland dysfunction in chronic blepharitis. *Cornea* 1991; 10(4):277–85.

72. Lemp MA, Hamill JR, Jr. Factors affecting tear film breakup in normal eyes. *Arch Ophthalmol* 1973; 89(2):103–5.

73. Carney LG, Hill RM. The nature of normal blinking patterns. *Acta Ophthalmol (Copenh)* 1982; 60(3):427–33.

74. Prydal JI, Campbell FW. Study of precorneal tear film thickness and structure by interferometry and confocal microscopy. *Invest Ophthalmol Vis Sci* 1992; 33(6):1996–2005.

75. Chen HB et al. Structure and composition of rat precorneal tear film. A study by an in vivo cryofixation. *Invest Ophthalmol Vis Sci* 1997; 38(2):381–7.

76. Zengin N et al. Meibomian gland dysfunction and tear film abnormalities in rosacea. *Cornea* 1995; 14(2):144–6.

77. Rolando M, Refojo MF, Kenyon KR. Tear water evaporation and eye surface diseases. *Ophthalmologica* 1985; 190(3):147–9.

78. Mathers WD. Ocular evaporation in meibomian gland dysfunction and dry eye. *Ophthalmology* 1993; 100(3):347–51.

79. Sullivan DA et al. Androgen regulation of the meibomian gland. *Adv Exp Med Biol* 1998; 438:327–31.

80. Sullivan DA et al. Does androgen insufficiency cause lacrimal gland inflammation and aqueous tear deficiency? *Invest Ophthalmol Vis Sci* 1999; 40(6):1261–5.

81. Botelho SY, Hisada M, Fuenmayor N. Functional innervation of the lacrimal gland in the cat. Origin of secretomotor fibers in the lacrimal nerve. *Arch Ophthalmol* 1966; 76(4):581–8.

82. Botelho SY. Tears and the lacrimal gland. *Sci Am* 1964; 211:78–86.

83. Baum J. A relatively dry eye during sleep [editorial]. *Cornea* 1990; 9(1):1.

84. Jordan A, Baum J. Basic tear flow. Does it exist? *Ophthalmology* 1980; 87(9):920–30.

85. Heigle TJ, Pflugfelder SC. Aqueous tear production in patients with neurotrophic keratitis. *Cornea* 1996; 15(2):135–8.

86. Gupta A, Heigle T, Pflugfelder SC. Nasolacrimal stimulation of aqueous tear production. *Cornea* 1997; 16(6):645–8.

87. Doane MG. Dynamics of the human blink. *Der Zusammenkunft Dtsch Ophthalmol Ges* 1979(77):13–7.

88. Doane MG. Blinking and the mechanics of the lacrimal drainage system. *Ophthalmology* 1981; 88(8):844–51.

89. Tsubota K, Nakamori K. Effects of ocular surface area and blink rate on tear dynamics. *Arch Ophthalmol* 1995; 113(2):155–8.

90. McEwen W. Secretion of tears and blinking. *The Eye*, ed. D. H. 1962, New York: Academic Press.

91. Ongerboer de Visser B. Anatomical and functional organization of reflexes involving the trigeminal system in man: jaw, blink reflex, corneal reflex and exteroceptive suppression. *Motor control mechanisms in health and disease*, ed. J Desmedt. 1983, New York: Raven. 727–738.

92. Yang HY et al. Lacrimal punctal occlusion for the treatment of superior limbic keratoconjunctivitis. *Am J Ophthalmol* 1997; 124(1):80–7.

93. Fujishima H et al. Corneal temperature in patients with dry eye evaluated by infrared radiation thermometry. *Br J Ophthalmol* 1996; 80(1):29–32.

94. Mori A et al. Efficacy and safety of infrared warming of the eyelids. *Cornea* 1999; 18(2):188–93.

95. Tsubota K et al. Quantitative videographic analysis of blinking in normal subjects and patients with dry eye. *Arch Ophthalmol* 1996; 114(6):715–20.

96. Mishima S et al. Determination of tear volume and tear flow. *Invest Ophthalmol* 1996; 5(3):264–76.

97. Van Best JA, Benitez del Castillo JM, Coulangeon LM. Measurement of basal tear turnover using a standardized protocol. European concerted action on ocular fluorometry. *Graefes Arch Clin Exp Ophthalmol* 1995; 233(1):1–7.

98. Xu KP et al. Tear function index. A new measure of dry eye. *Arch Ophthalmol* 1995; 113(1):84–8.

99. Xu KP, Tsubota K. Correlation of tear clearance rate and fluorophotometric assessment of tear turnover. *Br J Ophthalmol* 1995; 79(11):1042–9.

2

Classification of Ocular Surface Disease

Frederich E. Kruse

Pathophysiology of Ocular Surface Disease

During the past decade the number of options for the therapy of ocular surface diseases has greatly increased. This progress has been based on a better understanding of the pathophysiology of ocular surface disease. In order to choose from current conservative and surgical strategies, it is helpful for the physician to understand the pathophysiology and pathoanatomy of ocular surface disease.

Conjunctival Pathophysiology

Goblet Cell Dysfunction
One of the most important functional properties of the conjunctival epithelium is the secretion of specialized glycoproteins, especially mucins. Mucins are either secreted by apocrine-secreting goblet cells, or by secretory epithelial cells.[1] Mucins are of great importance for the interaction between the ocular surface epithelium and the tear film.

Two forms of dysfunction of the mucin-producing subset of conjunctival epithelial cells can be differentiated. *Hypersecretion* of mucins is associated with conjunctival inflammation and often leads to the formation of mucous strands in the tear film. In contrast, *hyposecretion* of mucins is a result of *goblet cell deficiency*. It is the common denominator of conjunctival scarring in the context of chronic conjunctival inflammation.

Hypersecretion of Mucins and Pseudoglandular Hyperplasia

A vast number of inflammatory mediators can cause transient increase of the number of conjunctival goblet cells as well as epithelial cells. Increased epithelial thickness leads to formation of crypts and ducts that are lined with goblet-cell-containing epithelium. Because of the similarity to true glands, these alterations are called pseudoglandular hyperplasia. Obstruction of crypts by cellular debris can cause thin-walled retention cysts visible by slit-lamp examination. They are predominantly located in the palpebral and forniceal conjunctiva. Pseudoglandular hyperplasia and increased goblet cells are found in the acute, as well as in the initial, stages of chronic conjunctivitis. Later stages of conjunctival inflammation are frequently characterized by cicatricial changes that lead to goblet cell deficiency.

Hyposecretion of Mucins Due to Goblet Cell Deficiency

A prerequisite for normal goblet cell function is coordinated cellular proliferation and differentiation. However, very little is known about factors regulating self-renewal and differentiation of goblet cells. On the basis of the underlying pathophysiology, goblet cell deficiency can be classified as shown in Table 2.1.

Goblet Cell Deficiency Due to Vitamin A Deficiency
Experimental evidence from other goblet-cell-containing tissues suggests that retinoids are essential for the normal differentiation of goblet cells. Furthermore, in vitro data suggest that retinoic acid may also be important for the differentiation of limbal progenitor cells of the corneal epithelium.[2] Systemic vitamin A deficiency due to malnutrition is common in the developing world. In contrast, malabsorption secondary to gastrointestinal and hepatic diseases (often in the context of chronic alcoholism), as well as surgical interventions, are the leading causes of vitamin A deficiency in industrialized countries. In vitamin A deficient animals, conjunctival goblet cells disappear over time, and the surface epithelium undergoes significant surface alterations and becomes keratinized.[3] In humans, early signs of vitamin A deficiency are reduction of goblet cells associated with increased cell proliferation.[4] The dull, irregular surface of the conjunctiva is due to squamous metaplasia with enlargement of epithelial cells and subsequent keratinization.[5] The histology of whitish, ele-

Table 2.1. Ocular surface disease associated with goblet cell deficiency.

Malnutrition
  Vitamin A deficiency
Oculocutaneous disease
  Cicatricial pemphigoid
  Bullous pemphigoid
  Linear IgA disease
  Dermatitis herpetiformis (Duhring)
  Epidermolysis bullosa acquisita
  Stevens–Johnson syndrome (Erythema multiforme majus)
  Toxic epidermal necrolysis (Lyell syndrome)
  Porphyria cutanea tarda
  Erythroderma ichthyosiform congenita
  Hydroa vacciniforme
  Atopic keratoconjunctivitis
  Acne rosacea
Drugs (pseudopemphigoid)
Miscellaneous conjunctival inflammations
  Sjögren's syndrome
  Systemic sclerosis (Scleroderma)
  Graft-versus-host disease
  Inflammatory bowel disease
  Reiter's syndrome
Infectious conjunctivitis
  Viral conjunctivitis (any cause of viral membranous conjunctivitis)
    Adenovirus
    Herpes simplex
    Varicella zoster
  Bacterial conjunctivitis (any cause of bacterial membranous conjunctivitis)
    Borrelia burgdorferi
    Corynebacterium diphteriae
    Beta-hemolytic streptococcus
    Staphylococcus
    Treponema pallidum (acquired and congenital syphilis)
  Chlamydial conjunctivitis
    Chlamydia trachomatis (trachoma)
Chemical-physical factors
  Acid burn
  Alkali burn
  Thermal burn
  Ionizing irradiation
  Trauma

vated Bitot spots shows loss of epithelial and goblet cells, basophilic intracellular granula, as well as keratinization of superficial cell layers.[6] In addition, impaired regeneration of the corneal epithelium can lead to persistent epithelial defects and ulceration.

Goblet Cell Deficiency Associated with Mucocutaneous Disease Conjunctivitis associated with mucocutaneous disorders is one of the leading causes of goblet cell dysfunction secondary to cicatricial changes. The common denominator of these diseases is hyperproliferation of fibroblasts resulting in subepithelial scarring. Many mucocutaneous diseases are based on cytotoxic type II and IV immune reactions. Furthermore, cicatricial pemphigoid, linear IgA disease, epidermolysis bullosa acquisita and heredita, erythema multiforme, and bullous pemphigoid share distinct histopathological changes in the basement membrane zone, such as linear deposition of antibodies and complement.

Cicatricial pemphigoid is a chronic, progressive bullous dermatosis characterized by vesiculobullous eruptions of the skin and mucosal erosions.[7,8] An association has been established between ocular pemphigoid and rheumatoid arthritis suggesting, at least in part, a common immunological mechanism.[9] The disease process is mediated by various autoantibodies that bind to antigens in the basement membrane zone.[10,11] Immunofluorescence shows a diagnostic linear pattern of deposition although a similar pattern can also be found in linear IgA disease and bullous pemphigoid.[12] Conjunctival inflammation is characterized by activation of the complement cascade through C3b and recruitment of macrophages, lymphocytes, plasma cells, and mast cells. The release of cytokines, especially during phases of acute inflammation, leads to activation of fibroblasts and scar formation.[10,13] Proliferation of conjunctival epithelial cells is significantly enhanced, but goes along with simultaneous reduction of the number of goblet cells, suggesting a dysregulation of goblet cell differentiation.[14,15] The early phase is characterized by subtle subconjunctival fibrosis that typically leads to a disappearance of the caruncle (Figure 2.1). The late phase of cicatricial pemphigoid is characterized by fibrosis and keratinization of the ocular surface epithelia with loss of goblet cells, as well as symblepharon formation (Figure 2.2).

In *bullous pemphigoid*, linear deposition of IgG and complement, together with inflammatory infiltrates, has been described. In contrast to the diseases mentioned above, fibrosis is usually minimal and biomicroscopic changes are limited to fine scars of the tarsal conjunctiva similar to those observed after acute infectious conjunctivitis.[16]

Pemphigus vulgaris is also characterized by subepithelial deposition of autoantibodies. However, involvement of the conjunctiva is rare and is characterized by hyperemia with mucoid discharge and the formation of conjunctival vesicles rather than conjunctival scarring.[17,18]

Linear IgA disease shows similar histopathological findings with the linear arrangement of antibodies in the basement membrane zone. Pathophysiological changes are characterized by deposition of IgA and complement, triggering inflammation. Mediators released from inflammatory cells lead to fibrosis, keratinization, goblet cell loss, and symblephara that is usually milder than in cicatricial pemphigoid.[19,20]

The histopathology of another chronic bullous, cutaneous disease, *dermatitis herpetiformis (Duhring)* is characterized by granular deposition of IgA along the basement membrane zone,[21] although the conjunctiva rarely develops secondary fibrosis.

Epidermolysis bullosa acquisita is a rare autoimmune mechanobullous disease that is also characterized by linear deposition of IgG and fibrin along basement

Figure 2.1. Cicatricial pemphigoid (early stage). Chronic inflammation, faint subconjunctival fibrosis with disappearance of the caruncle.

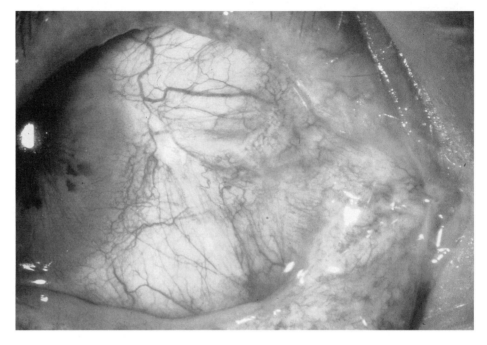

membranes, as well as by the accumulation of electron-dense amorphous material.[22,23]

Erythema multiforme, Stevens–Johnson syndrome and *toxic epidermal necrolysis (Lyell)* form another group of diseases with common clinical and pathophysiological characteristics. In contrast to the mucocutaneous diseases described above, they are characterized by acute onset of inflammation. The major form of erythema multiforme, also known as Stevens–Johnson syndrome, involves two or more mucosal surfaces together with vesiculobullous skin lesions. Toxic epidermal necrolysis (Lyell) is the most severe form of Stevens–Johnson syndrome, and clinical manifestations may resemble a thermal injury. In both forms, the acute inflammation can change into a chronic conjunctivitis (Figure 2.3).[24] Probably based on a specific genetic background,[25] most cases of Stevens–Johnson syndrome seem to be triggered by systemic, and sometimes even topical, medication, especially sulfonamides.[26–28] Stevens–Johnson syndrome has also been associated with a variety of infectious agents such as Herpes simplex or Mycoplasma pneumoniae.[29] The pathogenesis of toxic epidermal necrolysis might be based on an abnormal T-cell response,[30,31] impaired antigen presentation,[32] or alter-

Figure 2.2. Cicatricial pemphigoid (late stage). Vascularization, keratinization of the ocular surface, symblepharon formation.

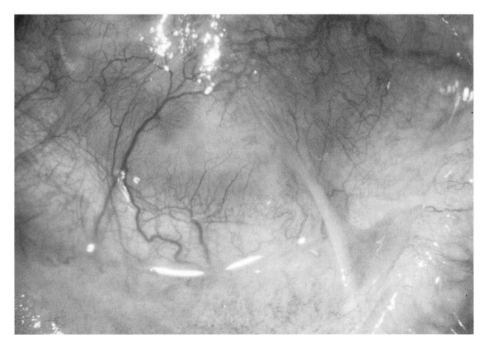

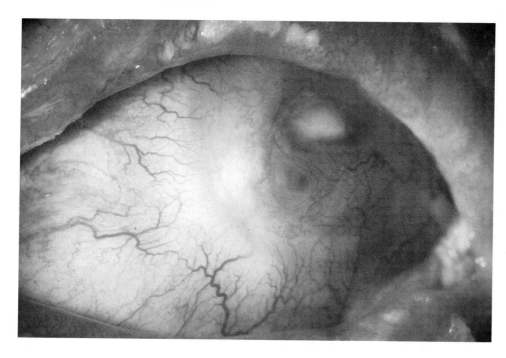

Figure 2.3. Chronic form of Stevens–Johnson syndrome. Chronic conjunctivitis, conjunctivalization of the corneal surface, stromal opacification.

ations in the cytokine production by subsets of inflammatory cells.[33] Histopathological changes can be classified as type III hypersensitivity reaction and represent an IgA-mediated necrotizing vasculitis with deposition of immune complexes.[34] During the acute phase, a diffuse, nonspecific inflammatory response has been described, and pseudomembranous or membranous conjunctivitis occurs. In the chronic conjunctivitis, the proliferation of basal conjunctival epithelial cells is increased while the number of goblet cells is continuously decreased, suggesting that goblet cell differentiation might be impaired.[35,36]

Porphyria cutanea tarda is based on abnormality of the porphyrin heme metabolism that renders the skin and ocular tissues sensitive to photochemical damage. In this very rare disease, conjunctival inflammation with formation of blisters and scarring occurs in response to sunlight. Other very rare causes of goblet cell deficiency in the context of cicatrizing oculocutaneous disease are erythroderma ichtyosiform congenita and hydroa vacciniforme. Conjunctival changes induced by atopic keratoconjunctivitis are described below (see Conjunctival Inflammation in Ocular Allergy).

Goblet Cell Deficiency in Drug-Induced Pseudopemphigoid Iatrogenic depletion of goblet cells may be caused by prolonged use of ophthalmic medications. In principle, any drug could cause pseudopemphigoid. However, it is most often due to preservatives or the prolonged use of glaucoma medication. Clinically, the subtle changes remain frequently unrecognized. Although based on a different mechanism, clinical and histopathological changes are almost indistinguishable from those in cicatricial pemphigoid.[37–39]

Goblet Cell Deficiency in Systemic Inflammatory Disease In secondary *Sjögren's syndrome*, connective-tissue disease is associated with aqueous tear deficiency. Mechanical alteration of the ocular surface epithelia, as well as chronic conjunctival inflammation in the context of keratoconjunctivitis sicca, results in progressive loss of goblet cells and epithelial stratification.[40]

Scleroderma is a chronic inflammatory disease leading to fibrosis of the skin and internal organs, possibly on the grounds of a systemic vasculitis. Chronic conjunctivitis is associated with microangiopathy including teleangiectasia, varicosis, and sludging. Histopathology shows loss of goblet cells, epithelial thinning and keratinization together with mild lymphocytic infiltrates.[41,42]

Graft-versus-host disease is a T-cell-mediated immunological reaction of transplanted hematopoetic stem cells against host antigens. The occurrence of acute conjunctivitis is associated with reduced life expectancy.[43] Conjunctival inflammation can be severe with subconjunctival hemorrhage, ulcerations, and pseudomembrane formation.[44] Aqueous tear deficiency is often present leading to severe keratoconjunctivitis sicca. Histopathological changes include epithelial necrosis with epithelial and stromal infiltrates. Keratinization, loss of goblet cells and conjunctival scarring occur in chronic forms.[43,44]

Although rare, *inflammatory bowel disease* can also cause conjunctival inflammation that can lead to cicatrization and goblet cell loss[45] that has also been observed in Reiter's syndrome.

Goblet Cell Deficiency Due to Conjunctival Infections Various pathogens can affect the conjunctival epithelium and cause severe conjunctival inflammation. As described below, membranous or pseudomembranous as well as necrotizing or ulcerative conjunctivitis can lead to conjunctival scarring and goblet cell loss.

Chronic conjunctivitis in *trachoma* is based on a T-cell-mediated type IV hypersensitivity response against chlamydial antigens.[46,47] Chronic follicular conjunctivitis leads to loss of goblet cells and keratinization of conjunctival epithelial cells as well as subepithelial scarring and cicatricial changes.

Goblet Cell Deficiency Due to Chemical and Physical Injury Numerous chemicals can cause surface damage with varying degrees of conjunctival scarring leading to mucin deficiency by reducing the number of goblet cells.

Acid burns cause denaturation of proteins and damage of the cell surface. Insoluble proteinates resulting from acid-protein interaction often prevent deeper penetration of the causative agent.[48] In contrast, *alkali burns* cause saponification of lipids that are present in cell membranes, and this reaction often reaches the basal layer. This process is augmented by the effects of collagenase and inflammatory mediators. Loss of conjunctival epithelial stem cells, chronic inflammation and subconjunctival fibrosis result in goblet cell loss and mucin deficiency.

Several forms of *irradiation* can cause dose-dependent damage to conjunctival epithelium with keratinization and subconjunctival scarring. In the acute phase, inflammatory changes are prevalent along with cell necrosis and obstruction of vessels. Loss of goblet cells along with telangiectatic vessels characterize the late phase.

Conjunctival Inflammation

The conjunctiva has a relatively simple histological structure that limits the response to inflammatory stimuli to very few pathophysiological changes. This explains why very different forms of conjunctival inflammation induce seemingly similar clinical pictures. Consequently, the diagnosis of conjunctival inflammations can be difficult. Knowledge of the different responses of the conjunctiva to inflammatory stimuli is essential for successful management of ocular surface disease.

Acute Conjunctival Inflammation

Hyperemia, Chemosis, Cellular Exudate Hyperemia is the most frequent acute response to inflammation and represents a dilation of blood vessels caused by inflammatory mediators. Increased permeability leads to *chemosis* secondary to the accumulation of fluid into the perivascular tissue. Increased adhesion of leukocytes to the wall of blood vessels allows for diapedesis and formation of a *cellular exudate* that is primarily confined to the subepithelial tissue and stroma. This exudate usually consists of leukocytes, plasma cells, lymphocytes and immunoglobulins. Hyperemia, chemosis and exudate represent nonspecific reactions that are found in various forms of conjunctival inflammation.

Pseudomembranous and Membranous Conjunctivitis Several variants of severe conjunctivitis can lead to the formation of *pseudomembranes*. These pseudomembranes are generated by coagulation of an exudate that contains fibrin and necrotic conjunctival cells. Pseudomembranes are deposited on the intact surface of an intact conjunctival epithelium and can, therefore, be removed without bleeding.

In contrast, true membranes are the result of coagulation of exudate with very high concentrations of fibrin within the epithelium and stroma. Consequently, the removal of pseudomembranes causes bleeding. The most common causes for membranous and pseudomembranous conjunctivitis are listed in Table 2.2.

Ulcerative, Necrotizing and Hemorrhagic Conjunctivitis During very severe conjunctival inflammation, necrosis of the conjunctival epithelium can lead to ulcerative changes and exposure of the stroma. Damage to stromal blood vessels not only causes formation of

Table 2.2. Ocular surface disease associated with formation of pseudomembranes and membranes.

Pseudomembranes
Viral
    Adenovirus
    Herpes simplex virus
    Herpes zoster
    Vaccinia
Bacteria
    Staphylococci
    S. pneumoniae
    Pneumococci
    Meningococci
    Pseudomonas aeruginosa
    E. Coli
    Mycobacterium tuberculosis
Fungi
    Candida albicans
Chemical and thermal burn
Immunological disease
    Cicatricial pemphigoid
    Linear IgA disease
    Bullous pemphigoid
    Epidermolysis bullosa acquisita
    Stevens–Johnson syndrome (Erythema multiforme majus)
    Toxic epidermal necrolysis (Lyell's syndrome)
    Conjunctivitis lignosa
Membranes
Viral
    Adenovirus
    Measles
    Herpes simplex
    Variola
Bacteria
    Corynebacterium diphtheriae
    Neisseria gonorrhoeae
    Pneumococcus
    Streptococci
    Pseudomonas aeruginosa
Immunological disease
    Stevens–Johnson syndrome (Erythema multiforme majus)
    Toxic epidermal necrolysis (Lyell's syndrome)
    Conjunctivitis lignosa

Table 2.3. Ocular surface disease associated with ulcerative, necrotizing and hemorrhagic conjunctivitis.

Virus
    Herpes zoster virus
    Adenovirus
    Enterovirus 70
Immunological disease
    Stevens–Johnson syndrome (Erythema multiforme majus)
    Toxic epidermal necrolysis (Lyell's syndrome)
Chemicals, toxins
    Chemical/thermal injury
    Bacterial toxins (staphylococci, neisseria)

significant leukocyte infiltration, but also induces bleeding. The most common forms of ulcerative conjunctivitis are shown in Table 2.3.

Follicular Conjunctivitis Conjunctival follicles are an important clinical sign that facilitates the differential diagnosis of conjunctival inflammation. The biomicroscopic appearance of conjunctival follicles is characterized by small, oval or round elevations that can have a pale, grayish color. The outline and direction of blood vessels on the follicle represent important criteria for the diagnosis: Vessels originate in the periphery of the follicle and are directed toward the center, without reaching it. Histology shows lymphoid hyperplasia with secondary vascularization from the periphery of the fol-

Table 2.4. Ocular surface disease associated with formation of follicles.

Infectious
    Acute
        Viral
            Adenovirus
            Herpes simplex virus
            Newcastle disease
            Enterovirus 70
        Chlamydia oculogenitalis
    Chronic
        Chlamydia
            C. trachomatis
            C. psittarcosis
        Bacteria
            Moraxella and other forms of bacterial conjunctivitis
            Borrelia burgdorferi
        Viral
            Epstein–Barr
            Measles
Noninfectious
    Drug-induced
        Iodine-desoxyuridine
        Eserine
        Atropine
        Various cosmetics
    Immunological reactions
        Molluscum contagiosum
        Antigens of exogenous origin (plants, animals, chemicals)
        Antigens of endogenous origin (measles, rubella)
    Uncorrected refractive errors

licle. In contrast to papillary hypertrophy, in which vessels originate in the center, the epithelium above the follicles is not thinned. Causes of follicular hypertrophy are listed in Table 2.4.

Chronic Conjunctival Inflammation
While acute conjunctivitis is generally self-limiting, it may also enter a chronic stage. Chronic conjunctivitis is characterized by persistent hyperemia. Increased production of mucous results from an increase of the number of goblet cells during the early phase of chronic conjunctivitis. The following histopathological changes develop in chronic conjunctivitis.

Papillary Hypertrophy Papillary hypertrophy is a result of chronic epithelial and stromal hyperplasia that causes round, hyperemic elevations of the conjunctival surface. Vessels originate in the center of the papillae, a sign that can serve to differentiate papillary hypertrophy from follicular changes. Initial changes are characterized by hyperemia and an inflammatory infiltrate in the stroma consisting of lymphocytes, plasma cells, mast cells, and granulocytes. In chronic forms, the conjunctival epithelium is pushed upward by the formation of stromal granulation tissue and fibrosis. The existence of fibrillary bands that reach from subepithelial tissue to the tarsal plate is responsible for the formation of indentations between papillae. The size of papillae is variable and reaches from small hyperemic changes to larger cobblestones and to giant papillary changes. The formation of papillary changes is a rather unspecific sign. However, such changes indicate the etiology of conjunctivitis, such as in certain forms of ocular allergy (Figure 2.4).

Subepithelial Scarring and Symblepharon Formation Persistent chronic inflammation leads to subepithelial fibrosis and deposition of collagen fibers that can be visible with the slit lamp as faint whitish lines. Chronic inflammation with destruction of the basement membrane and proliferation of the subepithelial tissue can cause significant fibrosis that results in foreshortening of the fornix and formation of symblepharon. Although symblepharon formation is a nonspecific sign of chronic inflammation, its presence is frequently induced by the disease entities listed in Table 2.5.

Granulomatous Conjunctivitis Inflammation associated with chalazion is the most frequent form of granulomatous conjunctivitis. Depending on the type of inflammation, the size of conjunctival granulomas can vary from very small and almost invisible lesions on slit lamp investigation (e.g., sarcoidosis) to large elevated nodules of yellow-whitish color surrounded by an area of hyperemic conjunctiva.

Depending on the underlying pathology, diffuse forms can be differentiated from zonular types. Diffuse granulomas result from an undirected infiltration of lymphocytes with proliferation of endothelial cells. In

Figure 2.4. Giant papillary conjunctivitis of the upper tarsus with mucoid discharge in vernal keratoconjunctivitis.

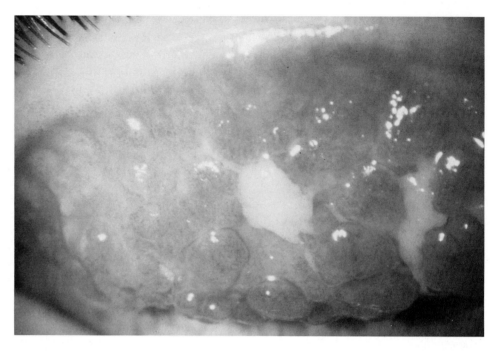

contrast, zonular granulomas are characterized by a specific architecture. The pathogenic substrate (e.g., a foreign body) is located in the center, surrounded by a ring of epitheloid cells and giant cells. The outermost zone of the granuloma is made up of lymphocytes, plasma cells, and eosinophilic granulocytes. Various forms of conjunctivitis associated with the formation of either diffuse or zonular granuloma are shown in Table 2.6.

Conjunctival Inflammation in Ocular Allergy
Based on the underlying pathomechanism, several forms of chronic conjunctivitis can be classified as related to allergy, as shown in Table 2.7.

Table 2.5. Ocular surface disease associated with formation of symblepharon.

Immunological disorders
   Cicatricial pemphigoid
   Stevens–Johnson syndrome (Erythema multiforme majus)
   Toxic epidermal necrolysis (Lyell's syndrome)
   Herpetiform dermatitis (Duhring)
   Linear IgA disease
   Acquired epidermolysis bullosa
   Atopic keratoconjunctivitis
Bacteria
   Corynebacterium diphtheriae
   Borrelia burgdorferi
Chlamydia
   Chlamydia trachomatis
Viral (rare, severe forms of inflammation)
   Adenovirus
   Herpes zoster
Chemicals, drugs, physical injury
   Chemical burn
   Thermal burn
   Drug-induced pseudopemphigoid

Perennial and *seasonal conjunctivitis* represent the most frequent manifestations of ocular allergy. These disorders are characterized by relatively benign pathological changes with mild epithelial hyperplasia and increased number of goblet cells. A characteristic, scant inflam-

Table 2.6. Ocular surface disease associated with formation of granuloma.

Bacteria
   Mycobacterium leprae or tuberculosis
   Treponema pallidum
   Hemophylus ducreii
   Yersinia
   Cat scratch disease (Afipia felis, Bartonella henselae)
   Listeria
   Franciscella tularensis
   Rickettsia
Chlamydia
Viral
   Epstein–Barr Virus
Other infectious organisms
   Actinomycosis
   Blastomycosis
   Sporotrichosis
   Leptospirosis
Systemic disease
   Sarcoidosis
   Wegener's granulomatosis
Allergic granulomas
   Parasites (toxocara canis, shistosoma, onchocerca)
   Caterpillar hairs
   Allergic granulomas without detectable antigen
Foreign-body granulomas
   Organic material (plants, insects)
   Nonorganic material
   Sutures
   Plastics (e.g., stuffed toys)

Table 2.7. Conjunctival inflammation in ocular allergy.

Seasonal conjunctivitis
Perennial conjunctivitis
Atopic keratoconjunctivitis
Vernal keratoconjunctivitis
Giant papillary conjunctivitis
Contact dermatitis

matory infiltrate is found in the substantia propria consisting of mast cells and esosinophils. The tarsal conjunctiva undergoes papillary hypertrophy. Upon contact with antigens, a type I hypersensitivity reaction results in synthesis of antibodies by B-lymphocytes. IgE and specific antibodies are increased in serum and tears.[49,50] Upon renewed contact, antigens are bound to IgE on the surface of mast cells, which leads to degranulation and the release of inflammatory mediators such as histamine, leucotriene and prostaglandins. These mediators cause dilation of vessels and secondary tissue damage by recruitment of inflammatory cells. The identification of the role of mast cells and the release of inflammatory mediators has enabled the development of powerful drugs for the treatment of seasonal/perennial conjunctivitis, such as mast cell stabilizers and antihistamines.

Atopic conjunctivitis is a chronic disease that is based on a number of deviations of the immune system, such as delayed hypersensitivity responses to pathogens (e.g., Candida albicans)[51] and defective T-cell function that include a possible failure to terminate the production of IgE in response to specific antigens.[52] In chronic type I and IV reactions, the conjunctival epithelium and stroma contain (degranulating) mast cells and eosino-

phils, as well as activated T-lymphocytes with an increased proportion of helper cells.[53] Inflammatory mediators induce the expression of MHC class II antigens as well as pseudoglandular hyperplasia.[54] The clinical picture is characterized by giant papillary conjunctivitis of the lower tarsus that can lead to linear tarsal scars, fornix foreshortening, and symblepharon. *Trantas* dots at the limbus represent focal accumulations of eosinophils. Keratitis associated with atopic dermatitis can be severe, including scarring and vascularization.

Vernal keratoconjunctivitis shares several clinical characteristics of atopic disease, and the immunological changes are also indicative of type I and IV hypersensitivity reactions. Similar to atopic disease, one of the most important pathophysiological mechanisms is the release of inflammatory mediators by degranulating mast cells and eosinophils (e.g., histamine or major basic protein).[55] Conjunctival plasma cells synthesize IgA, IgG and IgE.[56] Changes of the vascular endothelium such as hyperplasia, hypertrophy, and necrosis, together with the existence of basophilic granulocytes in epithelium and stroma, suggest a basophilic hypersensitivity reaction.[57] Increased vascular permeability, deposition of fibrin, and fibrovascular hypertrophy of subepithelial tissue leads to the formation of giant papillary changes that are predominantly located in the tarsal conjunctiva. In limbal vernal conjunctivitis, papillae are smaller and inflammatory degenerations of the epithelium cause formation of pseudocysts containing degenerated epithelial cells and eosinophilic granulocytes (*Trantas* dots) (Figure 2.5). Corneal changes include superficial keratitis, formation of (shield) ulcers, and stromal opacities that are frequently located at the limbus.

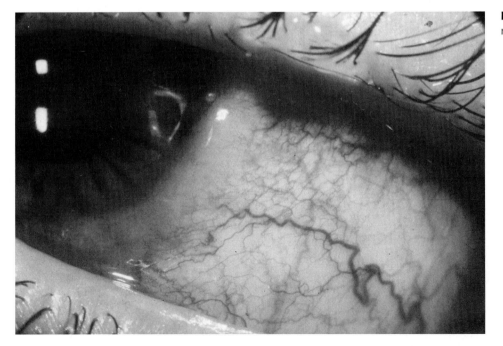

Figure 2.5. Limbal form of vernal keratoconjunctivitis.

Giant papillary conjunctivitis is caused by multiple immunological changes that are similar to those found in vernal or atopic keratoconjunctivitis.[55,58,59] This disease is mostly associated with the use of contact lenses, suggesting that plastic components or contents of storage/cleaning solutions might function as immunological stimuli. Conjunctivitis due to *allergic contact dermatitis* is based on a delayed type of hypersensitivity reaction.

Conjunctival Inflammation in Collagen Vascular Disease

The term collagen vascular disease is applied to a group of systemic disorders characterized by vasculitis and inflammation of connective tissue. Ocular surface disease related to collagen vascular disorder involves not only the conjunctiva, but also causes peripheral ulcerative disease of the cornea with damage to epithelium and stroma. The onset of ocular symptoms may be associated with increased activity of the systemic disease. Since ocular symptoms may precede systemic manifestation, the ophthalmologist is responsible for initiating a systemic workup and must also inform the rheumatologist about the association between ocular manifestations and potentially life-threatening disease activity.

The clinical picture of ocular surface disease in the different forms of collagen vascular disease is often very similar, and the differential diagnosis primarily involves the following disorders: rheumatoid arthritis, Wegener's granulomatosis, panarteriitis nodosa, systemic lupus erythematodes, and relapsing polychondritis.

The multifactorial etiology of *rheumatoid arthritis* seems to involve the presence of a special subset of histocompatibility antigens with possible cross-reactivity to bacterial or viral antigens.[60,61] Bacterial heat shock proteins can mimic human HLA antigens and are incriminated in the trigger of the onset of inflammation.[62] Keratoconjunctivitis sicca is the most common manifestation of rheumatoid arthritis and a part of secondary Sjögren's syndrome. Lymphocytic infiltration of the lacrimal glands is associated with acinar atrophy and proliferation of fibroblasts leading to glandular dysfunction.[63] The conjunctival epithelium undergoes stratification with subsequent loss of goblet cells and the stroma shows infiltration with T-cells and neutrophilic granulocytes.[64]

Wegener's granulomatosis is characterized by a triad consisting of necrotizing granulomas of the respiratory tract, generalized focal necrotizing vasculitis, and glomerulonephritis. As in other connective tissue diseases, a special HLA configuration seems to be present. Bacterial and viral infections are thought to trigger disease.[65] The discovery of antineutrophil cytoplasmic antibodies (ANCA) has greatly facilitated the diagnosis of Wegener's granulomatosis.[66] Although the role of the antibodies in the pathophysiology of the disease is unclear, they can be directed against proteolytic enzymes in the tissue.[67] Ocular manifestations involve most frequently the orbit and eyelids, as well as episclera and sclera. Conjunctival inflammation is found primarily in conjunction with scleritis, episcleritis, or with peripheral ulcerative disease of the cornea. Rare primary conjunctivitis is characterized by hyperemic, ulcerative lesions at the tarsus. Yellowish elevated areas of inflammation share similarities with granulomas or giant papillae. The conjunctiva contains inflammatory infiltrates composed of lymphocytes, plasma cells, giant cells and neutrophilic, as well as eosinophilic, granulocytes. Therefore, histology does not resemble the necrotizing vasculitis that is characteristic for Wegener's granulomatosis, but rather shows similarities to a pyogenic granuloma or chalazion.[68]

Periarteritis nodosa is a necrotizing vasculitis that can affect various organs. Conjunctival involvement causes chemosis, subconjunctival hemorrhage and yellowish, avascular zones.[69] Histology shows signs of vasculitis with fibrinoid necrosis of conjunctival vessels. Characteristically, necrotizing vasculitis is adjacent to almost normal segments of vessels with only moderate hyperplasia of endothelial cells and slight lymphocytic infiltration of the media. Immune complex deposition of IgG and IgM, as well as complement, is found in conjunctival vessels, and suggests that the disease might be an immune-complex-mediated vasculitis.[69]

Other Forms of Conjunctival Inflammation

Ligneous conjunctivitis is a rare membranous conjunctivitis primarily affecting infants and adolescents. Possibly based on a familial predisposition, the lymphocyte-mediated immune response is characterized by the formation of thick, yellowish membranes of the tarsal plate consisting of eosinophilic material, mucopolysaccharides, fibrin, and IgG.[70,71] The conjunctival epithelium is thickened with papillomatosis and dyskeratosis. The inflammatory infiltrate is composed of lymphocytes (more T-helper cells than suppresser cells), plasma cells, macrophages and polymorphonuclear granulocytes.[71] Vessels show thickened walls suggestive of vasculitis.[72]

Also of unknown origin, *superior limbic keratoconjunctivitis* is often bilateral in adults with characteristic rosebengal staining of the superior limbus. The pathogenesis might be based on environmental factors, or mechanical irritation of the surface. Keratinization, acanthosis, and dyskeratosis of the conjunctival epithelium occur together with alterations of cell nuclei.[73,74]

Conjunctivitis in *floppy eyelid syndrome* is characterized by papillary hypertrophy with thickening and partial keratinization of the epithelium. The subepithelial inflammatory infiltrate consists of lymphocytes and plasma cells.[75,76]

Disorders of the Tear Film

The integrity of the ocular surface depends on functional interaction with the tear film. This requires a defined quality and quantity of the three major components of the tear film, that is, the lipid phase, the aqueous phase, and the mucin phase. A poorly lubricated ocular surface is vulnerable to minute environmental challenges and can undergo various pathological changes. It has recently been established that the components of the ocular surface (e.g., lid margin and meibomian glands, conjunctiva and mucin secreting cells, as well as cornea) act as a functional unit together with the lacrimal gland and the interconnecting innervation.[77,78] In addition, tears need to be distributed on the ocular surface, a process that requires normal lid configuration. Alterations of each of the components of the ocular surface cause disturbances of the entire tear film system that can lead to pathological changes of the surface epithelia. Therefore, classification of the disorders of the tear film are necessarily artificial, and most diseases reflect disturbances of more than one component of the ocular surface.

The conventional classification used in most textbooks classifies tear film disorders on the basis of the organization of the tear film and differentiates between disorders of the lipid phase, the aqueous phase, and the mucin phase. Alternatively, two major categories have been suggested: evaporative dry eye and tear-deficient dry eye.[79,80] In this classification, *evaporative dry eye* consists of classic lipid deficiency such as meibomian gland dysfunction. Increased tear evaporation can also be caused by lid related disease, as well as by surface alterations due to contact lenses and metabolic dysfunction of the ocular surface epithelia. *Tear deficiency* is associated with Sjögren's syndrome as well as tear deficiency secondary to lacrimal disease, lacrimal obstruction and reflex block. Although tear dysfunction will be discussed in greater detail in Chapter 4, it is important to review these disorders from a pathophysiological viewpoint here.

Disorders of the Lipid Phase and Evaporative Tear Film Deficiency

Ocular surface abnormalities caused by increased evaporation of tears (Table 2.8) seem to be the most common reason for dry-eye-related problems. The major cause of increased tear evaporation is lipid deficiency. Various lipids and lipoproteins are secreted by meibomian glands and serve to stabilize the tear film and to reduce evaporation from the surface.[81] In lipid deficiency, the stability of the tear film is reduced and results in reduction of the tear breakup time, as well as the appearance of dry spots on the ocular surface.[82] As a consequence of lipid deficiency, the evaporation from the ocular surface is greatly enhanced and tear osmolarity is elevated.[83–84] Progressive alteration of the ocular surface epithelia results in specific staining patterns when vital dyes are applied.[85,86] Reduction of tear lipids can be due either to decreased synthesis, or to insufficient

Table 2.8. Lipid tear deficiency and evaporative dry eye.

Lipid deficiency
  Primary lipid deficiency
    Congenital absence of meibomian glands
  Secondary lipid deficiency
    Anterior blepharitis
      Staphylococcal blepharitis
    Posterior blepharitis
      Obstructive meibomian gland disease
      Rosacea
Lid-related evaporative dry eye
  Insufficient blink
  Increased lid aperture

delivery from meibomian glands. Relatively little is known about the synthesis of lipids in meibomian glands that might be under nervous regulation.[87] Meibomian oil delivery is dependent on a functional lid margin anatomy as well as blink action.[88,89] Consequently, diseases that alter the metabolism within meibomian glands, as well as alterations of meibomian gland orifices, are frequent causes of lipid deficiency.

Primary lipid deficiency is extremely rare and only occurs in the congenital absence of the meibomian glands that has been described in patients with anhidrotic ectodermal dysplasia. In contrast, the various forms of secondary lipid deficiency probably represent the most frequent cause of dry-eye-related complaints.

Anterior blepharitis can either be a primary disease, or associated with microbial infection. In the presence of chronic blepharitis, lid margins are frequently colonized by bacteria such as Staphylococci (aureus and coagulase negative), Corynebacterium and Propionibacterium.[90] Bacteria secrete various lipases that hydrolyse lipids (wax and sterol esters) into various kinds of fatty acids. These fatty acids destabilize the tear film and exert toxic effects on ocular surface epithelia resulting in chronic conjunctivitis and superficial punctate keratitis.[91] In addition, bacterial lipases may change the composition of lipids within the glands, leading to an increase in the viscosity of meibum, thus augmenting the obstruction of meibomian gland orifices. Bacteria on the lid margin also produce toxins that can induce the production of chemokines in corneal and conjunctival cells. Chemokines recruit inflammatory cells such as macrophages into the tissue and might, therefore, be important in the pathogenesis of blepharoconjunctivitis. Similarly, toxins are instrumental for the development of the marginal corneal ulcers and neovascularization associated with Staphylococci.

Posterior blepharitis is characterized by obstructive and inflammatory meibomian gland dysfunction. As a result, the composition and quantity of lipids in meibomian glands undergo significant changes.[92,93] Subsequent changes in tear film lipids can have toxic effects on the ocular surface epithelium. In addition, alterations of meibomian gland secretion are accompanied by decreasing melting point, but increasing thickness of the meibum. These changes lead to obstruction of the meibomian gland orifices which is augmented by keratinization of epithelial cells at the lid margin. Consequently, the process of meibomian oil secretion and delivery becomes impaired. Glands enlarge and finally degenerate. Rosacea is a major cause of meibomian gland disease and many of the pathological features of posterior blepharitis have been studied in the context of this disease.[82,94] (The clinical features of rosacea blepharitis will be described in Chapter 3.) Histology shows dilation of the blood vessels with perivascular infiltration of lymphocytes, plasma cells and histiocytes.[95] The presence of immune complexes in the skin and conjunctiva of patients with rosacea suggests an immune mediated disease.[96] By use of impression cytology "lytic changes" have been described in the superficial conjunctival epithelium of patients with meibomian gland disease.[97] These cellular abnormalities that can be well differentiated from squamous metaplasia (often present in aqueous tear deficiency), might be due to toxic effects exerted by pathological lipids or bacterial toxins.

Lid-related evaporative dry eye can be based on *insufficient blinking*. Lid blinking is important for spreading and clearing tears.[98] It has been established that the degree of tear evaporation is determined by the size of the ocular surface area that is not covered by eyelids.[99] Furthermore, the rate of blinking varies according to the occupation of the individual and decreases significantly during, e.g., reading.[100] Consequently, decreased blinking enhances the degree of tear evaporation from the surface, and dry eye symptoms can become evident during certain tasks in patients with compensated dry eye.

Similarly increased lid aperture goes along with increased evaporation of tears that can cause abnormalities of the surface epithelia.

Disorders of the Aqueous Phase

Common pathophysiological changes induced by aqueous tear deficiency are due to mechanical, osmotic and inflammatory alterations of the ocular surface epithelia. In prolonged aqueous tear deficiency, apical surface epithelia of both cornea and conjunctiva undergo ultrastructural changes that result in decreased binding of mucin. Cells not covered by mucin, or with an impaired expression of membranous mucin, can be stained with rose bengal (Figure 2.6).[101,102] Staining of the nasal conjunctiva is a characteristic change in early keratoconjunctivitis sicca.[103] In more severe cases, superficial punctate keratopathy develops that is characterized by intraepithelial edema and lymphocytic infiltration. Patients with aqueous tear deficiency in the context of Sjögren's syndrome may exhibit grayish peripheral corneal infiltrates that represent local deposits of immune complexes.

Although progressive reduction of the number of conjunctival goblet cells occurs in most patients with aqueous tear deficiency, an increase in goblet cells can be observed in the initial phase of the disease. Due to the reduction of the aqueous phase, the number of mucous and desquamated epithelial cells in the tear film is increased. This causes the formation of mucous threads that can adhere to the ocular surface. Filamentary keratopathy represent strands of degenerated epithelial cells combined with mucous and inflammatory cells. On impression cytology, the conjunctival epithelium shows a continuous decrease of the number of goblet cells and a continuous increase of the degree of squamous meta-

Figure 2.6. Staining of the nasal conjunctiva as characteristic change of early keratoconjunctivitis sicca.

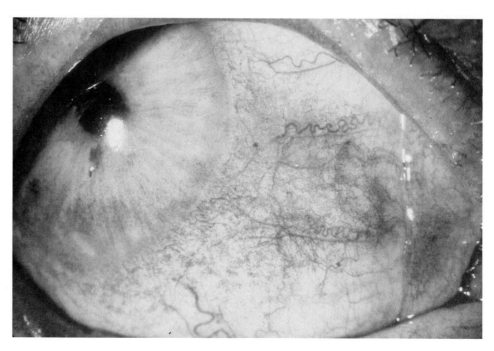

plasia. In advanced aqueous tear deficiency, complete loss of goblet cells and keratinization of the conjunctival epithelium occur. While conjunctival epithelial cells express condensations of nuclear chromatin, remaining goblet cells express no pathological ultrastructural changes.[40,104] The conjunctival stroma may contain inflammatory infiltrates of variable composition including polymorphonuclear granulocytes, lymphocytes and plasma cells.

Disorders that affect the main lacrimal gland and the accessory glands causing reduction of the quantity of the aqueous phase of the tear film are listed in Table 2.9. The clinical findings will be described in Chapter 4.

Sjögren's syndrome is an autoimmune disease that affects various glands.[105] Primary Sjögren's syndrome is characterized by insufficiency of the lacrimal and salivary glands, while secondary Sjögren's syndrome is accompanied by connective-tissue disease.[106,107] Sjögren's syndrome has long been interpreted solely as a result of a deficient tear production from lacrimal glands. Lymphocytic infiltration of the lacrimal gland containing CD-4-positive T-cells and B-cells has been described.[108,109] Cy-

tokines released from activated T-cells might be the cause of gland destruction and decreased responsiveness to neuronal stimuli necessary for reflex tear secretion. Subsequent pathological changes of conjunctival and corneal surfaces do not seem to be a consequence only of surface dryness, but rather represent an inflammatory disease of the ocular surface epithelia. Both human and canine conjunctivae are subjected to significant inflammatory changes, such as upregulation of class II HLA antigens and pro-inflammatory adhesion molecules.[110] Recent data obtained by conjunctival flow cytometry confirm upregulation of HLA-DR and demonstrate increased expression of surface markers related to inflammation (e.g., CD 40 and its ligand) or apoptosis (e.g., Fas).[111] Furthermore, the presence of increased levels of inflammatory cytokines such as interleukin (Il)-1 Beta, Il-6 and Il-8 have been documented in the conjunctiva of patients with Sjögren's syndrome.[112] These observations are suggestive of a true inflammatory disease of the ocular surface epithelium in Sjögren's syndrome tear deficiency.

Non-Sjögren tear deficiency can be divided into (1) primary and secondary disorders of the lacrimal gland, (2) obstruction of the lacrimal gland, and (3) a defective tear reflex.

Primary acquired lacrimal disease is the most common form of dry eye and has been seen as a primary, age-related condition. However, many patients show inflammatory changes of the conjunctiva that are similar to those in Sjögren's syndrome. For example, upregulation of HLA-DR and expression of adhesion molecules regulating leukocyte adhesion, such as ICAM-1, have been described.[113] Furthermore, the concept of primary atrophy has recently been challenged by the observation that reduction of the level of systemic androgens might be causative of the loss of lacrimal function and the induction of inflammation.[78] It has been proposed that reduced androgen levels might induce lacrimal gland atrophy.[114] Administration of androgens counteracts lacrimal gland necrosis and apoptosis, and prevents lymphocyte infiltration.[115] There is some evidence that androgens might also modulate the level of inflammatory cytokines in various tissues, and androgen receptors have recently been detected in ocular surface epithelia.[116] However, it is currently unclear whether androgens can also modulate conjunctival inflammation in the context of aqueous tear deficiency. Other causes of primary lacrimal gland disease are rare cases of congenital absence of the main lacrimal gland, as well as familial dysautonomia (Riley–Day syndrome).

Secondary lacrimal gland disease is caused by inflammatory infiltration, e.g., in the context of sarcoidosis or AIDS. Similarly, graft-versus-host disease and irradiation can cause dysfunction of the lacrimal glands. Most of these diseases go along with specific forms of conjunctivitis that have been described above, such as granulomatous inflammation in sarcoidosis.

Table 2.9. Aqueous tear deficiency.

Sjögren's syndrome
  Primary Sjögren's syndrome
  Secondary Sjögren's syndrome associated with
    Rheumatoid arthritis
    Panarteriitis nodosa
    Wegener's granulomatosis
    Systemic lupus erythematodes
    Scleroderma
    Primary biliary cirrhosis
    Thyreoiditis
    Pulmonary fibrosis
Non-Sjögren tear deficiency
  Lacrimal disease
    Primary lacrimal disease
      Primary acquired (senile) lacrimal deficiency
      Congenital lacrimal deficiency
      Riley–Day syndrome
    Secondary lacrimal disease
      Sarcoidosis
      AIDS
      Graft-versus-host disease
      Irradiation, injury to the lacrimal gland
  Lacrimal gland obstruction
    Cicatricial pemphigoid
    Drug-induced pseudopemphigoid
    Epidermolysis bullosa acquisita
    Stevens–Johnson syndrome (Erythema multiforme majus)
    Toxic epidermal necrolysis (Lyell's syndrome)
    Trachoma
    Chemical/thermal burns
  Impaired tear reflex
    Facial-nerve paralysis
    Neurotrophic keratitis
    Contact lens use
    Severe diabetes
    Drugs

Lacrimal gland obstruction is secondary to conjunctival inflammations that induce cicatricial changes of the conjunctiva, as well as mucin deficiency (Table 2.9).

Nervous feedback mechanisms are of importance for normal lacrimal function and secretion of aqueous tears.[77] The reflex system, consisting of the afferent trigeminal nerve (V) and the efferent facial nerve (VII), controls the secretion of aqueous tears from the lacrimal gland. The classic concept of basic tearing and reflex tearing has been challenged by the observation that tear production is reduced during general and local anesthesia, as well as during sleep.[117,118] In contrast, sensory signals deriving from corneal fibers of the trigeminal nerve play a substantial role in maintaining secretory lacrimal function.[77] *Impaired function of the reflex* arc occurs in primary acquired lacrimal disease, possibly as a consequence of decreased corneal sensitivity.[119] Furthermore, several diseases (e.g., contact lens wear that lead to decreased corneal sensitivity) are associated with aqueous tear deficiency.[120]

Disorders of the Mucin Phase

Mucins are essential components in tears, and have been thought to be an important interface between hydrophobic apical cell membranes of the ocular surface epithelia and the tear film.[121] Consequently, deficient mucin production should impair adhesion of the tear film and induce surface changes. This concept has been challenged by observations suggesting that not mucins, but the glycocalyx on the microvilli of epithelial cells, might be responsible for wetting of the ocular surface.[122,123] Various diseases can cause reduction in the number of goblet cells as previously reviewed. Nearly all these diseases go along with severe alterations of the ocular surface epithelia that also relate the microanatomy of its apical surface. Therefore, impaired interaction between surface epithelia and tear film in the context of mucin deficiency can also be explained by alterations of the surface epithelium.

Limbal Stem Cell Dysfunction

The corneal epithelium is characterized by a rapid and continuous cell turnover. A complicated process of self-renewal is necessary for the maintenance of a constant mass of corneal epithelial cells. Impairments of the self-renewing capacity of the corneal epithelium results in the clinical picture of limbal stem cell deficiency. During the past decades, a better understanding of several aspects of corneal pathophysiology, especially the concept of corneal epithelial stem cells, has revolutionized the clinical approach to these disorders.

Regeneration and Repair Requires
Functional Limbal Stem Cells

In a healthy eye, small corneal wounds heal by centripetal movement of neighboring corneal epithelium and closure of such wounds is independent of cell division. The subsequent adjustment of the depleted cell mass depends on cell proliferation, as well as on cell differentiation. Proliferation of corneal epithelial cells originates in stem cells that have an unlimited capacity for cell division. Corneal epithelial stem cells are segregated to the basal limbal epithelium and are not present in the peripheral or central epithelium. This hypothesis is of great importance for the understanding of corneal surface pathology, and the application of surgical strategies for the reconstruction of the abnormal corneal surface. Several functional studies have established that corneal regeneration is only possible in the presence of functional limbal stem cells, and that malfunction of these cells results in typical alterations of the corneal surface.

Dysfunction of Limbal Stem Cells
Results in Limbal Deficiency

When reviewing data concerning the pathology of corneal regeneration and wound healing, animal models can be differentiated from observations on human patients. In rabbits, the amount of stem-cell-containing limbal tissue that is sufficient for maintenance of the corneal epithelium has been quantified, and these studies rendered three major findings: (I) When only the superficial limbal epithelium is removed *together* with the peripheral and central epithelium, the remaining basal epithelium can maintain a corneal phenotype. Wound healing is normal even when the central cornea is wounded repeatedly.[124,125] (II) When the defect also includes the basal stem cells, less than two-thirds of the limbal tissue is sufficient to allow regrowth of the corneal epithelium. This observation seems to be of importance for the surgical correction of limbal stem cell dysfunction and suggests that 50% of the limbal tissue can be harvested from a normal human eye without jeopardizing the capacity for self-renewal. However, rabbit eyes with less than 50% of their stem cells have been shown to suffer from delayed wound healing in the case of severe or repeated injury. When transposed to the human situation, care should be taken when dealing with eyes that have suffered from previous insult to limbal stem cells as, for example, in chemical injury. These eyes seem to have an increased risk for developing problems with wound healing following iatrogenic stem cell depletion for stem cell transplantation.[124,126] (III) When the entire limbal epithelium is removed *together* with the peripheral and central epithelium, more than 90% of the rabbits develop delayed wound healing with subsequent vascularization of the corneal surface. Re-epithelialization is slow, and may take weeks to complete. The resulting epithelium has a dull, irregular appearance and tends to exhibit areas of recurrent epithelial breakdown. The underlying stroma shows varying degrees of superficial haze and opacification.

Subepithelial and superficial stromal vascularization is present. Microscopically, the epithelium is indistinguishable from conjunctival epithelium and contains numerous goblet cells.[125,127] This conjunctivalization of the corneal surface in the absence of limbal stem cells has been termed *limbal stem cell deficiency*.

Limbal Stem Cell Deficiency versus Conjunctival Transdifferentiation

Decades before the development of the stem cell model, clinical observations had shown that complete destruction of the corneal epithelium and the limbus results in conjunctivalization.[128,129] Nevertheless, some patients did not develop neovascularization and healed with a seemingly normal corneal surface despite severe damage to both corneal epithelium and limbus. Subsequent investigations suggested that the absence of corneal neovascularization allows the conjunctival epithelium on the corneal surface to alter its histological appearance and to become cornea-like.[129–131] The transition of the conjunctival phenotype into a corneal phenotype has been termed *conjunctival transdifferentiation*. This phenomenon has led to the hypothesis that the conjunctival epithelium can actually change its phenotype and become corneal epithelium.[132–135] Furthermore, it was thought that the conjunctiva is the proliferative source of the corneal epithelium even under normal circumstances.[136]

However, detailed investigations have proved that transdifferentiated corneal epithelium is significantly different from genuine corneal epithelium.[137–139] It is presently not known whether transdifferentiated epithelium represents atypical corneal or conjunctival epithelium. The latter hypothesis seems to be supported by the observation that occlusion of the vessels in conjunctivalized epithelium induces conjunctival transdifferentiation.[140] This suggests that the vasculature supplies the conjunctival epithelium on the corneal surface with substances that are necessary for the maintenance of the conjunctival phenotype. Retinoic acid is important for the differentiation of goblet cells, and treatment with retinoic acid can prevent conjunctival transdifferentiation.[141–144] It was, therefore, tempting to speculate that a localized deficiency of retinoic acid (and other unidentified factors) results in a loss of goblet cells and a modulation of conjunctival epithelium into a cornea-like epithelium. On the contrary, in vitro data have shown that conjunctival epithelium cannot change its phenotype into corneal epithelium. In humans, longitudinal studies of patients have confirmed that true transdifferentiation did not occur over the course of several months, and that a process of replacement of the corneal epithelium, rather than transdifferentiation, can be observed.[145] In addition, experimental studies suggest that transdifferentiation, at least in animal models, might be a phenomenon that results from a *subtotal loss*

of limbal stem cells.[127,146] Incomplete removal of the limbal epithelium may allow the reconstruction of the corneal epithelium after a certain period that is needed for recovery of the damaged epithelium and can be interpreted as the time sequence of conjunctival transdifferentiation.

Common Pathological Features of Limbal Stem Cell Deficiency

The hallmark of limbal stem cell deficiency is the presence of *goblet cells on the corneal surface*. Histology shows an irregular epithelium of variable thickness that contains numerous cells that can be stained both with alcian blue and PAS. These goblet cells may be prevalent not only in the periphery but in all parts of the cornea including the center. Since the presence of goblet cells is the only certain diagnostic criterion for limbal deficiency, it is important that their existence on the corneal surface be proved. This seems to be mandatory when patients are subjected to any of the forms of allogeneic stem cell transplantation that requires immunosuppression with the inherent risk of significant side effects. Proof of goblet cells can be obtained either by a small (invasive) biopsy or, more elegantly, by (noninvasive) impression cytology.[147] Immunohistochemically, both the absence of a cornea-type differentiation (such as the absence of keratin K-3) as well as the presence of mucin in goblet cells has been shown by monoclonal antibodies.[148,149]

The pathophysiological characteristics of conjunctival epithelium on the corneal surface, in comparison with genuine corneal epithelium, can explain several of the biomicroscopical features of limbal deficiency that are visible on slit-lamp investigation. While the lateral connection of corneal epithelial cells is established by firm tight junctions, the interconnection of genuine conjunctival epithelium is relatively loose. Although no ultrastructural investigations have been performed in limbal deficiency, this could explain the dull, irregular aspect of the corneal surface. The observation that conjunctival epithelium is more permeable than corneal epithelium explains increased staining with fluorescein in limbal stem cell disease that can be appreciated as *delayed fluorescence staining*.[150,151] Increased permeability may also contribute to the generation of calcification in corneas with limbal deficiency. Loose intercellular contact might favor the influx of leukocytes from the tear film, thus explaining chronic inflammatory changes that are prevalent in many patients with limbal deficiency. Genuine corneal epithelium is attached to the basement membrane by hemidesmosomal structures that are not formed by conjunctival basal cells. This lack of hemidesmosomes might explain the tendency of the patients with limbal deficiency to develop recurrent epithelial defects. Furthermore, numerous reports have shown that the integrity and function of the corneal stroma depends on a healthy corneal epithelium. On a cellular level, crosstalk between these two cell types is mediated by polypeptide growth factors that are known to govern cellular differentiation.[152,153] Each cell type seems to express a unique set of cytokines. Therefore, when the corneal epithelium is replaced by conjunctival cells, the cytokine repertoire in the epithelial compartment is most likely changed. This could, in part, explain stromal pathology such as opacification, and haze that might be due to prolonged activation of myofibroblasts. Subepithelial and stromal vascularization is another important histopathological feature of limbal deficiency. As mentioned, the presence of blood vessels seems to be important for the maintenance of the conjunctival phenotype, possibly by supplying retinoids that are crucial for the differentiation of goblet cells. Although it is not known how corneal neovascularization develops, several angiogenic and antiangiogenic growth factors have been identified, and there seems to be some evidence to suggest that the corneal epithelium might contain antiangiogenic factors, while the conjunctiva expresses angiogenic factors.[154] Furthermore, inflammatory cytokines play a major role in corneal angiogenesis. In an experimental setting, limbal deficiency with vascularization of the corneal surface recurred much more frequently in severely inflamed eyes than in eyes with full immunosuppression.[155]

Diseases Associated with Limbal Deficiency

The clinical manifestations of limbal stem cell deficiency can be classified according to the extent of severity, as well as origin (Table 2.10).

Partial limbal deficiency is characterized by various degrees of peripheral conjunctivalization while the visual axis is still covered by corneal epithelium. Sequential observations of patients with corneal and limbal injuries have established that limbal epithelial wounds heal by circumferential movement of small buds of remaining limbal epithelium.[150] In large defects, these migrating limbal sheets cannot meet and instead, conjunctival epithelium can cross the compromised limbal barrier, resulting in partial limbal deficiency. Partial limbal deficiency can be anticipated in most patients with large limbal and corneal defects. It has been established that the conjunctival epithelium can cross the limbal barrier in such patients and that such areas tend to increase with time.[145,150,151] Consequently, mechanical scraping of the invading conjunctival epithelium to allow the neighboring limbal epithelium to cover the defect has been suggested.[151]

Total or *diffuse limbal deficiency* is characterized by conjunctivalization of the entire corneal surface. In some instances, the corneal surface can still contain islands of functional corneal epithelium, and the borders between these two cell types may not be clearly demarcated from each other. This mixed phenotype represents a mosaic pattern.[145]

Depending on the cause of the disease, *primary limbal deficiency* can be differentiated from *secondary limbal deficiency*. Primary limbal deficiency is characterized by the absence of external factors such as injuries, mechanical damage, or medication. Although rare, three disease entities can be attributed to loss or functional impairment of stem cells: aniridia, multiple endocrine deficiency, and congenital erythrokeratodermia. The extent of corneal changes in aniridia is highly variable. A subset of patients expresses irregular and hazy epithelium with neovascularization. In such eyes, goblet cells in the corneal epithelium have been observed by use of impression cytology, suggesting an ingrowth of conjunctival epithelium due to loss of the limbal barrier.[147,156] Two patients with multiple endocrine deficiency also showed goblet cells on the corneal surface.[147] In congenital erythrokeratodermia that was initially described by Burns,[157] a clear but irregular corneal epithelium that contains goblet cells is traversed by blood vessels (Figure 2.7).[158]

The majority of ocular surface disorders that are caused by the absence or dysfunction of corneal stem cells are of secondary origin (Figure 2.8). Most important, chemical and thermal burns cause damage to limbal epithelium and vasculature. The extent of this damage is the cornerstone of various classifications for prognosis after the acute injury.[159–162] Increased permeability of the limbal vasculature leads to an influx of leukocytes that can alter cellular proliferation and differentiation.[160,163,164] In contrast to minor injuries, in which a loss of corneal epithelium is combined with minor limbal damage, larger defects of the limbal circumference cannot heal by sliding of the adjacent healthy limbal epithelium.[150] In partial limbal damage and in severe inflammation, a localized loss of the limbal barrier occurs with conservative invasion of conjunctival epithelium.[128,150,165] Exposure to *irradiation* can also induce limbal stem cell dysfunction. Depending on the dose and the recovery of limbal stem cells, damage can either be permanent or transient.[166]

Table 2.10. Limbal stem cell deficiency.

Primary limbal stem cell deficiency
  Aniridia
  Multiple endocrine deficiency
  Erythrokeratodermia
Secondary limbal stem cell deficiency
  Chemical burns
  Thermal burns
  Irradiation
  Contact lens
  Iatrogenic limbal deficiency
    Multiple limbal surgeries
  Inflammation
    Stevens–Johnson syndrome
    Cicatricial pemphigoid
    Bacterial keratitis

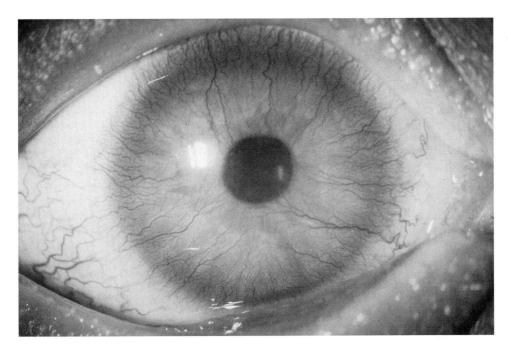

Figure 2.7. Primary limbal deficiency in congenital erythrokeratodermia burns.

Mechanical alteration, toxic factors, and inflammatory mediators combined with hypoxia may lead to limbal deficiency in *contact lens wearers*.[167,168] The clinical triad of corneal neovascularization, epithelial abnormalities (such as indolent ulceration and irregularities with whorled pattern), and stromal opacities has been called contact lens-related epithelial dysfunction.[169] Although there is little information regarding eyes with this disorder, successful surface reconstruction after limbal transplantation further supports that dysfunction of limbal stem cells is the key pathogenic factor.[169,170]

Repeated surgical manipulation at the limbus can also cause permanent dysfunction of limbal stem cells. This entity has been termed *iatrogenic stem cell deficiency*.[171,172] Examples for causative manipulations are excisions of limbus-based malformations such as squamous cell carcinoma or corneal intraepithelial neoplasms, surgery for recurrent pterygium and cryotherapy of the ciliary body.[171,172] The resulting dysfunction of the limbal epithelium has been treated by limbal transplantation.[170,173]

Chronic inflammatory disease can also affect limbal stem cells and cause limbal deficiency. Most patients suffer from long-standing disease frequently aggra-

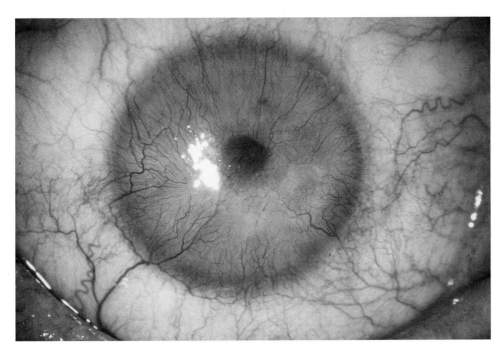

Figure 2.8. Secondary limbal deficiency after chemical burn. Conjunctivalization of the cornea with dull, irregular surface.

vated by the continuous use of topical medication. Important clinical entities in this context are Stevens–Johnson syndrome, cicatrical pemphigoid and other forms of immune-mediated conjunctival inflammation resulting in scarring, as well as microbial keratitis.

In addition to generally accepted forms of stem cell disease, a number of diseases have been attributed to stem cell failure, but this hypothesis is a matter of controversy. It has been suggested that the pathophysiology of *pterygium* is based on malfunction of limbal stem cells.[174,175] Furthermore, this disease has been repeatedly cured by limbal transplantation.[176–178] However, several features of limbal stem cell deficiency are not present in pterygium, and numerous other theories have been proposed to explain the pathology.

Similarly conjunctival intraepithelial neoplasia originates from the limbus and has been interpreted as limbal stem cell disease.[177] Finally *dystrophies of the corneal epithelium and stroma* have been shown to be based on gene mutations.[179,180] Therefore, diseased corneal epithelial cells originate from host stem cells. Based on this assumption, several corneal dystrophies might be interpreted as stem cell disease, and consequently treated by transplantation of healthy limbal tissue.[181]

We have explored disorders of the ocular surface from the viewpoint of pathophysiology. Subsequent chapters will emphasize clinical manifestations, as well as medical and surgical management.

References

1. Greiner JV, Weidman TA, Korb DR, Allansmith MR. Histochemical analysis of secretory vesicles in nongoblet conjunctival epithelial cells. *Acta Ophthalmol* (Copenh) 1985; 63:89–92.
2. Kruse FE, Tseng SCG. Retinoic acid regulates clonal growth and differentiation of cultured limbal and peripheral corneal epithelium. *Invest Ophthalmol Vis Sci* 1994; 35:2405–2420.
3. Wolbach SB, Howe PR. Tissue changes following deprivation of fat-soluble A vitamin. *J Exp Med* 1925; 42: 753–777.
4. Rao V, Friend J, Thoft RA, Underwood BA, Reddy PR. Conjunctival goblet cells and mitotic rate in children with retinol deficiency and measles. *Arch Ophthalmol* 1987; 105:378–380.
5. Pfister RR, Renner ME. The corneal and conjunctival surface in vitamin A deficiency: A scanning electron microscopic study. *Invest Ophthalmol Vis Sci* 1978; 17:874–883.
6. Sommer A, Green WR, Kenyon KR. Bitot's spots responsive and nonresponsive to vitamin A. Clinicopathologic correlations. *Arch Ophthalmol* 1981; 99:2014–2027.
7. Zaltas MM, Ahmed R, Foster CS. Association of HLA-DR4 with ocular cicatricial pemphigoid. *Curr Eye Res* 1989; 8:189–193.
8. Mondino BJ, Brown SI, Rabin BS. HLA antigens in ocular cicatricial pemphigoid. *Arch Ophthalmol* 1979; 97:479.
9. Olsen KE, Holland EJ. The association between ocular

10. cicatricial pemphigoid and rheumatoid arthritis. *Cornea* 1998; 17:504–507.
11. Foster CS. Cicatricial pemphigoid. *Trans Am Ophthalmol Soc* 1986; 84:527–663.
12. Smith EP, Taylor TB, Meyer LJ, Zone JJ. Identification of a basement membrane zone antigen reactive with circulating IgA antibody in ocular cicatricial pemphigoid. *J Invest Dermatol* 1993; 101:619–623.
13. Leonard JN, Hobday CM, Haffenden GP, Griffiths CEM, Powles AV, Wright P, Fry L. Immunofluorescence studies in ocular cicatricial pemphigoid. *Br J Dermatol* 1988; 118:209–217.
14. Bernauer W, Wright P, Dart JK, Leonard JN, Lightman S. The conjunctiva in acute and chronic mucous membrane pemphigoid. An immunohistochemical analysis. *Ophthalmology* 1993; 100:339–346.
15. Roat MI, Sossi G, Lo CY, Thoft RA. Hyperproliferation of conjunctival fibroblasts from patients with cicatricial pemphigoid. *Arch Ophthalmol* 1989; 107:1064–1067.
16. Thoft RA, Friend J, Kinoshita S, Nicolic L, Foster CS. Ocular cicatricial pemphigoid associated with hyperproliferation of the conjunctival epithelium. *Am J Ophthalmol* 1984; 98:37–42.
17. Frith PA, Venning VA, Wojnarowska F, Millard PR, Bron AJ. Conjunctival involvement in cicatricial and bullous pemphigoid: a clinical and immunopathological study. *Br J Ophthalmol* 1989; 73:52–56.
18. Hodak E, Kremer I, David M, Hazaz B, Rothem A, Feuerman P, Sandbank M. Conjunctival involvement in pemphigus vulgaris: a clinical, histopathologic and immunofluorescence study. *Br J Dermatol* 1990; 123:615–620.
19. Schwab IR, Plotnik RD, Mannis MJ. Pemphigus and pemphigoid. *Arch Ophthalmol* 1992; 110:171.
20. Aultbrinker EA, Starr MB, Donnenfeld ED. Linear IgA disease. The ocular manifestations. *Ophthalmology* 1988; 95:340–343.
21. Webster GF, Raber I, Penne R, Jacoby RA, Beutner EH. Cicatrizing conjunctivitis as a predominant manifestation of linear IgA bullous dermatosis. *J Am Acad Dermatol* 1994; 30:355–357.
22. Chorzelski TP, Beutner EH, Jablonska S, Blaszcyk M, Tviftshauser C. Immunofluorescence studies in the diagnosis of dermatitis herpetiformis and its differentiation from bullous pemphigoid. *J Invest Dermatol* 1971; 65: 373–380.
23. Zierhut M, Thiel HJ, Weidle EG, Steuhl KP, Sonnichsen K, Schaumburg-Lever G. Ocular involvement in epidermolysis bullosa acquisita. *Arch Ophthalmol* 1989; 107:398–401.
24. Lin AN, Murphy F, Brodie SE, Carter DM. Review of ophthalmic findings in 204 patients with epidermolysis bullosa. *Am J Ophthalmol* 1994; 118:384–390.
25. Foster CS, Fong LP, Azar D, Kenyon KR. Episodic conjunctival inflammation after Stevens–Johnson syndrome. *Ophthalmology* 1988; 95:453–462.
26. Mondino BJ, Brown SI, Biglan AW. HLA antigens in Stevens–Johnson syndrome with ocular involvement. *Arch Ophthalmol* 1982; 100:1453–1554.
27. Chan HL, Stern RS, Arndt KA, Langlois J, Jick SS, Jick H, Walker AM. The incidence of erythema multiforme, Stevens–Johnson syndrome, and toxic epidermal necrol-

ysis. A population-based study with particular reference to reactions caused by drugs among outpatients. *Arch Dermatol* 1990; 126:43–47.

27. Bianchine JR, Macaraeg PVJ Jr, Lasagna L, Azarnoff DL, Brunk SF, Hvidberg EF, Owen JA Jr. Drugs as etiologic factors in the Stevens–Johnson syndrome. *Am J Med* 1968; 44:390–405.

28. Rubin Z. Ophthalmic sulfonamide-induced Stevens–Johnson syndrome. *Arch Dermatol* 1977; 113:235–236.

29. Shelley WB. Herpes simplex as a cause for erythema multiforme. *JAMA* 1967; 201:153–156.

30. Correia O, Delango L. Cutaneous T-cell recruitment in toxic epidermal necrolysis. *Arch Dermatol* 1993; 129:466–468.

31. Moncada B, Delgado C, Quevedo ME, Lorinez AL. Abnormal T-cell response in toxic epidermal necrolysis. *Arch Dermatol* 1994; 130:116–117.

32. Bagot M, Charue D, Heslan M, Wechsler J, Roujeau JC, Revuz J. Impaired antigen presentation in toxic epidermal necrolysis. *Arch Dermatol* 1993; 129:721–727.

33. Paquet P, Nikkels A, Arrese JE, Vanderkelen A, Pierad GE. Macrophages and tumor necrosis factor alpha in toxic epidermal necrolysis. *Arch Dermatol* 1994; 130:605–608.

34. Wuepper KD, Watson PA, Kazmierowski JA. Immune complexes in erythema multiforme and the Stevens–Johnson syndrome. *J Invest Dermatol* 1980; 74:368–371.

35. Weisman SS, Char DH, Herbort CP, Ostler HB, Kaleta-Michaels S. Alteration of human conjunctival proliferation. *Arch Ophthalmol* 1992; 110:357–359.

36. Nelson JD, Wright JC. Conjunctival goblet cell densities in ocular surface disease. *Arch Ophthalmol* 1984; 102:1049–1051.

37. Hirst LW, Werblin T, Nowak M. Drug induced cicatrizing conjunctivitis simulating ocular pemphigoid. *Cornea* 1982; 1:121–128.

38. Pouliquen Y, Patey A, Foster CS, Goichot L, Savoldelli M. Drug-induced cicatricial pemphigoid affecting the conjunctiva: light and electron microscopic features. *Ophthalmology* 1986; 93:775–781.

39. Fiore PM, Jacobs IH, Goldberg DH. Drug induced ocular pemphigoid. A spectrum of diseases. *Arch Ophthalmol* 1987; 105:1660–1663.

40. Abdel-Khalek LMR, Williamson J, Lee WR. Morphological changes in the human conjunctival epithelium. II in keratoconjunctivitis sicca. *Br J Ophthalmol* 1978; 62:800–806.

41. Hogan EC. Ophthalmic manifestations of progressive systemic sclerosis. *Br J Ophthalmol* 1969; 53:388–392.

42. West RH, Barnett AJ. Ocular involvement in scleroderma. *Br J Ophthalmol* 1979; 63:845–847.

43. Jabs DA, Wingard J, Green WR, Farmer ER, Vogelsang G, Saral R. The eye in bone marrow transplantation. III. Conjunctival graft-vs-host disease. *Arch Ophthalmol* 1989; 107:1343–1348.

44. Jack MK, Jack GM, Sale GE, Shulman HM, Sullivan KM. Ocular manifestation of graft versus host disease. *Arch Ophthalmol* 1983; 103:1080–1084.

45. Wright P. Conjunctival changes associated with inflammatory disease of the bowel. *Trans Ophthalmol Soc UK* 1980; 100:96–97.

46. Whittum-Hudson JA, Taylor HR, Farazdaghi M, Prendergast RA. Immunhistological study of the local inflammatory response to chlamydial infection. *Invest Ophthalmol Vis Sci* 1986; 27:64–69.

47. Taylor HR, Johnson SL, Schachter J, Caldwell HD, Prendergast RA. Pathogenesis of trachoma: the stimulus for inflammation. *J Immunol* 1987; 138:3023–3027.

48. Friedenwald JS, Hughes WF, Hermann H. Acid burns of the eye. *Arch Ophthalmol* 1946; 108:98–108.

49. Ballow M, Mendelson L, Donshik P, Rooklin A, Rapacz P. Pollen-specific IgG antibodies in the tears of patients with allergic-like conjunctivitis. *J Allergy Clin Immunol* 1984; 73:376–380.

50. Dart JKG, Buckley RJ, Monnickendan P, Prasad J. Perennial allergic conjunctivitis: definition, clinical characteristics and prevalence. A comparison with seasonal allergic conjunctivitis. *Trans Ophthalmol Sco UK* 1986; 105: 513–520.

51. McGready SJ, Buckley RH. Depression of cell-mediated immunity in atopic eczema. *J Allergy Clin Immunol* 1975; 56:393–406.

52. Rachelefsky GS, Opelz G, Mickey MR, Kiuchi M, Terasaki P, Siegel S, Stiehm ER. Defective T cell function in atopic dermatitis. *J Allergy Clin Immunol* 1976; 57:569–576.

53. Foster CS, Rice BA, Dutt JE. Immunopathology of atopic keratoconjunctivitis. *Ophthalmology* 1991; 98:1190–1196.

54. Roat MI, Ohij M, Hunt LVE, Thoft RA. Conjunctival epithelial hypermitosis and goblet cell hyperplasia in atopic keratoconjunctivitis. *Am J Ophthalmol* 1993; 116:456–463.

55. Trocme SD, Kephart GM, Allensmith MR, Bourne WM, Gleich GS. Conjunctival deposition of eosinophil granule major basic protein in vernal conjunctivitis and contact lens-associated giant papillary conjunctivitis. *Am J Ophthalmol* 1989; 108:57–63.

56. Allensmith MR, Hahn GS, Simon MA. Tissue, tear and serum IgE concentrations in vernal conjunctivitis. *Am J Ophthalmol* 1977; 81:506–511.

57. Collin HB, Allensmith MA. Basophils in vernal conjunctivitis in humans: An electron microscopic study. *Invest Ophthalmol Vis Sci* 1977; 16:858–864.

58. Allensmith MR, Baird RS, Greiner JV. Vernal conjunctivitis and contact lens-associated giant papillary conjunctivitis compared and contrasted. *Am J Ophthalmol* 1979; 87:544–555.

59. Allensmith MR, Baird RS, Greiner JV. Density of goblet cells in vernal conjunctivitis and contact lens-associated giant papillary conjunctivitis. *Arch Ophthalmol* 1981; 99: 884–885.

60. McMichael AJ, Sazuki T, McDevitt HO, Payne RO. Increased frequency of HLACw3 and HLADw4 in rheumatoid arthritis. *Arthritis Rheum* 1977; 20:1037–1042.

61. Harris ED Jr. Mechanism of disease: rheumatoid arthritis—pathophysiology and implications for therapy. *N Engl J Med* 1990; 322:1277–1289.

62. Ford DK, Schulzer M. Synovial lymphocytes indicate "bacterial" antigens may cause some cases of rheumatoid arthritis. *J Rheum* 1994; 21:1447–1449.

63. Williamson J, Gibson AAM, Wilson T, Forrester JV, Whaley K, Dick WC. Histology of the lacrimal gland in keratoconjunctivitis sicca. *Br J Ophthalmol* 1973; 57:852–855.

64. Raphael M, Bellefqih S, Piette JC, LeHoang P, Debre P,

Chomette G. Conjunctival biopsy in Sjögren's syndrome: Correlations between histological and immunohistochemical features. *Histopathology* 1988; 13:191–202.

65. Pinching AJ, Rees AJ, Pussell BA, Lockwood CM, Mitchison RS, Peters DK. Relapses in Wegener's granulomatosis: the role of infection. *Br Med J* 1980; 281:836–838.

66. Van der Woude FJ, Rasmussen N, Lebatto S, Wiik A, Permin H, van Es LA, van der Giessen M, van der Hem, GK, The TK. Autoantibodies against neutrophils and monocytes: Tool for diagnosis and marker for disease activity in Wegener's granulomatosis. *Lancet* 1985; 1:425–429.

67. Ludemann J, Utrecht B, Gross WL. Anti-neutrophil cytoplasm antibodies in Wegener's granulomatosis recognize an elastolytic enzyme. *J Exp Med* 1990; 171:357–362.

68. Jordan DR, Addison DJ. Wegener's granulomatosis. Eyelid and conjunctival manifestations as the presenting features in two individuals. *Ophthalmology* 1994; 101:602–607.

69. Purcell JJ, Bikenkamp R, Tsai CC. Conjunctival lesions in panarteritis nodosa. A clinical and immunopathologic study. *Arch Ophthalmol* 1984; 102:736–738.

70. Eagle RC, Brooks JSJ, Katowitz JA, Weinberg JC, Perry HC. Fibrin is a major constituent of ligneous conjunctivitis. *Am J Ophthalmol* 1986;101:493–504.

71. Holland EJ, Chan CC, Kuwabara T, Palestine AG, Rowsey JJ, Nussenblatt RB. Immunohistologic findings and results of treatment with cyclosporine in ligneous conjunctivitis. *Am J Ophthalmol* 1989; 107:160–166.

72. Kosik D, Landolt E, Speiser P. Conjunctivitis lignosa. *Klin Mbl Augenheilk* 1980; 176:640–643.

73. Theodore FH, Ferry AP. Superior limbic keratoconjunctivitis. Clinical and pathological correlations. *Arch Ophthalmol* 1970; 84:481–484.

74. Wander AH, Mukusawa T. Unusual appearance of condensed chromatin in conjunctival cells in superior limbic keratitis. *Lancet* 1981; 2:42.

75. Culbertson W, Ostler JB. The floppy eyelid syndrome. *Am J Ophthalmol* 1981; 92:568–575.

76. Arocker-Mettinger E, Haddad R, Konrad K, Steinkogler FJ. Floppy eyelid syndrome. Light and electron microscopic observations. *Klin Mbl Augenkeilk* 1986; 188:596–598.

77. Tseng SC, Tsubota K. Important concepts for treating ocular surface and tear disorders. *Am J Opthalmol* 1997; 124: 825–835.

78. Stern ME, Beurman RW, Fox RI, Gao J, Austin KM, Pflugfelder SC. The pathology of dry eye: The interaction between the ocular surface and lacrimal glands. *Cornea* 1998; 17:584–598.

79. Lemp MA. Report of the National Eye Institute/Industry workshop on clinical trials in dry eyes. *CLAO J* 1995; 21:221–232.

80. Bron AJ. The Doyne lecture. Reflections on the tears. *Eye* 1997; 11:583–602.

81. Chen H, Yamabayashi S, Tanaka Y, Ohno S, Tsukahara S. Structure and composition of rat precorneal tear film: a study by an in vitro cryofixation. *Invest Ophthalmol Vis Sci* 1997; 38:381–387.

82. Zenigin N, Tol H, Gunduz K, Okudan S, Balevi S, Endogru H. Meibomian gland dysfunction tear film abnormalities in rosacea. *Cornea* 1995; 14:144–146.

83. Rolando M, Refojo MF, Kenyon KR. Tear water evaporation and eye surface diseases. *Ophthalmologica* 1985; 190:147–149.

84. Mathers WD, Shields WJ, Sachdev MS, Petroll WM, Jester JV. Meibomian gland dysfunction in chronic blepharitis. *Cornea* 1991; 10:277–285.

85. Mathers WD. Ocular evaporation in meibomian dysfunction and dry eye. *Ophthalmology* 1993; 100:347–351.

86. Shimazaki J, Sakata M, Tsubota K. Ocular surface changes and discomfort in patients with meibomian gland dysfunction. *Arch Ophthalmol* 1995; 113:1266–1270.

87. Chung CW, Tigges M, Stone RA. Peptidergic innervation of the primate meibomian gland. *Invest Ophthalmol Vis Sci* 1996; 37:238–245.

88. Lintron RG, Curnow DH, Riley WJ. The meibomian gland: an investigation into secretion and some aspects of the physiology. *Br J Ophthalmol* 1961; 66:905–909.

89. McDonald JE. Surface phenomena of tear films. *Trans Am Ophthalmol Soc* 1968; 66:905–909.

90. Dougherty JM, McCulley JP, Silvany RE, Meyer DR. The role of tetracycline in chronic blepharitis. *Invest Ophthalmol Vis Sci* 1991; 32:2970–2975.

91. Smolin G, Okumoto M. Staphylococcal blepharitis. *Arch Ophthalmol* 1977; 95:812–816.

92. Shine WE, McCulley JP. The role of cholesterol in chronic blepharitis. *Invest Ophthalmol Vis Sci* 1991; 32:2272–2280.

93. Dougherty JM, Osgood JK, McCulley JP. The role of wax and sterol ester fatty acids in chronic blepharitis. *Invest Ophthalmol Vis Sci* 1991; 32:1932–1937.

94. Browning DJ, Prioa AD. Ocular rosacea. *Surv Ophthalmol* 1986; 31:145–186.

95. Marks R, Harcourt-Webster JN. Histopathology of rosacea. *Arch Dermatol* 1969; 100:683–691.

96. Manna V, Marks R, Holt P. Involvement of immune mechanisms in the pathogenesis of rosacea. *Br J Dermatol* 1982; 107:20–208.

97. Lee S-H, Tseng SCG. Rose bengal staining and cytologic characteristics associated with lipid tear deficiency. *Am J Ophthalmol* 1997; 124:736–750.

98. Doane MG. Interaction of eyelids and tears in corneal wetting and the dynamics of the normal human eyeblink. *Am J Ophthalmol* 1980; 89:507–516.

99. Tsubota K, Yamada M. Tear evaporation from the ocular surface. *Invest Ophthalmol Vis Sci* 1992; 33:2942–2950.

100. Tsubota K, Nakamori K. Dry eyes and video display terminals. *New Engl J Med* 1993; 328:584.

101. Feenstra RPC, Tseng SCG. What is actually stained by rose bengal? *Arch Ophthalmol* 1992; 110:984–993.

102. Feenstra RPC, Tseng SCG. Comparison of fluorescein and rose bengal staining. *Ophthalmology* 1992; 99:605–617.

103. Norm MS. Vital staining of the cornea and conjunctiva. *Acta Ophthalmol Scand* 1969; 99:605–617.

104. Marner K. "Snake-like" appearance of nuclear chromatin in conjunctival epithelial cells from patients with keratoconjunctivitis sicca. *Acta Ophthalmol* (Copenh) 1980; 58: 849–53.

105. Sjögren HS. Zur Kenntnis der Keratokonjunctivitis Sicca. *Acta Ophthalmol* (Copenh) 1933; 11:1–151.

106. Manthorpe R, Oxholm P, Prause JU, Schiöde M. The Copenhagen criteria for Sjögren's syndrome. *Scand J Rheumatol Suppl* 1986; 61:19–21.

107. Shimazaki J. Definition and criteria for dry eye. Report of the Dry Eye research/Diagnostic Standards Committee. *Ophthalmology* (Japan) 1995; 37:765–770.

108. Pflugfelder SC, Wilhelmus KR, Osato MS, Matoba AY, Fond RL. The autoimmune nature of aqueous tear deficiency. *Ophthalmology* 1986; 93:1513–1517.

109. Pepose JS, Akata RF, Pflugfelder SC, Vorgt W. Mononuclear cell phenotypes and immunoglobulin gene rearrangements in lacrimal gland biopsies from patients with Sjögren's syndrome *Ophthalmology* 1990; 97:1599–1605.

110. Jones DT, Monroy D, Ji Z, Atherton SS, Pflugfelder SC, Sjögren's syndrome: cytokine and Epstein-Barr viral gene expression within the conjunctival epithelium. *Invest Ophthalmol Vis Sci* 1994; 35:3493–3504.

111. Brignole F, Pisella PJ, Goldschild M, DeSaint JM, Goguel A, Baudin C. Flow cytometric analysis of inflammatory markers in conjunctival epithelial cells of patients with dry eyes. *Invest Ophthalmol Vis Sci* 2000; 41:1356–1363.

112. Pflugfelder SC, Ji Z, Naqui R. Immune cytokine RNA expression in normal and Sjögren's syndrome conjunctiva. *Invest Ophthalmol Vis Sci* 1996; 37:S358.

113. Pisella PJ, Brignole F, Debbasch C, Lozato PA, Creuzot-Garcher C, Bara J, Saiag P, Warnet JM, Baudin C. Flow cytometric analysis of conjunctival epithelium in ocular rosacea and keratoconjunctivitis sicca. *Invest Ophthalmol Vis Sci* 2000; 107:1841–1849.

114. Mircheff AK, Warren DW, Wood RL. Hormonal support of lacrimal gland function, primary lacrimal gland deficiency, autoimmunity, and peripheral tolerance in the lacrimal gland. *Ocul Immunol Inflamm* 1996; 4:145–172.

115. Azzarolo AM, Wood RL, Mircheff AK, Richters A, Olsen E, Berkowitz M, Bachmann M, Huang ZM, Zolfagari R, Warren DW. Androgen influence on lacrimal gland apoptosis, necrosis, and lymphocytic infiltration. *Invest Ophthalmol Vis Sci* 1999; 40:592–602.

116. Rocha EM, Wickham LA, da Silveira LA, Krenzer KL, Yu FS, Toda I, Sullivan BD, Sullivan DA. Identification of androgen receptor protein and 5alpha-reductase mRNA in human ocular tissues. *Br J Ophthalmol* 2000; 84:76–84.

117. Jordan A, Baum J. Basic tear flow: does it exist? *Ophthalmology* 1980; 87:920–930.

118. Baum J. A relative dry eye during sleep. *Cornea* 1990; 9:1.

119. Xu K, Yagi Y, Tsubota K. Decrease in corneal sensitivity and change in tear function in dry eye. *Cornea* 1996; 15:235–239.

120. Gilbard JP, Gray KL, Rossi SR. A proposed mechanism for increased tear film osmolarity in contact lens wearers. *Am J Ophthalmol* 1986; 102:505–507.

121. Holly FJ, Lemp MA. Wettability and wetting of corneal epithelium. *Exp Eye Res* 1971; 11:239–250.

122. Cope C, Dilly PN, Kaura R, Tiffany JM. Wettability of the corneal surface: a reappraisal. *Curr Eye Res* 1986; 195:119–124.

123. Liotet S, van Bijsterfeld OP, Kogbe O, Laroche L. A new hypothesis on tear film stability. *Ophthalmologica* 1987; 195:119–124.

124. Chen JJY, Tseng SCG. Corneal epithelial wound healing in partial limbal deficiency. *Invest Ophthalmol Vis Sci* 1990; 31:1301–1314.

125. Huang AJW, Tseng SCG. Corneal epithelial wound healing in the absence of limbal epithelium. *Invest Ophthalmol Vis Sci* 1991; 32:96–105.

126. Chen JJY, Tseng SCG. Abnormal corneal epithelial wound healing in partial-thickness removal of limbal basal epithelium. *Invest Ophthalmol Vis Sci* 1991; 32:2219–2233.

127. Kruse FE, Chen JJY, Tsai RJF, Tseng SCG. Conjunctival transdifferentiation is due to incomplete removal of limbal basal epithelium. *Invest Ophthalmol Vis Sci* 1990; 31:1903–1913.

128. Mann I, Pullinger BD. A study of mustard gas lesions of the eyes of rabbits and man. *Proc R Soc Med* 1942; 35:229–244.

129. Maumenee AE, Scholz RO. Histopathology of the ocular lesions produced by sulfur and nitrogen mustard. *Johns Hopk Hosp Bull* 1948; 82:121–147.

130. Friedenwald JS, Buschke W, Scholz RO. Effects of mustard and nitrogen mustard on mitotic and wound healing activities of the corneal epithelium. *Johns Hopk Hosp Bull* 1948; 82:148–160.

131. Friedenwald J. Growth pressure and metaplasia of conjunctival and corneal epithelium. *Doc Ophthalmol* 1951; 5–6:184–192.

132. Friend J, Thoft RA. Functional competence of regeneration ocular surface epithelium. *Invest Ophthalmol Vis Sci* 1978; 17:134–139.

133. Shapiro MS, Friend J, Thoft RA. Corneal re-epithelialization from the conjunctiva. *Invest Ophthalmol Vis Sci* 1981; 21:135–142.

134. Kinoshita S, Kiorpes TC, Friend J, Thoft RA. Limbal epithelium in ocular surface wound healing. *Invest Ophthalmol Vis Sci* 1982; 23:73–80.

135. Kinoshita S, Friend J, Thoft RA. Biphasic cell proliferation in transdifferentiation of conjunctival to corneal epithelium in rabbits. *Invest Ophthalmol Vis Sci* 1983; 24:1008–1014.

136. Buck RC. Ultrastructure of conjunctival epithelium replacing corneal epithelium. *Curr Eye Res* 1986; 5:149–159.

137. Thoft RA, Friend J. Biochemical transformation of regenerating ocular surface epithelium. *Invest Ophthalmol Vis Sci* 1977; 16:14–20.

138. Kinoshita S, Friend J, Kiorpes TC, Thoft RA. Keratin-like proteins in corneal and conjunctival epithelium are different. *Invest Ophthalmol Vis Sci* 1983; 24:577–581.

139. Harris TM, Berry ER, Pakurar AS, Sheppard LB. Biochemical transformation of bulbar conjunctiva into corneal epithelium: an electrophoretic analysis. *Exp Eye Res* 1985; 41:597–606.

140. Huang AJW, Watson BD, Hernandez E, Tseng SCG. Induction of conjunctival transdifferentiation on vascularized corneas by photothrombotic occlusion of corneal neovascularization. *Ophthalmology* 1988; 95:228–235.

141. Tseng SCG, Hatchell D, Tierney N. Expression of specific keratin markers by rabbit corneal, conjunctival and esophageal epithelium during vitamin A deficiency. *J Cell Biol* 1984; 99:2279–2286.

142. Tseng SCG, Hirst LW, Faradzaghi M, Green WR. Inhibition of conjunctival transdifferentiation by topical retinoids. *Invest Ophthalmol Vis Sci* 1987; 28:538–542.

143. Tseng SCG, Farazdaghi M, Ryder AA. Conjunctival transdifferentiation induced by systemic vitamin A defi-

ciency in vascularized rabbit corneas. *Invest Ophthalmol Vis Sci* 1987; 28:1497–1504.

144. Tseng SC, Farazdaghi M. Reversal of conjunctival transdifferentiation by topical retinoic acid. *Cornea* 1988; 7: 273–279.

145. Dua HS. The conjunctiva in corneal epithelial wound healing. *Br J Ophthalmol* 1998; 82:1407–1411.

146. Cintron C, Hassinger L, Kublin CL, Friend J. A simple method for removal of rabbit corneal epithelium utilizing n-heptanol. *Ophthalmic Res* 1979; 11:90–97.

147. Puangsricharern V, Tseng SCG. Cytologic evidence of corneal diseases with limbal stem cell deficiency. *Ophthalmology* 1995; 102:1476–1485.

148. Huang AJW, Tseng SCG. Development of monoclonal antibodies to rabbit ocular mucin. *Invest Ophthalmol Vis Sci* 1987; 28:1483–1491.

149. Kenyon KR, Bulusoglu G, Zieske JD. Clinical pathologic correlations of limbal autograft of limbal autograft transplantation. *Invest Ophthalmol Vis Sci* 1990; 31:S1.

150. Dua HS, Forrester JV. The corneoscleral limbus in human corneal wound healing. *Am J Ophthalmol* 1990; 110:646–656.

151. Dua HS, Gomes JA, Singh A. Corneal epithelial wound healing. *Br J Ophthalmol* 1994; 78:401–408.

152. Li D-Q, Tseng SCG. Three patterns of cytokine expression involved in epithelial-fibroblast interaction of human ocular surface. *J Cell Phys* 1995; 163:61–79.

153. You L, Kruse FE, Pohl J, Völcker H. Bone morphogenetic proteins and growth and differentiation factors in the human cornea. *Invest Ophthalmol Vis Sci* 1999; 40:296–311.

154. Chang JH, Azar DT, Hernandez-Quintela HC, Lin T, Kato T, Kure T, Lu PC, Ye HQ. Characterization of angiostatin in the mouse cornea. *Invest Ophthalmol Vis Sci* 2000; 41:S832.

155. Tsai RJ, Tseng SCG. Effect of stromal inflammation on the outcome of limbal transplantation for corneal surface reconstruction. *Cornea* 1995; 14:439–49.

156. Nishida K, Kinoshita S, Ohashi Y, Kuwayama Y. Ocular surface abnormalities in aniridia. *Am J Ophthalmol* 1995; 120:368–375.

157. Burns FS. A case of generalized congenital keratodermia *J Cutan Dis* 1915; 33:255–261.

158. Kruse FE, Rohrschneider K, Blum M, Völcker HE, Tilgen M, Longère G, Anton-Lamprecht I. Ocular findings in progressive erythrokeratodermia. *Ger J Ophthalmol* 1993; 2:368.

159. Hughes WR Jr. Alkali burns of the eye I. Review of the literature and summary of the present knowledge. *Arch Ophthalmol* 1946; 35:423.

160. Hughes WR Jr. Alkali burns of the eye II. Clinical and pathologic course. *Arch Ophthalmol* 1946; 36:189–214.

161. Roper-Hall MJ. Thermal and chemical burns. *Trans Ophthalmol Soc UK* 1965; 85:631–646.

162. Thoft RA. Chemical and thermal injury. *Int Ophthalmol Clin* 1979; 19:243–256.

163. Brown SI, Wassermann HE, Dunn MW. Alkali burns of the cornea. *Arch Ophthalmol* 1969; 82:91–94.

164. Matsua H, Smelser GK. Epithelium and stroma in alkali-burned corneas. *Arch Ophthalmol* 1973; 89:396–401.

165. Faulkner WJ, Kenyon KR, Rowsey JJ, Hanninen L, Gipson IK, Gayler J. Chemical burns of the human ocular surface: clinicopathological studies in 14 cases. *Invest Ophthalmol Vis Sci* 1981; 20:S8.

166. Fujishima H, Shimazaki J, Tsubota K. Temporary corneal stem cell dysfunction after radiation therapy. *Br J Ophthalmol* 1996; 80:911–914.

167. Schecter DR, Emery JM, Soper JW. Corneal neovascularization in therapeutic soft lens wear. *Contact Intraocul Lens Med J* 1975; 1:141–146.

168. Weinberg RJ. Deep corneal vascularization caused by aphasic soft contact lens wear. *Am J Ophthalmol* 1977; 83: 121–122.

169. Clinch TE, Goins KM, Cobo LM. Treatment of contact lens-related ocular surface disorders with autologous conjunctival transplantation. *Ophthalmology* 1992; 99:634–638.

170. Kenyon KR, Tseng SCG. Limbal autograft transplantation for ocular surface disorders. *Ophthalmology* 1989; 96:709–722.

171. Schwartz GS, Holland EJ. Iatrogenic limbal stem cell deficiency. *Cornea* 1998; 17:31–37.

172. Holland EJ, Schwartz GS. Iatrogenic limbal stem cell deficiency. *Trans Am Ophthalmol Soc* 1997; 95:95–107.

173. Copeland RA Jr, Char DH. Limbal autograft reconstruction after conjunctival squamous cell carcinoma. *Am J Ophthalmol* 1990; 110:412–415.

174. Kwok LS, Coroneo MT. A model for pterygium formation. *Cornea* 1994; 13:219–224.

175. Dushku N, Reid TW. Immunohistochemical evidence that human pterygia originate from an invasion of vimentin-expressing altered limbal epithelial basal cells. *Curr Eye Res* 1994; 13:473–81.

176. Guler M, Sobaci G, Ilker S, Ozturk F, Mutlu FM, Yildirim E. Limbal-conjunctival autograft transplantation in cases with recurrent pterygium. *Acta Ophthalmol* (Copenh) 1994; 72:721–726.

177. Dua HS, Azuara-Blanco A. Autologous limbal transplantation in patients with unilateral corneal stem cell deficiency. *Br J Ophthalmol* 2000; 84:273–278.

178. Gris O, Guell JL, del Campo Z. Limbal-conjunctival autograft transplantation for the treatment of recurrent pterygium. *Ophthalmology* 2000; 107:270–273.

179. Nishida K, Honma Y, Dota A, Kawasaki S, Adachi W, Nakamura T, Quantock AJ, Hosotani H, Yamamoto S, Okada M, Shimomura Y, Kinoshita S. Isolation and chromosomal localization of a cornea-specific human keratin 12 gene and detection of four mutations in Meesmanns corneal epithelial dystrophy. *Am J Hum Genet* 1997; 61: 1268–1275.

180. Munier FL, Korvatska E, Djemai A, Le Paslier D, Zografos L, Pescia G, Schorderet DF. Kerato-epithelin mutations in four 5q31-linked corneal dystrophies. *Nat Genet* 1997; 15:247–251.

181. Sundmacher R, Spelsberg H, Reinhard T. Homologous penetrating central limbokeratoplasty in granular and lattice corneal dystrophy. *Cornea* 1999; 18:664–70.

Part II

Diseases of the Ocular Surface

3
Blepharitis: Lid Margin Disease and the Ocular Surface

Gary N. Foulks

Clinical Classification of Blepharitis

Overview of Blepharitis

Blepharitis is, by definition, inflammation of the eyelids. Broadly, this includes cutaneous disorders and infectious diseases affecting the skin of the eyelid and the eyelashes. More common clinical use of the term blepharitis refers to lid margin disease, including involvement of the accessory glands of the eyelid margin, the mucocutaneous junction, and the meibomian glands. A global representation of the spectrum of blepharitis is depicted in Figure 3.1. While certain cutaneous disorders can be associated with ocular surface disease, it is lid margin disease that is most frequent and most commonly associated with ocular surface damage.

Cutaneous Disease

Probably the most common and dramatic cutaneous expression of blepharitis occurs with allergic or hypersensitivity disease. Contact dermatitis is the most common cause of cutaneous inflammation of the eyelid and can be of two types, irritant or allergic.[1,2] The irritant form is due to physical or chemical insult to the skin. The allergic form is most common (72%) and is a hypersensitivity response often related to cosmetics or topically applied agents.[1] The inflammation can be a type I hypersensitivity reaction with signs of edema and erythema and symptoms of itch and excess tearing.[2] More often, the inflammation is a type IV delayed hypersensitivity reaction or medication reaction with erythema, edema and occasionally desquamation[2] (Figure 3.2). Atopic disease often causes dermatitis of the skin of the eyelid, inflammation of the eyelid margin, and conjunctivitis (Figure 3.3). Conjunctivitis, superficial keratitis, and subsequent corneal vascularization may frequently occur.

Cutaneous infection of the skin of the eyelid is most commonly bacterial (staphylococcal) or viral (herpetic).

Staphylococcal infection can be purulent or ulcerative and often causes angular blepharitis, a focal infection in the skin of the lateral canthus.[3] Herpetic infection classically begins as grouped vesicles on an erythematous base that subsequently ulcerates. Eyelid involvement is one of the most common expressions of recurrent herpetic disease,[4,5] and recurrent angular blepharitis has been documented.[6]

Parasitic infestations of the eyelashes are uncommon, but can also produce chronic inflammation of the eyelids. Phthirus pubis, the pubic louse, has long been recognized as an occasional parasitic inhabitant of the eyelashes and can be associated with blepharitis in both adults[7] and children.[8,9] A curious and somewhat problematic inhabitant of the eyelashes is Demodex, the hair-follicle mite (*D. folliculorum* and *D. brevis*). It is a much more common parasite whose prevalence increases with the age of the patient.[10,11] Infestation has been identified in almost everyone over age 70 and more often in patients with blepharitis, but a causative relationship to blepharitis has not been established.[10,12] Chronic repeated trauma, such as eyelid rubbing, can also provoke cutaneous inflammation and potential ulceration of the eyelid skin.

Lid Margin Disease

Lid margin disease is perhaps the most commonly encountered clinical form of blepharitis. Although well-controlled epidemiologic studies are lacking, surveys indicate that the predominant ocular problems encountered in general practice are the external inflammatory conditions of conjunctivitis and blepharitis.[13] Acute infection of the eyelid margin is usually located in the glands of the eyelid and is most frequently caused by bacteria (Staphylococcus) as manifested in an acute hordeolum, but acute infection of the eyelid margin can occur with Herpes simplex virus producing an ulcerative lesion on the lid border.

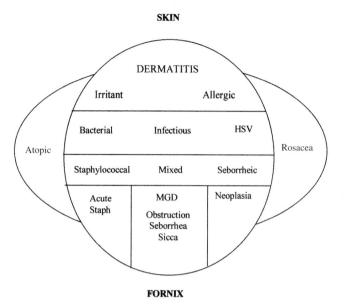

Figure 3.1. The spectrum of blepharitis.

The more problematic condition is chronic blepharitis, which is commonly seen and yet less well understood. Most reviews document the multifactorial etiology of the condition and the difficulty in eradicating the problem with our present treatment options.[14,15,16] The importance of bacterial infection of the lid margin, particularly with Staphylococcus organisms, is well recognized;[17,18,19] yet the frequent colonization of the eyelid by staphylococcal species without frank clinical disease indicates a more complex situation than simple bacterial presence alone.[20]

Historically, the clinical description of chronic lid margin disease (blepharitis) was divided by Thygeson into two types: (1) the squamous type manifested as lid border hyperemia associated with dry or greasy scales at the lash margin (Figure 3.4); and (2) the ulcerative type manifested by small pustules of the lid margin and hair follicles that would subsequently ulcerate (Figure 3.4).[16] Through further microbiologic investigations, Thygeson classified blepharitis as seborrheic, staphylococcic, and mixed seborrheic/staphylococcic, documenting the frequent association of Staphylococcus bacteria and the underlying sebaceous glandular disease. Indeed, recognition of the importance and chronicity of the meibomian gland component was identified as the main obstacle to the successful treatment of blepharitis. A classification of meibomian gland disease was proposed by Gifford in the early 1920s based upon the clinical characteristics of the meibomian secretion and sequelae of disease (Figure 3.5; p. 42), but the system did not clarify pathogenesis of the disease process.[21] Clinical parlance in the early 1970s would refer to anterior versus posterior lid margin disease, but real progress in understanding the disease process came in the late 1970s. This understanding developed from investigations more focused on the meibomian gland secretions, the alterations produced by sebaceous gland dysfunction, and the interactions of the lid margin microflora with those secretions.[21–26] The deleterious effects of lid margin disease on the ocular surface also became more clearly understood as a result of these investigations, which revealed the disturbance of tear film function in such afflictions.[21,26,27,28,29]

Figure 3.2. Allergic blepharitis: contact dermatitis due to topically applied cosmetic.

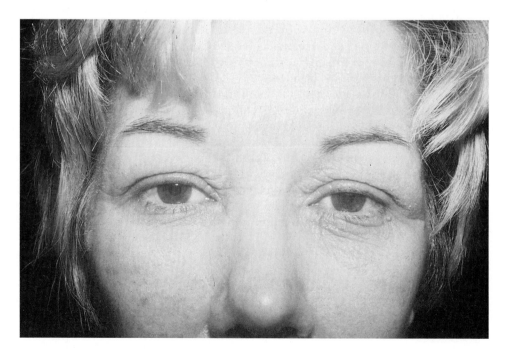

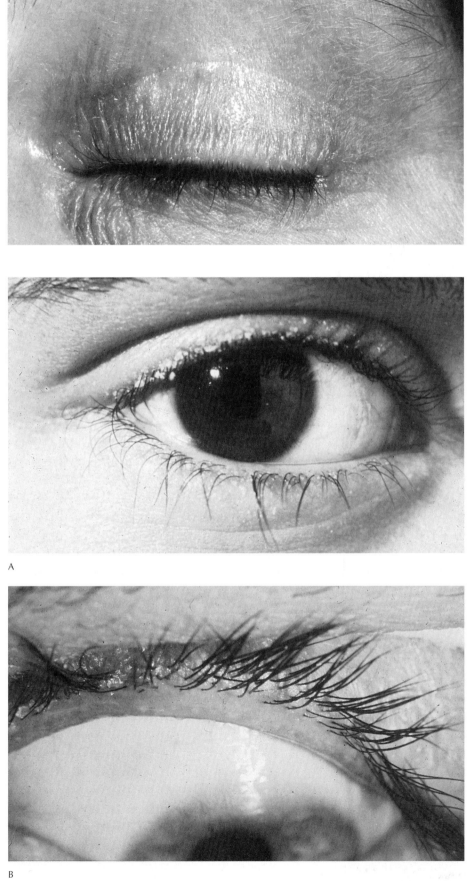

Figure 3.3. Atopic blepharocon-junctivitis.

Figure 3.4. Squamous blepharitis with scaling of the base of the eyelashes (A) and ulcerative bleph-aritis with erosion at the base of the eyelash follicle (B).

A

B

Figure 3.5. Abnormal meibomian secretions. Progressively thicker secretion with clear seborrhea (A), turbid secretion (B), and thick, toothpaste-like secretion requiring expression (C).

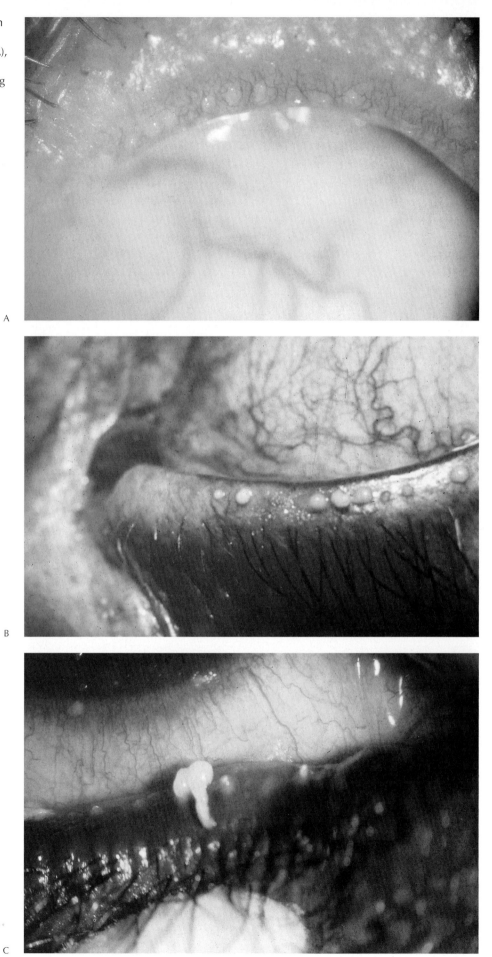

A

B

C

Table 3.1. McCulley classification of blepharitis.

Group	Clinical features
1. Staphylococcal	Lid/lash crust: dry scale, collarettes, more inflammation, short history, little associated seborrheic dermatitis
2. Seborrheic alone	Lid/lash crust: greasy scales, less inflammation, longer course, frequent associated seborrheic dermatitis
3. Seborrheic/staph mixed	Lid/lash crust: greasy scales, more inflammation, exacerbations, frequent associated seborrheic dermatitis
4. Seborrheic/meibomian seborrhea	Lid/lash crust: greasy scales, meibomian secretion normal but increased, frequent associated seborrheic dermatitis
5. Seborrheic/secondary meibomitis	Lid/lash crust: greasy scales, meibomian inflammation patchy with clusters, frequent associated seborrheic dermatitis
6. Primary meibomitis	Lid/lash crust: minimal, meibomian inflammation diffuse, frequent associated seborrheic dermatitis or rosacea
7. Other	Associated with atopy, psoriasis, fungal infection

Based upon extensive analysis of the interaction of bacteria with the secretions of the meibomian glands, McCulley and associates proposed a classification system for chronic blepharitis, identifying six major groups based on clinical signs of disease, and including a seventh group associated with other disorders (Table 3.1).[27] Working from a different perspective, Mathers and associates evaluated the anatomy and function of the meibomian glands in relation to tear film function and characterized the abnormalities of these glands by clinical observations, special photographic techniques, and measurement of tear film characteristics (Table 3.2).[28,30,31] These investigations confirmed the association between blepharitis and dry eye,[32] demonstrating a threefold increase in prevalence of dry eye in patients with blepharitis and verifying increased evaporation of the tear film that had previously been postulated as a contributing factor to dry eye.[33] Bron and associates comprehensively reviewed the anatomy and clinical presentation of abnormalities of the meibomian glands and suggested a grading system for describing anomalies of the glands in an attempt to better characterize meibomian gland disease (Tables 3.3 and 3.4).[34] Although considerable progress has been made in classifying and describing blepharitis and the abnormalities of meibomian gland disease, there is as yet no universal consensus on a definitive classification schema that uniquely categorizes all clinical presentations of blepharitis and meibomian gland disease.[35] An attempt to reach such consensus is being undertaken by a group of investigators active in the field.

Another clinical aspect of meibomian gland dysfunction is based on a growing body of evidence suggesting that hormonal control of the meibomian gland determines its functional capability. Sebaceous glands are very active from birth until about three months of age, possibly due to influence of placental hormones.[36] Activity subsides until puberty when hormones, particularly testosterone, stimulate activity on into adult life. Identification of androgen receptors in the meibomian glands and response of meibomian glands to exogenously administered androgens in animal models indicate an active role for androgen stimulation of structure and function.[37,38] The identification of abnormal tear stability in patients taking anti-androgen therapy and findings of abnormal meibomian gland anatomy and tear instability in female patients with a unique condition of complete androgen insensitivity syndrome offer clinical support to the concept that androgen support is critical for meibomian gland function.

Table 3.2. Mathers classification of meibomian gland dysfunction.

Group	Clinical features
1. Seborrheic	Normal gland morphology but hypersecretion, normal tear film osmolality
2. Obstructive	High gland dropout, low secretion, elevated tear film osmolality
3. Obstructive with sicca	High gland dropout, low secretion, elevated tear film osmolality, reduced Schirmer test
4. Sicca	Normal gland morphology elevated tear film osmolality, reduced Schirmer test

Table 3.3. Bron classification of meibomian gland disease.

1. Absent or deficient
   a. primary
      Congenital
      Anhidrotic ectodermal dysplasia
      Ectrodactyly, ectodermal dysplasia, cleft lip and palate
      Ichthyosis
   b. secondary to lid disease
2. Replacement
   a. primary: dystichiasis
   b. secondary: dystichiasis due to dysplasia
3. Meibomian seborrhea
4. Meibomitis
5. Meibomian neoplasia

Table 3.4. Bron modification of the McCulley classification of blepharitis.

Anterior Blepharitis
  Staphylococcal
  Seborrheic
    Alone
    With staphylococci
    With seborrhea
    With secondary meibomitis
Posterior Blepharitis
  Meibomian seborrhea
  Primary Meibomitis
  Secondary Meibomitis
    secondary to seborrheic blepharitis
    secondary to other disorders (e.g., atropy, cicatrizing
      conjunctivitis, etc.)

Associated Clinical Problems

As might be expected from the previous discussion, certain systemic clinical conditions have a frequent association with blepharitis. The occurrence of blepharoconjunctivitis with dermatologic disease is seen with atopic dermatitis (eczema), epidermolysis bullosa, and sebaceous gland disease (acne rosacea, seborrheic dermatitis).[39] A recent summary of 407 European patients documented associated dermatological disease in 73% of patients (seborrheic dermatitis present in 33%, acne rosacea occurring in 27%, and atopic dermatitis found in 12% of patients).[40] Acute and chronic inflammatory diseases such as cicatricial pemphigoid, Stevens–Johnson syndrome, and toxic epidermal necrolysis also can produce an acute, and sometimes chronic, blepharitis. It is prudent to remember that neoplastic disease can also masquerade as inflammatory blepharitis and that recalcitrant cases of blepharoconjunctivitis demand exclusion of sebaceous carcinoma of the meibomian gland as a cause of chronic and progressive disease.[41,42]

Relationship to Ocular Surface Disease

The adverse effects of lid margin disease on the ocular surface are due to disturbances in the tear film, the action of any participating micro-organisms on the ocular surface, the inflammatory mediators stimulated in the tears and the tissues, and the host immune response.

Relation to the Tear Film

The frequent association of dry eye with blepharitis and meibomian gland disease (MGD) has been documented by several investigators to include not only instability of the tear film, but also lowered tear production.[16,30,31,43,44] The frequency of dry eye is as high as 56% in patients with blepharitis, 48% of patients with obstructive MGD, and 79% of patients with seborrheic MGD.[31] Mathers found a high correlation between presence of reduced Schirmer testing, tear volume, tear flow, and many pa-

rameters of blepharitis or MGD, including gland dropout, lipid viscosity, and lipid volume.[31] Since the tear film provides protection and nutrition to the ocular surface, it is not surprising that disturbance in the quality and quantity of the tears would result in epitheliopathy, susceptibility to superinfection, and the sequelae of scarring and vascularization.

Chronic Inflammation and Immune Responses

The hallmark of blepharitis is inflammation, and such inflammation can affect the ocular surface (Figure 3.6). The contribution of bacterial damage to the ocular surface is multifactorial and probably includes, in addition to lipolytic changes in meibomian gland secretion,[25,45] release of exotoxins, as well as stimulation and release of pro-inflammatory cytokines and chemo-attractants that further provoke inflammation.[16,46] The role of exotoxins has not been well established,[47] but evidence is increasing that pro-inflammatory cytokines and chemo-attractants are produced in patients with ocular rosacea.[16,48] The inflammatory cascade can lead to formation of reactive oxygen species, such as hydrogen peroxide, superoxide free radicals and hydroxyl radicals, all of which can damage cellular membranes.[16]

It is well known that chronic or repeated exposure to bacteria such as Staphylococcus can provoke hypersensitivity reactions resulting in conjunctival inflammation, surface epitheliopathy, corneal limbal infiltrates, and phlyctenular disease with corneal vascularization.[2] With recurrent episodes of phlyctenular disease, hypertrophic scarring of the corneal surface may result (Salzmann's nodular degeneration). More severe and protracted inflammation can damage the periphery of the cornea and the limbal stem cells, resulting in secondary surface failure and progressive vascularization.

Treatment Guidelines

Control of Infectious Organisms

Since the participation of bacterial organisms, particular Staphylococcus species, is frequently associated as a primary or secondary offender in blepharitis, control of any infectious agent is a first step in treatment. This is particularly true of those patients exhibiting ulcerative lesions on the eyelid margin, or other signs suggestive of bacterial growth. Antibiotic coverage for Staphylococcus is advisable with topical agents that are nontoxic and well tolerated, such as erythromycin, bacitracin or trimethoprim/polymyxin delivered three or four times a day for five to seven days. In vitro comparison of susceptibilities of bacterial isolates from patients with conjunctivitis and blepharitis suggests that, while no single antibiotic drug provides 100% broad-spectrum coverage, both established and newly available antibiotics

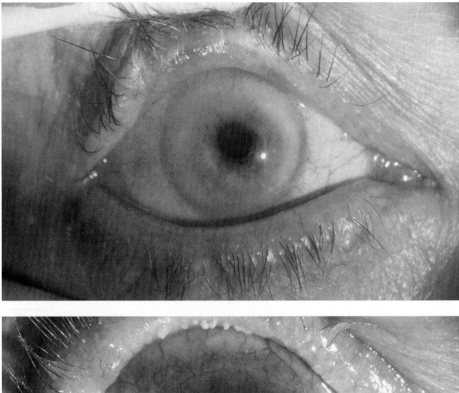

A

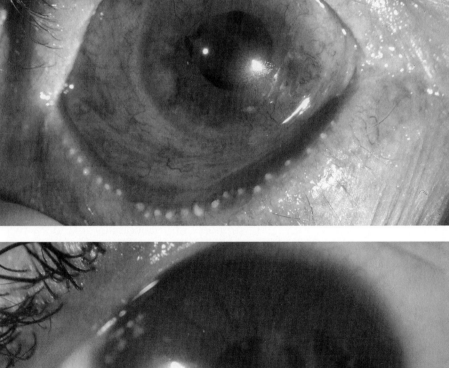

B

C

Figure 3.6. Chronic lid margin scarring and loss of lashes and peripheral corneal vascularization with lipid deposits (A). Conjunctival scarring and peripheral corneal opacities from repeated bouts of blepharoconjunctivitis (B). (Note meibomian gland inspissation.) Central corneal scarring from repeated bouts of phlyctenular keratoconjunctivitis (C).

provide comparable coverage, such that therapy can be based upon the practitioner's clinical experience and cost-effectiveness of therapy.[49] Obviously, if Herpes is a suspected organism, treatment with antiviral agents is appropriate either as topical or systemic medication depending on extent and severity, as well as history of recurrent disease. Topical antibiotic therapy alone will not control chronic blepharitis, but eradication of contributing organisms by a short course of topical therapy is reasonable when bacteria are suspected from clinical signs. Should a suspected microbial agent not respond to initial treatment, culture and sensitivity determination would be appropriate. Systemic tetracycline and the tetracycline family of drugs have been effective therapy for blepharitis. Some of this effectiveness is probably due to the antibiotic properties of the drug, although a greater effect may be due to chemical alteration of lipids and lipases that contribute to lid margin inflammation.[45]

Cleansing of the eyelid margin with dilute solutions of baby shampoo has long been advocated for control of the scaling and debris that accumulates on the eyelid margin. New commercial eyelid wipes impregnated with alkaline detergent solutions are available as convenient packets for patient use. It is important to instruct the patient in the use of such devices to be sure they achieve maximum effect. While such cleansing is helpful in controlling eyelash debris, it does not effectively express the secretions from the meibomian glands. Massage of the eyelids on a daily basis is important in managing chronic blepharitis and lid margin disease.

Treatment of the Meibomian Glands

There are essentially four modalities available to treat meibomian gland disease: physical, medicinal, nutritional, and hormonal. The first two modalities are immediately available and time-tested; the second two modalities are suggested by preliminary work reported, but have not yet been fully evaluated in clinical trials. Nevertheless, such modalities represent future options for consideration in therapy.

Physical methods of treatment include thermal and mechanical approaches. Application of heat to the eyelid facilitates the melting of the secretion and greater expressibility of the secretion from the meibomian glands. The simplest method is direct application of a warm cloth to the eyelid preceding mechanical massage. It is important to instruct the patient in the goal and method of such treatment in order to avoid misapplication of the heat or mechanical measures. While some patients prefer techniques such as heating rice in a sock in the microwave, misadventures can occur when patients become too creative in their technique.[50] Application of heat through infrared or other thermal application devices is effective, but the devices are not always readily available.[51] The mechanical expression of the meibomian gland is probably the most important aspect of physical therapy. Occasionally, the patient is not able to achieve full expression of the glands and requires expression of the eyelids in the office. The expression is easily accomplished with topical anesthesia and application of cotton-tipped applicators to the front and back of the eyelid, expressing the gland between the two applicators in a rolling motion.

The medicinal method of treating meibomian gland disease is predominantly the oral administration of the tetracycline family of drugs (tetracycline, doxycycline, or minocycline) to alter the character of the meibomian gland secretion and inhibit lipase activity of any attendant microorganism.[45] For example, oral doxycyline 100 mg twice daily may be used, with treatment continued for at least two months. The dosage can be tapered to 100 mg daily if maintenance therapy is needed for a longer period of treatment.

Nutritional supplements may have a role in the modification of meibomian gland secretion. A preliminary report of an uncontrolled, unmasked study of oral supplementation of linoleic and linolenic essential fatty acids in eight patients reported symptomatic improvement in intractable, chronic meibomitis.[52] While placebo effect must be considered as responsible for improvement in this anecdotal report, the clinical value of nutritional supplements should be evaluated, especially since these particular fatty acids may have a pharmacologic effect as well in modulating inflammation.[53]

The use of androgen hormone therapy either topically or systemically is under evaluation for treatment of dry-eye disease. A beneficial effect on the anatomy and function of meibomian glands may be possible given the accumulating information about the role of androgen support of meibomian gland activity. Whether the virilizing features of the present generation of androgen congeners can be avoided, or if precursors of androgenic hormones can be appropriately directed as therapy, is yet to be determined, but the possibilities are exciting. The potential anti-inflammatory effects of androgen therapy may also hold promise.

Summary

Great strides have been made in our understanding of the interactions of the eyelid microflora, meibomian gland function, tear film function, and the inflammatory mediators responsible for the clinical manifestations of blepharitis and lid margin disease. While a fully comprehensive and universally accepted classification system is not yet defined to uniquely categorize all aspects of blepharitis and meibomian gland dysfunction, significant advances appear forthcoming to enhance therapy of this common and often vexing condition.

References

1. Shah M, Lewis FM, and Gawkrodger DJ. Facial dermatitis and eyelid dermatitis: a comparison of patch test results and final diagnosis. *Contact Dermatitis* 1996; 34:140–1.

2. Friedlander MH. *Allergy and Immunology of the Eye.* Hagerstown: Harper & Row, 1979.

3. Glover AT. Eyelid infections. In Albert DM, Jakobiec FA, editors. *Principles and Practice of Ophthalmology*, Volume 3. Philadelphia: W. B. Saunders Co., 1994.

4. Liesegang TJ. Epidemiology of ocular herpes simplex: natural history in Rochester, MN, 1950 through 1982. *Arch Ophthalmol* 1989; 107:1160–1165.

5. Egerer I, Stary A. Erosive-ulcerative herpes simplex blepharitis. *Arch Ophthalmol* 1980; 98:1760–1763.

6. Jakobiec FA, Srinivasan BD, Gamboa ET. Recurrent herpetic angular blepharitis in an adult. *Amer Jour Ophthalmol* 1979; 88:744–7.

7. Wingate JR. Phthiriasis palpebrarum—an unusual cause of blepharitis. *Journ Royal Naval Med Service* 1981; 67:29–31.

8. Baker RS, Feingold M. Phthirus pubis (pubic louse) blepharitis. *Amer Jour Dis Child* 1984; 138:1079–80.

9. Turow VD. Phthiriasis palpebrarum: an unusual course of blepharitis. *Arch Ped Adoles Med* 1995; 149:704–5.

10. Norn MS. Demodex folliculorum. Incidence and possible pathogenic role in the human eyelid. *Acta Ophthalmol* 1970; 108:85–9.

11. Roth AM. Demodex folliculorum in the hair follicles of the eyelid skin. *Ann Ophthalmol* 1979; 11:37–45.

12. Coston TM. Demodex folliculorum blepharitis. *Trans Am Ophthalmol Soc* 1967; 65:361–8.

13. McDonnel PJ. How do general practitioners manage eye disease in the community? *Brit Jour Ophthalmol* 1988; 72: 733–42.

14. Raskin EM, Speaker MG, Laibson PR. Blepharitis. *Infectious Disease Clinics of North America* 1992; 6:777–87.

15. Smith RE, Flowers CW Jr. Chronic blepharitis: a review. *CLAO Journal* 1995; 21:200–7.

16. McCulley JP, Shine WE. Changing concepts in the diagnosis and management of blepharitis. *Cornea* 2000; 19:650–7.

17. Thygeson P. Etiology and treatment of blepharitis. *Arch Ophthalmol* 1946; 36:445–77.

18. Smolin G, Okumoto M. Staphylococcal blepharitis. *Arch Ophthalmol* 1976; 95:812–20.

19. Groden LR, Murphy B, Rodnite J, et al. Lid flora in blepharitis. *Cornea* 1991; 10:50–3.

20. Baum J. Current concepts in ophthalmology: ocular infections. *N Eng Jour Med* 1978; 299:28–38.

21. Gifford SR. Meibomian glands in chronic blepharoconjunctivitis. *Amer Journ Ophthalmol* 1921; 4:489–94.

22. Tiffany JM. Individual variations in human meibomian lipid composition. *Exp Eye Res* 1978; 27:289–300.

23. Dougherty JM, McCulley JP. Comparative bacteriology of chronic blepharitis. *Br Jour Ophthalmol* 1984; 68:524–8.

24. McCulley JP, Dougherty JM. Bacterial aspects of blepharitis. *Trans Ophthalmic Soc UK* 1986; 105:314–8.

25. Dougherty JM, McCulley JP. Bacterial lipases and chronic blepharitis. *Invest Ophthalmol Vis Sci* 1986; 27:486–91.

26. Shine WE, Silvany R, McCulley JP. Relation of cholesterol-stimulated staphylococcus aureus growth to chronic blepharitis. *Invest Ophthalmol Vis Sci* 1993; 34:2291–6.

27. McCulley JP, Dougherty JM, Deneau DG. Classification of chronic blepharitis. *Ophthalmology* 1982; 89:1173–80.

28. Mathers WD, Shields WJ, Sachdev MS, et al. Meibomian gland dysfunction in chronic blepharitis. *Cornea* 1991; 10: 277–85.

29. Bron AJ, Tiffany JM. The meibomian glands and tearfilm lipids. Structure, function, and control. *Adv Exp Med Biol* 1998; 438:281–95.

30. Mathers WD, Lane JA, Sutphin JE, et al. Model for ocular tearfilm function. *Cornea* 1996; 15:110–119.

31. Mathers WD. Why the eye becomes dry. *CLAO Journal* (in press).

32. Bowman RW, Dougherty JM, McCulley JP. Chronic blepharitis and dry eyes. *Int Ophthalmol Clinics* 1987; 27:27–35.

33. Rolando M, Refojo MF, Kenyon KR. Increased tear evaporation in eyes with keratoconjunctivitis sicca. *Arch Ophthalmol* 1983; 101:557–8.

34. Bron AJ, Benjamin L, Snibson GR. Meibomian gland disease: classification and grading of lid changes. *Eye* 1991; 5:395–411.

35. Driver PJ, Lemp MA. Meibomian gland dysfunction. *Survey Ophthalmol* 1996; 40:343–67.

36. Duke EMC. Infantile acne associated with transient increases in plasma concentration of luteinizing hormone, follicle-stimulating hormone, and testosterone. *Br Med Jour* 1981; 282:1275–9.

37. Rocha EM, Wickam LA, deSilveira LA, et al. Identification of androgen receptor protein and 5 alpha reductase mRNA in human ocular tissues. *Br Jour Ophthalmol* 2000; 84:76–84.

38. Sullivan DA, Rocha EM, Ullman MD, Krenzer KL, et al. Androgen regulation of the meibomian gland. *Adv Exp Med Biol* 1998; 438:327–31.

39. McCulley JP, Dougherty JM. Blepharitis associated with acne rosacea and seborrheic dermatitis. *Internat Ophthalmol Clinics* 1985; 25:159–72.

40. Huber-Spitzy V, Baumgartner I, Bohler-Sommeregger K, et al. Blepharitis—a diagnostic and therapeutic challenge. *Graefes Archiv fur Clin Exper Ophthalmol* 1991; 229:224–7.

41. Jakobiec FA. Sebaceous tumors of the ocular adnexa. In Albert DM, Jakobiec FA, editors. *Principles and Practice of Ophthalmology*, Chapter 156, Volume 3. Philadelphia: W. B. Saunders Co., 1994.

42. Akpek EK, Polcharoen W, Chan R, et al. Ocular surface neoplasia masquerading as chronic blepharoconjunctivitis. *Cornea* 1999; 18:282–8.

43. McCulley JP, Sciallis GF. Meibomian keratoconjunctivitis. *Amer Jour Ophthalmol* 1977; 84:788–93.

44. Mathers WD, Lane JA. Meibomian gland lipid, evaporation and tear film stability. In Sullivan DA, Dartt DA, Meneray M, editors. *Lacrimal Gland, Tear Film, and Dry Eye Syndromes 2.* New York: Plenum Press, 1998.

45. Dougherty JM, McCulley JP. The role of tetracycline in chronic blepharitis-inhibition of lipase production in staphylococci. *Invest Ophthalmol Vis Sci* 1991; 32:2970–5.

46. Song CH, Choi JS, Kim DK, et al. Enhanced secretory group II PLA2 activity in the tears of chronic blepharitis patients. *Invest Ophthalmol Vis Sci* 1999; 40:2744–8.

47. Seal D, Ficker L, Ramakrishnana M, et al. Role of staphylococcal toxins production in blepharitis. *Ophthalmology* 1990; 97:1684–8.

48. Barton K, Monroy DC, Nava A, et al. Inflammatory cytokines in the tears of patients with ocular rosacea. *Opthalmology* 1997; 104:1868–74.

49. Everett SL, Kowalski RP, Karenchak LM, et al. An in vitro comparison of the susceptibilities of bacterial isolates from patients with conjunctivitis and blepharitis to newer and established topical antibiotics. *Cornea* 1995; 14:382–7.

50. Harrison DA, Lawlor D. Experiences in treating patients for blepharitis. *Arch Ophthalmol* 1998; 116:1133–4.

51. Mori A, Oguchi Y, Goto E, et al. Efficacy and safety of infrared warming of the eyelids. *Cornea* 1999; 18:188–93.

52. Lahners, Palay D, Jones D. Improvement in chronic meibomitis with essential fatty acid supplementation. *Invest Ophthal Vis Sci* 1999;40:S541.

53. Brown NA, Bron AJ, Harding JJ, et al. Nutritional supplements and the eye. *Eye* 1998; 12:127–33.

4
Dry Eye

Stephen C. Pflugfelder and Abraham Solomon

Dry eye is the second most common complaint of patients presenting to ophthalmologists.[1] Despite the prevalence of this condition, physicians use a variety of criteria to diagnose dry eye. These include complaints of eye irritation, rapid tear breakup time, the presence of corneal fluorescein staining, or a low Schirmer test score. More often than not, doctors will say that they know a dry eye when they see it. The lack of a universally accepted gold standard for diagnosis of dry eye stems from the fact that until recently there have not been formal diagnostic criteria for dry eye.

The NEI/Industry workshop held on the campus of the National Eye Institute in Bethesda, Maryland, in 1992 proposed a diagnostic classification for dry eye. That workshop stratified dry eye into conditions resulting from decreased aqueous tear production due to lacrimal gland disease or dysfunction, or from increased tear evaporation, primarily due to meibomian gland disease (Figure 4.1).[2] In clinical practice, segregation of patients into one of these disease categories is complicated by the coexistence of aqueous tear deficiency and meibomian gland disease in many patients.[3] Determining the relative contribution of either of these conditions to a particular patient's discomfort or ocular surface disease is often difficult. This may be due to the fact that the lacrimal gland and ocular surface function as an integrated unit connected by sensory and autonomic nerves.[4] A common feature of all types of dry eye is reduced ocular surface sensation.[3,5] This relative anesthesia reduces the sensory-stimulated drive of tear production by the lacrimal glands. Therefore, perturbations of the ocular surface environment in dry eye from any number of causes may create an escalating disease cycle. This concept helps to explain the considerable clinical overlap that is observed between different dry eye conditions.

The components of this integrated unit consist of the main and accessory lacrimal glands that secrete tear fluid and proteins, the meibomian glands that secrete the lipid evaporative barrier of the tear film, the blink mechanism to spread tears, the drainage system that removes used tears, and the afferent and efferent nerves that interconnect these components. Disease or dys-

function of any of these components can lead to ocular irritation and/or ocular surface disease. This chapter will review an algorithm for diagnosing dysfunction of this integrated unit.

Algorithm for Diagnosis of Dry Eye

Patient History

We have proposed an algorithm for diagnosis of dry eye based on symptoms, signs, and select diagnostic tests (Figure 4.2). Because the majority of patients who present with dry eye disease express subjective complaints of discomfort, the entry point to this diagnostic algorithm is symptoms of ocular irritation. A detailed history should be obtained from patients regarding the nature of their irritation symptoms, conditions that exacerbate their discomfort (such as air travel, forced-air heating, air-conditioning, and prolonged visual efforts such as reading or working on a computer), the duration of their symptoms and their symptomatic response to artificial tears. The most common complaints of dry eye patients are foreign-body sensation, burning, redness, itching, blurred vision, and light sensitivity.[2,3] Other commonly reported symptoms include heavy or tired eyes, soreness, frequent blinking, excessive mucous secretion and intolerance to air drafts or dry environments. Patients with aqueous tear deficiency tend to have worse irritation symptoms in the evening, whereas those with meibomian gland disease and delayed tear clearance tend to have worse symptoms upon awakening in the morning.

A complete past ocular and medical history should be taken. The ocular history should include information about current or prior contact lens use, corneal or anterior segment surgery, allergy, eyelid trauma or surgery, facial nerve (Bell's) palsy, and topical medication use. The medical history should inquire about systemic conditions that may cause or exacerbate dry eye, including dermatological disease (e.g., atopy, Stevens–Johnson syndrome), menopause, nerve trauma and disease (e.g., Parkinson's disease, autonomic dysfunction), neuro-

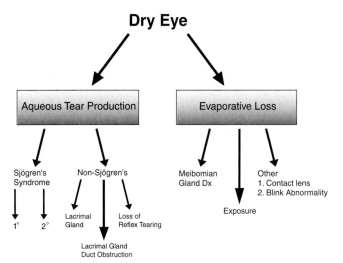

Figure 4.1. Classification scheme proposed by the National Eye Institute (NEI)/Industry workshop for diagnosis of dry eye disease (Reprinted with permission from Murillo-Lopez F, Pflugfelder SC. Dry Eye in *Cornea*, Krachmer J, Mannis M, Holland E editors, Mosby, St. Louis, 1997 p. 664). This scheme stratifies these conditions into those associated with decreased lacrimal function and those with increased evaporative loss.

surgery, autoimmune disease (such as rheumatoid arthritis, systemic lupus erythematosus and scleroderma) and the use of systemic medications with anticholinergic side effects that decrease lacrimal gland tear secretion (such as antidepressants, antihistamines, and agents that suppress bowel and bladder spasms and tremors).[6,7]

Diagnostic Tests

The patient examination should include a careful evaluation of the face, eyelids, and ocular surface for signs of dry eye or non-tear-film related causes of ocular irritation such as staphylococcal blepharitis, ecotropion, entropion, floppy eyelid syndrome or allergy. Patients with irritation symptoms due to dysfunction of the integrated ocular surface/lacrimal gland unit share three common features: an unstable tear film with a rapid tear breakup time, elevated tear osmolarity, and delayed tear fluorescein clearance. If entry-level diagnostic tests identify any of these findings, then patients should undergo tests to identify the specific cause(s) of their problems. These include a Schirmer test to identify aqueous tear deficiency and meibomian gland evaluation to diagnose meibomian gland disease or dysfunction. Aqueous tear deficiency can be classified as Sjögren's-syndrome-related or non-Sjögren's, based on the presence of serum auto-antibodies, a dry mouth, the severity of ocular surface staining with diagnostic dyes, and loss of the nasal-lacrimal reflex. The methods for performing these tests and their endpoints are presented below.

Entry Level Tests

Tear Breakup Time

A reduced tear breakup time (TBUT), indicative of tear film instability, is shared by all the different conditions that can cause dry eye.[3] TBUT is measured using a technique originally described by Norn,[8] and later by Lemp and Holly.[9] The tear film is stained with fluorescein dye and the interval between a complete blink and the appearance of the first randomly distributed black dry spot, hole or streak in the precorneal fluorescein layer is evaluated. An alternative method for measuring tear film stability is by reflecting a regular pattern (such as a grid or rings) off the precorneal tear layer and measuring the time it takes before the pattern distorts or breaks up after a blink.[3,10] This noninvasive tear breakup time, or NIBUT,[10] can be measured with a xeroscope or keratometer.[10,11] Alternatively, corneal surface regularity can be evaluated with the surface regularity index (SRI) of the Tomey TMS-1 videokeratoscopy instrument (Tomey, Cambridge, Mass.).[12] The main advantage of the NIBUT techniques is that they minimize the effect

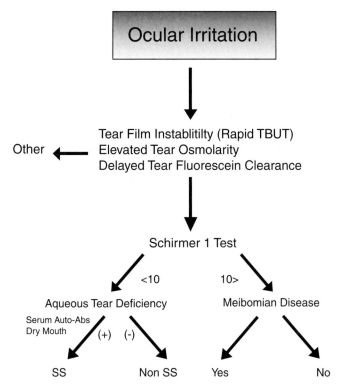

Figure 4.2. Algorithm for diagnosis of dry eye disease. Patients with ocular irritation due to a tear film disorder will have tear film instability with a rapid tear breakup time (TBUT), elevated tear film osmolarity, and delayed tear fluorescein clearance. If one or more of these findings are identified, patients should undergo a Schirmer tear test. Patients with Schirmer tests scores >10 mm should be examined for signs of meibomian gland disease. SS = Sjögren's syndrome; Non SS = Non-Sjögren's syndrome.

of any confounding factors that affect the tear film, such as fluorescein itself or the reflex tearing caused by the instilled fluorescein.[8,13]

Fluorescein TBUT has been reported previously to be rapid in different types of dry eye, including aqueous tear deficiency, mucin deficiency, and meibomian gland disease.[3,8,14–16] Clearly there is wide variability in the tear breakup times of normal subjects, but a time of 10 seconds or less for both fluorescein-added and noninvasive techniques, if consistently obtained, appears to indicate the presence of tear film instability.[3,17]

Fluorescein Clearance Test

Delayed clearance of fluorescein dye instilled onto the ocular surface has been reported in the two most commonly encountered dry eye conditions, aqueous tear deficiency and meibomian gland disease.[3,5] Evaluation of tear fluorescein clearance can be performed using a variety of techniques.[3,5,18,19] Recently, our group developed a fluorophotometric method that provides accurate quantitative assessment of tear fluorescein clearance,[5] as well as a more clinically useful standardized visual scale to evaluate the tear fluorescein concentration.[20]

The standardized visual scale test was shown to be equivalent to fluorometric assessment of tear clearance in its correlation with irritation symptoms, ocular surface sensitivity, and the severity of ocular surface, eyelid, and meibomian disease.[20] Indeed, both methods of assessing delayed tear clearance show greater correlation with symptoms and signs of dry eye than the Schirmer 1 test. The ability of the fluorescein clearance test to separate healthy subjects from patients with meibomian gland disease and aqueous tear deficiency can be further improved by applying a correction factor based on the Schirmer 1 test score.[21]

Tear Film Osmolarity

The relationship between decreased tear secretion and elevated tear film osmolarity was first proposed in 1941.[22] Elevated tear film osmolarity may be secondary to decreased lacrimal gland tear secretion and/or increased tear film evaporation from exposure, blink abnormalities, or the lipid tear deficiency of meibomian gland disease.[23]

Because of the lack of standardization and the high cost of instruments to measure tear osmolarity, this is not a routine clinical test.

Tests to Determine the Specific Causes of Dry Eye

Schirmer Test

The most commonly used technique for measuring aqueous tear secretion is the Schirmer test that was originally described in 1903.[24] This test can be performed with or without topical anesthesia; the latter is known as the Schirmer 1 test. A Schirmer 1 test value of ≤5.5 mm of strip wetting in 5 minutes was recommended by Van Bijsterveld for diagnosis of aqueous tear deficiency.[25] Using this cutoff value, he reported that the correct diagnosis was made in 83% of dry eye patients tested. Jones popularized the method of instilling a topical anesthetic drop prior to performing the Schirmer test for the purpose of measuring "basal" tear secretion, independent of reflex tearing, and defined a value of less than 10 mm of strip wetting in 5 minutes as abnormal.[26] It has been observed that even the Schirmer test with anesthesia is not completely free of reflex components.[27]

The Schirmer test has been criticized for its variability and poor reproducibility. However, significant differences in Schirmer 1 values were noted between patients with aqueous tear deficiency, patients with meibomian gland disease, and normal controls.[3] All eyes of the normal controls and patients with meibomian gland disease had Schirmer 1 values greater than 5 mm in both eyes, whereas only 5% of eyes in subjects with Sjögren's syndrome aqueous tear deficiency and 33% of eyes in subjects with non-Sjögren's aqueous tear deficiency had Schirmer 1 values greater than 5 mm.[3]

If aqueous tear deficiency is demonstrated with a Schirmer test, then the integrity of the nasal-lacrimal reflex, the severity of ocular surface dye staining with rose bengal or fluorescein dyes, and the presence of serum antibodies may be helpful in differentiating Sjögren's syndrome from non-Sjögren's etiologies.[3]

Diagnostic Dye Staining

The most commonly used dyes to detect the ocular surface disease associated with dry eye (termed keratoconjunctivitis sicca) are fluorescein and rose bengal. Fluorescein stains the ocular surface epithelium by penetrating intercellular spaces. The normal corneal epithelium does not stain with fluorescein; however, this dye readily penetrates the corneal epithelium when the mucous layer is removed.[28] Rose bengal dye stains devitalized epithelial cells as well as healthy epithelial cells that are not coated with mucous.[29] Therefore, these dyes can be used clinically to evaluate the integrity of the pre-ocular mucous layer. It is now recognized that an intact mucous layer is a marker of normal ocular surface epithelial function. Rose bengal also stains lipid-contaminated mucous strands and corneal epithelial filaments. The use of a mixture of fluorescein and rose bengal dyes has been reported for clinical use to take advantage of the unique staining properties of both dyes with instillation of a single drop.[30,31] The classic location of rose bengal staining in aqueous tear deficiency is the interpalpebral conjunctiva. The staining appears in the shape of two triangles whose bases are at the limbus.[32] The conjunctiva usually shows stronger staining than the cornea, but in severe cases of keratoconjunctivitis sicca the entire cornea can stain with rose bengal. Lissamine green B dye has been reported to stain dead or degenerated cells, and it produces less irritation after topical administration than rose bengal.[33]

Sjögren's Syndrome
Certain tests are useful for distinguishing Sjögren's syndrome aqueous tear deficiency from non-Sjögren's causes.

Absence of Nasal-Lacrimal Reflex Tearing
The nasal-lacrimal reflex can be elicited by stimulating the nasal mucosa under the middle turbinate with a cotton-tipped applicator. It was reported that the nasal-lacrimal reflex is preserved in most patients with non-Sjögren's aqueous tear deficiency; however, it is typically lost early in the course of the disease in patients with the syndrome.[3,34] This may be due to the presence in a high percentage of Sjögren's syndrome patients of circulating anti-M3 muscarinic cholinergic receptor antibodies. These receptor antibodies inhibit cholinergic-stimulated tear secretion by the lacrimal gland secretory acini.[35,36]

Severity of Ocular Surface Dye Staining
In a study performed by our group, subjects with Sjögren's aqueous tear deficiency had significantly greater Van Bijsterveld rose bengal staining scores and ocular surface fluorescein staining scores than normal control patients and patients with non-Sjögren's aqueous tear deficiency and meibomian gland disease.[3]

Serum Antibodies
Certain diagnostic criteria for Sjögren's syndrome require the presence of one or more of the following serum autoantibodies: antinuclear antibodies (ANA, titer ≥ 1:160), rheumatoid factor (titer ≥ 1:160), or Sjögren's syndrome specific antibodies such as anti-Ro (SS-A) or anti-La (SS-B).[37] A prospective evaluation of our patients with Sjögren's syndrome found ANA positivity in 63%, rheumatoid factor in 76%, SS-A in 67%, and SS-B in 47%.[3]

Meibomian Gland Evaluation
Meibomian gland disease may be due to atrophy of the lipid-secreting acini, obstruction of glandular ducts from epithelial hyperplasia/keratinization, or other structural changes.[38,39] Diagnosis of meibomian gland disease is made by biomicroscopic identification of the following pathologic signs: ductal orifice metaplasia (white shafts of keratin in the orifices), reduced expressibility of meibomian gland secretions, and increased turbidity or decreased fluidity of the expressed secretions. Furthermore, the percentage of meibomian gland acinar dropout can be quantified by transilluminating the inferior tarsus with a halogen Finhoff transilluminator (Welch Allyn, Inc., Schenectady, N.Y.).[3]

Relationship of Tear Function to the Ocular Surface

The importance of the tear film in maintaining ocular surface health has been recognized for centuries. Clini-

cians have also recognized that patients with decreased aqueous tear production may develop keratoconjunctivitis sicca (KCS). There is no direct relationship between the levels of aqueous tear production and the severity of KCS. Some patients with low Schirmer test scores have minimal or no KCS, while others with moderate levels of aqueous tear production develop severe KCS. Two measures of tear function have been found to show better correlation with the severity of KCS than the Schirmer test. These are loss of the ability to reflex tear in response to sensory stimulation (nasal-lacrimal reflex) and delayed clearance of tears from the ocular surface (measured by the tear fluorescein clearance test). When the correlation between Schirmer 1 test scores and ocular surface rose bengal staining scores (graded 0–12) was evaluated, a significant correlation was observed between these two parameters. However, patients with Schirmer 1 test scores less than 10 mm could be segregated into two groups, those with minimal or no dye staining (scores ≤5) and those with staining scores greater than 5.[3] Over 80% of the patients in the latter group had lost their nasal-lacrimal reflex.[3] Indeed, the most severe KCS is observed in dry eye conditions where the ability to reflex tear is lost, such as Sjögren's syndrome and neurotrophic disease.[3,40] It has been demonstrated in several studies that the clearance of tear fluid from the ocular surface shows better correlation with the severity of KCS than the level of aqueous tear production.[5,21] These findings suggest that the tear film must be refreshed constantly in order to maintain the health of the ocular surface. This may be due to the fact that the concentration of pathogenic factors in the tear fluid, such as the inflammatory cytokine IL-1 and the matrix degrading enzyme MMP-9, increase as tear clearance decreases.[41] It is possible that certain of these factors produce a toxic or inflammatory effect on the ocular surface epithelium that leads to abnormal differentiation and altered mucin production by the epithelium or ocular surface, the hallmark of KCS.

Taken together, these findings suggest that ocular surface health is maintained by an intact ocular surface lacrimal gland integrated unit that appropriately responds to ocular surface insults with delivery of fresh tear fluid onto the ocular surface on demand. This system also requires the proper clearance of used tears through the conjunctiva and lacrimal drainage system. Disruption of any of these mechanisms can lead to ocular surface disease.

Medical Therapy of Dry Eye

Treatment Strategies

A number of treatment modalities are available for dry eye disease. The specific treatment should be tailored to the cause or causes of dry eye that were identified through use of the diagnostic algorithm presented above. Most commonly, patients will be found to have aqueous tear deficiency, meibomian gland disease, or a combination of both. If intrinsic irritation stimuli such as allergy, atopy, infection, mechanical problems (lid and lashes abnormalities), and medication toxicity are identified in the workup, they should be treated first. A stepwise approach may be followed for treatment of aqueous tear deficiency.

1. Lubricate the ocular surface with artificial tears, gels, ointments, or autologous serum drops.
2. Suppress inflammation with topically applied corticosteroids or cyclosporin A.
3. When there is severe aqueous tear deficiency, conserve endogenously produced aqueous tear fluid by punctal occlusion.
4. Minimize exposure. When the lid position causes ocular surface exposure, tarsorrhaphy or Botulinum-toxin-induced ptosis should be considered.
5. Reduce tear evaporation with moisture chamber glasses or protective goggles.
6. Stimulate lacrimal tear secretion by suppressing lacrimal gland lymphocytic reaction with cyclosporin A, or stimulating tear secretion with cholinergic agonists (oral pilocarpine or cevimeline).

Meibomian gland disease may be treated in the following manner:

1. Suppress inflammation with topical corticosteroids or systemic tetracyclines.
2. Treat secondary aqueous deficiency with artificial tears.

Aqueous Enhancement Therapy

1. Tear Substitutes
Artificial tears are aqueous solutions containing polymers or macromolecules that increase the retention time or adherence of the preparation to the ocular surface. These solutions contain materials such as cellulose derivatives (methylcellulose, ethylcellulose, hydroxyethylcellulose), polyvinyl derivatives (polyvinyl alcohol, polyvinylpyrolidone, polyvinylcarboxylic acid), chondroitin sulfate, sodium hyaluronate, and glycerol.[42–47] Lubricant gels contain viscous polymers such as carbomer 940 and polyacrylic acid, and ointments contain oily substances (lanolin, white petrolatum).[46]

Unfortunately, there are no true therapeutic tear replacements with biological activities that mimic the tear film. None of the currently available tear substitutes has proved to be clinically superior. Aqueous enhancement therapies often decrease irritation symptoms and improve ocular surface disease in patients with mild to moderate disease, but they may have a minimal effect in patients with severe dry eye, as typically seen in Sjögren's syndrome. Furthermore, they do not improve conjunctival squamous metaplasia.[47,48]

It is now recognized that frequent use of artificial tears preserved with benzalkonium chloride may produce ocular surface epithelial toxicity.[49] The introduction of preservative-free tear preparations, marketed in unit-dose vials, has eliminated this problem, allowing patients to use drops as frequently as they desire without causing epithelial toxicity.[50] Non-preserved tear substitutes should be recommended for patients with moderate to severe aqueous tear deficiency who feel the need to administer these drops more than 4 times a day. Third generation multidose artificial tears with disappearing preservatives, such as sodium perborate that decomposes to water and oxygen upon contact with the tear fluid, have been released. Ointments and gels may be used to supplement artificial tears because of their greater viscosity and longer residence time. Patients often complain that ointments feel sticky and blur vision and as a consequence are best tolerated when instilled before sleep. Non-blurring gels that rapidly dissipate are better tolerated during the day.

2. Autologous Serum
The beneficial effect of autologous serum in KCS was reported in the mid-1980s.[51,52] A rationale for using serum to treat dry eyes is that it contains fibronectin, vitamin A, epidermal growth factor (EGF), and other growth factors that may have a beneficial effect on the ocular surface epithelium. A recent study found that patients with Sjögren's syndrome had a significant decrease of rose bengal and fluorescein staining following application of 20% autologous serum diluted in normal saline.[53] This treatment also showed efficacy for treating ocular graft-versus-host disease.[54]

Anti-Inflammatory Agents

1. Corticosteroids
Based on increasing evidence that inflammation may be an important factor in the pathogenesis of KCS, topically applied corticosteroids have been evaluated for treatment of dry eye disease. Topical administration of a 1% solution of nonpreserved methylprednisolone, given 3–4 times daily for 2 weeks to patients with Sjögren's syndrome KCS, resulted in moderate or complete relief of symptoms in all patients. In addition, there was a decrease of fluorescein staining and complete resolution of filamentary keratitis.[55] This therapy was effective even for patients suffering from severe KCS who had no improvement from maximum aqueous enhancement therapies. To prevent steroid-related complications with their long-term use, it is recommended that they be used only for short-term "pulse" treatment of exacerbations of KCS.[55] A separate study performed in patients with delayed tear clearance found that topical nonpreserved 1% methylprednisolone resulted in subjective (83%) and objective (80%) improvement and improved tear clearance.[18]

2. Cyclosporin A

Cyclosporin A (CSA) has been evaluated for treating various forms of KCS. Cyclosporin is a peptide that prevents activation and nuclear translocation of cytoplasmic transcription factors that are required for T-cell activation and inflammatory cytokine production. A pilot study performed in 1993 found symptomatic relief and decreased rose bengal staining in patients with KCS treated with topical 1% CSA.[56] Two large multicenter placebo-controlled studies have confirmed the efficacy and safety of topical CSA for the treatment of dry eye disease. In an FDA Phase 2 study, CSA was administered in an oil-in-water emulsion formulation to 129 patients with moderate to severe dry eye disease, in various concentrations, twice daily for 12 weeks. A significant improvement in ocular surface rose bengal staining, superficial punctate keratitis, and a number of irritation symptoms was observed. The 0.1% concentration was found to be the most effective.[57] A Phase 3 trial evaluation of 877 patients with moderate to severe dry eye disease found that CSA, 0.05% or 0.1%, produced significantly greater improvement than vehicle in corneal staining and Schirmer test scores. CSA 0.05% treatment also gave significantly greater improvements in parameters such as blurred vision, need for concomitant artificial tears, and the physician's evaluation of global response to treatment. CSA was found to be safe, without significant topical or systemic adverse effects.[58] A decrease in the number of activated T-lymphocytes infiltrating the conjunctiva and a decrease in expression of the inflammatory cytokine IL-6 in the conjunctival epithelium were noted after 6 months of topical CSA treatment, but not after treatment with the vehicle.[59,60]

3. Tetracyclines

Tetracyclines are compounds that have traditionally been used as antibiotics. More recently, they have been observed to have numerous anti-inflammatory properties, including decreased production and activity of inflammatory cytokines, decreased nitric oxide production, decreased expression of HLA class II antigens, and inhibited metalloproteinase production and activation.[61–63] With regard to the ocular surface, they have been observed to decrease production of IL-1 and MMP-9 by human corneal epithelial cells.[64,65] They have also produced significant improvement in symptoms and joint destruction in patients with rheumatoid arthritis.[66]

Systemically administered tetracycline antibiotics have long been recognized as effective therapies for ocular surface inflammatory diseases. The semisynthetic tetracycline, doxycycline, has been reported to successfully treat the common dry eye condition acne rosacea,[67,68] as well as recurrent corneal erosions[69] and phlyctenular keratoconjunctivitis.[70]

4. Secretogogues

Several therapeutic agents have been reported to stimulate tear secretion. The cholinergic agonist, pilocarpine, has been reported to stimulate tear secretion and decrease the severity of KCS irritation symptoms and artificial tear use when taken orally.[71] This agent is not selective for glandular M3 acetylcholine receptors. Patients may, therefore, experience side effects from excessive cholinergic stimulation such as sweating and intestinal cramping. Cevimeline is another orally administered cholinergic agonist that may have fewer systemic side effects than pilocarpine.[72]

Extracellular UTP and other nucleotides that stimulate P2Y2 purinergic receptors have been reported to increase chloride, fluid, and mucin secretion by the conjunctiva.[73,74] They are being investigated in FDA Phase 3 clinical trials.

Indications for Surgical Treatment of Dry Eye

Surgical therapy of dry eye is reserved for rare patients who do not respond to medical therapy. These therapies can be segregated into three groups: (1) punctal occlusion to conserve endogenously produced tears, (2) tarsorrhaphy and Botulinum A toxin induced ptosis to protect the ocular surface from desiccation and environmental insults, and (3) salivary gland transplantation to supply aqueous fluid to the ocular surface.

Punctal Occlusion

Punctal occlusion is one of the most useful and practical therapies for conserving endogenous tear fluid. Electrocauterization of the tear drainage apparatus was initially described in 1935 by Beetham.[75] Prosthetic punctal plugs were initially reported in 1971.[76] Since that time, a variety of styles of punctal and canalicular plugs have been described, including collagen plugs for temporary occlusion that dissolved in 24 to 72 hours and a thermolabile plug that is injected into the tear canaliculus and solidifies as it reaches body temperature. Although no controlled studies have evaluated the effectiveness of punctal occlusion, clinical series have reported an improvement in signs and symptoms of dry eye.[77–79] One study by Willis and associates reported that the majority of patients experienced an improvement in irritation symptoms, an increase in Schirmer test scores, and a decrease in ocular surface rose bengal and fluorescein staining following punctal occlusion.[79] It appears that punctal occlusion is most effective for patients with markedly reduced aqueous tear production and moderate to severe KCS, as occurs in Sjögren's syndrome. In addition to improving KCS, punctal occlusion also appears to be helpful in treating filamentary keratitis and superior limbic keratoconjunctivitis.[78,80] Punctal occlusion must be used with caution in patients with delayed tear clearance and moderate eyelid or ocular surface inflammation, since this combination of factors may further increase the concentration of pathogenic inflammatory factors in the tear fluid.

Tarsorrhaphy and Botulinum-Toxin-Induced Ptosis

These procedures are indicated for patients with reduced aqueous tear production, with or without altered blinking and ocular surface exposure, who have developed severe epitheliopathy, nonhealing corneal epithelial defects, or frank stromal ulceration. Tarsorrhaphy can be performed on the medial or lateral aspects of the eyelids and can be done temporarily or permanently. This procedure is often effective in healing corneal epithelial defects that have been refractory to other treatment modalities. Type A Botulinum toxin injected into the levator palpebrae muscle induces a temporary (6–8 week) complete ptosis of the upper eyelid that can serve as an alternative to tarsorrhaphy. This therapy has been reported to be successful in healing corneal epithelial defects in several clinical series.[81–83]

Salivary Gland Transplantation

Salivary gland transplantation has been reported to be successful in dry eye conditions with severe permanent lacrimal gland dysfunction, particularly those not associated with systemic autoimmune disease, such as Sjögren's syndrome. These include cases of Stevens–Johnson syndrome (after resolution of the acute inflammation), surgical removal of the lacrimal gland and radiation-induced lacrimal gland atrophy. Two strategies have been employed. The first, reported by Murube, involves transplanting excised minor salivary glands into the inferior tarsal conjunctiva or the conjunctival fornix. These glands remain viable and secrete fluid with the composition of saliva in certain patients.[84] The second approach is transplantation of a portion of the submandibular salivary gland with its attached duct into a pocket made in the temporal fossa. The duct is then directed subcutaneously into the superotemporal conjunctival fornix. This procedure lessened the severity of KCS in almost 100% of the patients with vital grafts one year after the procedure was done.[85] Surgical techniques of this type suffer the disadvantages of technical complexity, as well as the altered consistency of a "tear" film produced by the salivary gland.

References

1. Hikichi T, Yoshida A, Fukui Y, et al. Prevalence of dry eye in Japanese eye centers. *Graefes Arch Clin Exp Ophthalmol* 1995; 223:555–8.
2. Lemp MA: Report of the National Eye Institute/Industry workshop on clinical trials in dry eyes. *CLAO J* 1995; 21: 221–232.
3. Pflugfelder SC, Tseng SC, Sanabria O, et al. Evaluation of subjective assessments and objective diagnostic tests for diagnosing tear-film disorders known to cause ocular irritation. *Cornea* 1998; 17:38–56.
4. Stern ME, Beuerman RW, Fox RI, et al. The pathology of dry eye: The interaction between ocular surface and lacrimal glands. *Cornea* 1998; 17:584–589.
5. Afonso AA, Monroy D, Stern ME, et al. Correlation of tear fluorescein clearance and Schirmer test scores with ocular irritation symptoms. *Ophthalmology* 1999; 106:803–10.
6. Koffler BH, Lemp MA. The effect of an antihistamine (chlorpheniramine maleate) on tear production in humans. *Am Ophthalmol* 1980; 12:217.
7. Mader TH, Stulting RD. Keratoconjunctivitis sicca caused by diphenoxylate hydrochloride with atropine sulfate (Lomotil) [letter]. *Am J Ophthalmol* 1991; 111:377–378.
8. Norn MS. Desiccation of the precorneal film. II. Permanent discontinuity and dellen. *Acta Ophthalmol* (Copenh) 1969; 47:881–9.
9. Lemp MA, Holly FJ. Recent advances in ocular surface chemistry. *Am J Optom Arch Am Acad Optom* 1970; 47:669–72.
10. Mengher LS, Bron AJ, Tonge SR, Gilbert DJ. A non-invasive instrument for clinical assessment of pre-corneal tear film stability. *Curr Eye Res* 1985; 4:1–7.
11. Madden RK, Paugh JR, Wang C. Comparative study of two non-invasive tear film stability techniques. *Curr Eye Res* 1994; 13:263–9.
12. Liu Z, Pflugfelder SC. Corneal surface regularity and the effect of artificial tears in aqueous tear deficiency. *Ophthalmology* 1999; 106:939–943.
13. Mengher LS, Bron AJ, Tonge SR, Gilbert DJ. Effect of fluorescein instillation on the pre-corneal tear film stability. *Curr Eye Res* 1985; 4:9–12.
14. Lemp MA, Dohlman CH, Kuwabara T et al. Dry eye secondary to mucous deficiency. *Trans Am Acad Ophthalmol Otolaryngol* 1971; 75:1223–7.
15. McCulley JP, Sciallis GF: Meibomian keratoconjunctivitis. *Am J Ophthalmol* 1977; 84:788–93.
16. Zengin N, Tol H, Gunduz K et al. Meibomian gland dysfunction and tear film abnormalities in rosacea. *Cornea* 1995; 14:144–6.
17. Paschides CA, Kitsios G, Karakostas KX. Evaluation of tear break-up time, Schirmer's-I test and rose bengal staining as confirmatory tests for keratoconjunctivitis sicca. *Clin Exp Rheumatol* 1989; 7:155–7.
18. Prabhasawat P, Tseng SC. Frequent association of delayed tear clearance in ocular irritation. *Br J Ophthalmol* 1998; 82: 666–75.
19. Xu KP, Tsubota K. Correlation of tear clearance rate and fluorophotometric assessment of tear turnover. *Br J Ophthalmol* 1995; 79:1042–9.
20. Macri A, Rolando M, Pflugfelder SC. A standardized visual scale for evaluation of tear fluorescein clearance. *Ophthalmology* 2000; 107:1338–1343.
21. Macri A, Pflugfelder SC. Correlation of the Schirmer 1 and fluorescein clearance tests with the severity of corneal epithelial and eyelid disease. *Arch Ophthalmol* 2000; 118: 1632–1638.

22. Von Bahr G. Konnte der Flussigkeitsabgang durch die cornea von physiologischer bedengtung sein. *Acta Ophthalmol* (Copenh) 1941; 19:125–134.

23. Gilbard JP, Farris RL, Santamaria II J. Osmolarity of tear microvolumes in keratoconjunctivitis sicca. *Arch Ophthalmol* 1978; 96:677–681.

24. Schirmer O. Studien zur Physiologie und Pathologie der Tränenabsonderdung und Tränenabfuhr. *Graefes Arch Clin Exp Ophthalmol* 1903; 56:197.

25. Van Bijsterveld OP. Diagnostic tests in sicca syndrome. *Arch Ophthalmol* 1969; 82:10–14.

26. Jones LT. The lacrimal secretory system and its treatment. *Am J Ophthalmol* 1966; 62:47–60.

27. Clinch TE, Benedetto DA, Felberg NT, Laibson PR. Schirmer's test: a closer look. *Arch Ophthalmol* 1983; 101: 1383–6.

28. Dursun D, Monroy D, Knighton R, et al. The effects of experimental tear removal on corneal surface regularity and barrier function. *Ophthalmology* 2000; 107:1754–60.

29. Feenstra RP, Tseng SCG. Comparison of fluorescein and rose bengal staining. *Ophthalmology* 1992; 99:605–17.

30. Norn MS. Vital staining of the cornea and conjunctiva; with a mixture of fluorescein and rose bengal. *Am J Ophthalmol* 1967; 64:1078–80.

31. Toda I, Tsubota K. Practical double vital staining for ocular surface evaluation. *Cornea* 1993; 12:366–7.

32. Sjögren HS. Zur kenntnis der keratoconjunctivitis sicca (keratitis folliformis bei hypofunktion der tranendrusen) *Acta Ophthalmol* (Copenh) 1933; 11:1–151.

33. Norn MS. Lissamine green. Vital staining of cornea and conjunctiva. *Acta Ophthalmol* (Copenh) 1973; 51:483–91.

34. Tsubota K. The importance of the Schirmer test with nasal stimulation. *Am J Ophthalmol* 1991; 111:106–8.

35. Robinson CP, Brayer J, Yamachika S, et al. Transfer of human serum IgG to non-obese diabetic Igmu null mice reveals a role for autoantibodies in the loss of secretory function of exocrine tissues in Sjögren's Syndrome. *Proc Natl Acad Sci USA* 1998; 95:7538–43.

36. Waterman SA, Gordon TP, Rischmueller M. Inhibitory effects of muscarinic receptor autoantibodies on parasympathetic neurotransmission in Sjögren's Syndrome. *Arthritis Rheum* 2000; 43:1647–54.

37. Pflugfelder SC, Whitcher JP, Daniels T. Sjögren's Syndrome. In Pepose J, Holland G, Wilhelmus K, editors: *Ocular infection and immunity*, Mosby, St. Louis, 1996, pp. 1043–1047.

38. Gutgesell VJ, Stern GA, Hood GI. Histopathology of meibomian gland dysfunction. *Am J Ophthalmol* 1982; 94:383–7.

39. Jester JV, Nicolaides N, Kiss-Palvolgyi I, Smith RE. Meibomian gland dysfunction. II. The role of keratinization in a rabbit model of MGD. *Invest Ophthalmol Vis Sci* 1989; 30:936–45.

40. Heigle TJ, Pflugfelder SC. Aqueous tear production in patients with neurotrophic keratitis. *Cornea* 1996; 15:135–138.

41. Afonso A, Sobrin L, Monroy DC, et al. Tear fluid gelatinase B activity correlates with tear IL-1α concentration and fluorescein tear clearance. *Invest Ophthalmol Vis Sci* 1999; 40:2506–12.

42. Sand BB, Marner K, Norn MS. Sodium hyaluronate in the treatment of keratoconjunctivitis sicca. A double masked clinical trial. *Acta Ophthalmol* (Copenh) 1989; 67:181–183.

43. Laroche L, Arrata M, Brasseur G, Lagoutte F, Le Mer Y, Lumbroso P, Mercante M, Normand F, Rigal D, Roncin S. Treatment of dry eye syndrome with lacrimal gel: a randomized multicenter study. *J Fr Ophthalmol* 1991; 14:321–326.

44. Solomon A, Merin S. The effect of a new tear substitute containing glycerol and hyaluronate on keratoconjunctivitis sicca. *J Ocul Pharmacol Ther* 1998; 14:497–504.

45. Toda I, Shinozaki N, Tsubota K. Hydroxypropyl methylcellulose for the treatment of severe dry eye associated with Sjögren's Syndrome. *Cornea* 1996; 15:120–8.

46. Murube J, Murube A, Chen A. Classification of artificial tears. II. Additives and commercial formulas. *Adv Exp Med Bio* 1998; 438:705–715.

47. Nelson JD, Farris RL. Sodium hyaluronate and polyvinyl artificial tear preparations: a comparison on patients with keratoconjunctivitis sicca. *Arch Ophthalmol* 1988; 106:484–487.

48. Holly FJ, Lemp MA. Tear physiology and dry eyes. *Surv Ophthalmol*, 1977; 22:69–87.

49. Pfister RR, Burstein N. The effects of ophthalmic drugs, vehicles, and preservatives on corneal epithelium: a scanning electron microscope study. *Invest Ophthalmol* 1976; 15:246–259.

50. Adams J, Wilcox MJ, Trousdale MD, Chien DS, Shimizu RW. Morphologic and physiologic effects of artificial tear formulations on corneal epithelial derived cells. *Cornea* 1992; 11:234–241.

51. Fox RI, Chan R, Michelson JB, Belmont JB, Michelson PE. Beneficial effect of artificial tears made with autologous serum in patients with keratoconjunctivitis sicca. *Arthritis Rheum* 1984; 27:459–461.

52. Kono I, Kono K, Narushima K, Akama T, Suzuki H, Yamane K, Kashiwagi H. Beneficial effect of the local application of plasma fibronectin and autologous serum in patients with the keratoconjunctivitis sicca of Sjögren's syndrome. *Ryumachi* 1986; 26:339–343.

53. Tsubota K, Goto E, Fujita H, Ono M, Inoue H, Saito I, Shimmura S. Treatment of dry eye by autologous serum application in Sjögren's syndrome [see comments]. *Br J Ophthalmol* 1999; 83:390–395.

54. Rocha EM, Pelegrino FS, de Paiva CS, Vigorito AC, de Souza CA. GVHD dry eyes treated with autologous serum tears. *Bone Marrow Transplant* 2000; 25:1101–1103.

55. Marsh P, Pflugfelder SC. Topical nonpreserved methylprednisolone therapy for keratoconjunctivitis sicca in Sjögren's syndrome. *Ophthalmology* 1999; 106:811–816.

56. Laibovitz RA, Solch S, Andriano K, O'Connell M, Silverman MH. Pilot trial of cyclosporine 1% ophthalmic ointment in the treatment of keratoconjunctivitis sicca. *Cornea* 1993; 12:315–323.

57. Stevenson D, Tauber J, Reis BL. Efficacy and safety of cyclosporin A ophthalmic emulsion in the treatment of moderate-to-severe dry eye disease: a dose-ranging, randomized trial. The Cyclosporin A Phase 2 Study Group. *Ophthalmology* 2000; 107:967–974.

58. Sall K, Stevenson OD, Mundorf TK, Reis BL. Two multicenter, randomized studies of the efficacy and safety of

cyclosporine ophthalmic emulsion in moderate to severe dry eye disease. CsA Phase 3 Study Group. *Ophthalmology* 2000; 107:631–639.

59. Kunert KS, Tisdale AS, Stern ME, et al. Analysis of topical cyclosporin treatment of patients with dry eye syndrome: effect on conjunctival lymphocytes. *Arch Ophthalmol* 2000; 118:1489–96.

60. Turner K, Pflugfelder SC, Ji Z, et al. Interleukin-6 levels in the conjunctival epithelium of patients with dry eye disease treated with cyclosporin ophthalmic emulsion. *Cornea* 2000; 19:492–6.

61. Shapiro L, Houri Y, Barak V, Soskolne WA, Halabi A, Stabholz A. Tetracycline inhibits porphyromonas gingivalis lipopolysaccharide lesions in vivo and TNF alpha processing in vitro. *J Periodontal Res* 1997; 32:183–188.

62. Golub LM, Ramamurthy NS, McNamara TF, Greenwald RA, Rifkin BR. Tetracyclines inhibit connective tissue breakdown: New therapeutic implications for an old family of drugs. *Crit Rev Oral Biol Med* 1991; 2:297–322.

63. Golub LM, Sorsa T, Lee HM, Ciancio S, Sorbi D, Ramamurthy NS, Gruber B, Salo T, Konttinen YT. Doxycycline inhibits neutrophil (PMN)-type matrix metalloproteinases in human adult periodontitis. *J Clin Periodontol* 1995; 22: 100–109.

64. Solomon A, Rosenblatt M, Li DQ, et al. Doxycycline inhibition of interleukin-1 in the corneal epithelium. *Invest Ophthalmol Vis Sci* 2000; 41:2544–57.

65. Sobrin L, Liu Z, Monroy DC, et al. Regulation of MMP-9 activity in human tear fluid and corneal epithelial cell culture supernatant. *Invest Ophthalmol Vis Sci* 2000; 41:1703–9.

66. Greenwald RA. Treatment of destructive arthritic disorders with MMP inhibitors: Potential role of tetracyclines. *Ann NY Acad Sci* 1994; 732:181–198.

67. Frucht-Pery J, Sagi E, Hemo I, Ever-Hadani P. Efficacy of doxycycline and tetracycline in ocular rosacea. *Am J Ophthalmol* 1993; 116:88–92.

68. Akpek EK, Merchant A, Pinar V, Foster CS. Ocular rosacea: patient characteristics and follow-up. *Ophthalmology* 1997; 104:1863–1867.

69. Hope-Ross MW, Chell PB, Kervick GN, McDonnell PJ, Jones HS. Oral tetracycline in the treatment of recurrent corneal erosions. *Eye* 1994; 8(Pt 4):384–388.

70. Culbertson WW, Huang AJ, Mandelbaum SH, Pflugfelder SC, Boozalis GT, Miller D. Effective treatment of phlyctenular keratoconjunctivitis with oral tetracycline. *Ophthalmology* 1993; 100:1358–1366.

71. Nelson JD, Friedlaender M, Yeatts RP, et al. Oral pilocarpine for symptomatic relief of keratoconjunctivitis sicca in patients with Sjögren's Syndrome. The MGI Pharma Sjögren's Syndrome study group. *Adv Exp Med Biol* 1998; 438:979–83.

72. Fox RI, Stern M, Michelson P. Update on Sjögren's Syndrome. *Curr Opin Rheumatol* 2000; 12:391–8.

73. Jumblatt JE, Jumblatt MM. Regulation of ocular mucin secretion by P2Y2 nucleotide receptors in rabbit and human conjunctiva. *Exp Eye Res* 1998; 67:341–6.

74. Hoyasa K, Veda H, Kim KJ, et al. Nucleotide stimulation of Cl(−) secretion in the pigmented rabbit conjunctiva. *J Pharmacol Exp Ther* 1999; 291:53–9.

75. Beetham WP. Filamentary keratitis. *Trans Am Ophthalmol Soc* 1936; 33:413–416.

76. Freeman JM. Punctal plug: evaluation of a new treatment for dry eye. *Trans Am Acad Ophthalmol* 1975; 79:874–76.

77. Dohlman DH. Punctal occlusion in keratoconjunctivitis sicca. *Ophthalmology* 1978; 85:1277–81.

78. Tuberville AW, Frederick WR, Wood P. Punctal occlusion in tear deficiency syndromes. *Ophthalmology* 1982; 89:1170–1172.

79. Willis RM, Folberg R, Krackmer JH, Holland EJ. The treatment of aqueous-deficient dry eye with removable punctal plugs: a clinical and impression cytology study. *Ophthalmology* 1987; 84:514–518.

80. Yang HY, Fujishima H, Toda I, Shimazaki J, Tsubota K. Lacrimal punctal occlusion for the treatment of superior limbic keratoconjunctivitis. *Am J Ophthalmol* 1997; 124: 80–7.

81. Gusek-Schneider GC, Erbguth F. Protective ptosis by botulinum A toxin injection in corneal affections. *Klin Monatsbl Augenheilkd* 1998; 213:15–22.

82. Wuebbolt GE, Drummond G. Temporary tarsorrhaphy induced with type A botulinum toxin. *Can J Ophthalmol* 1991; 26:383–5.

83. Kirkness CM, Adams GG, Dilly PN, Lee JP. Botulinum toxin A-induced protective ptosis in corneal disease. *Ophthalmology* 1988; 95:473–80.

84. Murube J, Marcos MG, Javate R. Amylase in mare lacrimale in patients with submandibular salivary gland transplantation to the lacrimal basin. *Adv Exp Med Biol* 1994; 350:565–570.

85. Geerling G, Sieg P, Bastian GO, Laqua H. Transplantation of the autologous submandibular gland for most severe cases of keratoconjunctivitis sicca. *Ophthalmology* 1998; 105:327–35.

5
Epithelial Adhesion Disorders

Larry F. Rich and Frederick W. Fraunfelder

Pathoanatomy of Epithelial Adhesion

The maintenance of the corneal surface is critical for the normal physiologic function of the cornea as a biodefense mechanism and as a refractive surface. Smooth, uninterrupted epithelium is essential for clear vision. Because the cornea faces the external environment directly, it is vulnerable to changing external stimuli including biologic, physical, and chemical agents. Although the cornea is protected by the eyelids, tear film, and blinking action, it also has a maintenance system that renews the corneal epithelium and provides a mechanism for wound healing.

Wound Healing

The initial step in wound healing is epithelial cell migration.[1] Epithelial cells are constantly renewed vertically from the basal cell layer. In addition, there is centripetal movement of new cells from the pluripotential limbal stem cells. When the epithelial cell population at the limbus is traumatized, the first event is the sliding and migration of the adjacent viable epithelial cells to the defective area.[2–5] Once the newly migrated cells cover the denuded area, they begin to proliferate and form wing and surface epithelial cells. Those cells remaining in the basal layer begin to form adhesion complexes with the underlying structures.

There are two mechanisms responsible for keeping cells adherent to neighboring cells and to the extracellular matrix: (1) receptor-mediated adhesion to cells or cellular matrix and (2) formation of an adhesion junctional complex between the epithelium and the underlying stroma.[6]

The Adhesion Complex

Abnormal adhesions from defective junctional complexes result in recurrent corneal erosions. Khodadoust et al.,[7] when examining rabbit corneal epithelium and stroma, described the importance of the adhesion complex in maintaining tight cellular adherence. Abrasive removal of the corneal epithelium left an intact under-lying basement membrane that remained firmly attached to the stroma with the debris of ruptured basal cells. New epithelium migrated to the wound area, utilizing the old basement membrane. The epithelium was initially nonadherent and did not develop tight adhesions until seven days after the initial scraping. Conversely, when the corneal epithelium was removed along with its corresponding basement membrane and superficial stroma, the regenerating epithelium did not cover the defect for four days and did not adhere normally to the underlying stroma for eight weeks. This reinforced the notion that delayed adhesion between epithelium and underlying structures may be a significant factor in recurrent corneal erosions, and led to further studies of this clinical entity.

Electron microscopy shows the thickness of the corneal epithelial basement membrane to be approximately 480 Å. in thickness and to contain fine fibrils and a mucoprotein matrix. The basal epithelial cell is separated from the adjacent basement membrane by a very narrow space measuring 110 Å. Numerous hemidesmosomes, major constituents of the adhesion complex, are scattered along the basal cell membrane, and fine osmophilic fibrils radiate from them across the space between the cell membrane and the basement membrane to join them together.[8]

Studies at the ultrastructural level indicate that the adhesion complex is made up of the following: intermediate filaments (keratin), the hemidesmosome, anchoring filaments, anchoring fibrils, and an anchoring plaque.[9,10] The major cell-matrix adhesion junction of the corneal epithelium is the hemidesmosome. The hemidesmosome consists of a plaque on the cytoplasmic side of the cell membrane that acts as an anchoring site for bundles of intermediate filaments. On the external side, anchoring filaments extend from the electron-dense plaque through the lamina lucida to the lamina densa region of the basement membrane. Anchoring fibrils insert from the stromal extensions into the basement membrane opposite the hemidesmosome (Figure 5.1).

The most common electron microscopic finding in patients with recurrent erosion syndrome is reduplica-

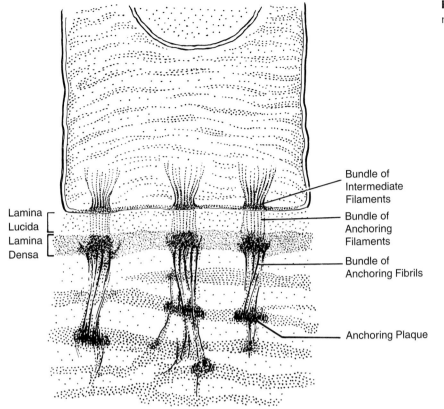

Figure 5.1. Diagram of the corneal anterior basement membrane complex.

Bundle of
Intermediate
Filaments

Bundle of
Anchoring
Filaments

Bundle of
Anchoring Fibrils

Anchoring Plaque

Lamina
Lucida
Lamina
Densa

tion of the basement membrane with loculated connective tissue. Absence of basement membrane and hemidesmosomes is a predictive finding in electron microscopy for severe clinical symptoms.[11]

Attempts at biochemical characterization are under way that may shed light on other mechanisms responsible for abnormal epithelial adhesion. The bullous pemphigoid antigen and the alpha-6 beta-4 integrin heterodimer are two components of the hemidesmosome that have been identified.[6,12] The anchoring filament may be composed of kalinin, and the anchoring fibrils consist of both a globular and helical form of type VII collagen.[13–16]

Normal adhesion between the epithelium and stroma can be affected by many mechanisms, including trauma, ocular, or systemic disease, and inherited corneal dystrophies.

Recurrent Erosion Syndrome

Recurrent corneal erosion is a relatively common condition characterized by repeated episodes of breakdown of the corneal epithelium. Patients typically describe awakening from sleep with a foreign body sensation, photophobia, tearing, and decreased vision. A history of eye trauma dating even years earlier is not uncommon. The trauma is often a minor abrasion, such as a glancing blow caused by a fingernail, or a leaf from a

tree. If the condition is present without a history of eye trauma, then a corneal dystrophy, especially anterior basement membrane dystrophy, should be suspected.

Etiology

Apart from trauma and genetically mediated corneal dystrophies, causes for recurrent erosion include degenerations (Salzmann's nodular degeneration, band keratopathy), herpetic infection, lagophthalmos, keratoconjunctivitis sicca, neurotrophic disease, microbial ulcers, and systemic disease (diabetes mellitus, epidermolysis bullosa).[17]

Given the multiple causes of recurrent erosion syndrome, it is helpful to categorize the condition as either primary or secondary depending on whether the basement membrane complex abnormalities are intrinsic or acquired. The corneal dystrophies (primary dystrophic disorders) frequently cause recurrent erosion syndrome and are more prone to cause recurrent erosion syndrome the more anteriorly they occur in the cornea. Secondary erosive disorders encompass all of the conditions described above except corneal dystrophies.

Anterior Corneal Dystrophies

Anterior epithelial basement membrane dystrophy (map-dot-fingerprint dystrophy, Cogan's dystrophy) is the most common dystrophic cause of recurrent corneal erosion syndrome.[18] This dystrophy appears to occur more often in adults (women > men), usually during the fourth decade of life or later. The condition is bilateral and is characterized by various patterns of subepithelial dots, map-like lines, and random linear fingerprint-like patterns often in the visual axis (Figure 5.2).[19–21] Recurrent erosions or irregular corneal astigmatism frequently bring the dystrophy to the attention of the eye-care professional, although many patients have no symptoms with this type of dystrophy. The erosions may occur because of inherent structural weakness of the thickened, redundant corneal epithelial basement membrane with respect to the synthesis and deposition of type IV collagen.[22]

Meesman's juvenile epithelial dystrophy is characterized by multiple fine epithelial vesicles and often appears earlier in life. Patients rarely experience recurrent erosion syndrome with this entity, but can have recurrent irritation from micro-erosions in the cornea.

Reis-Bücklers' dystrophy is associated with recurrent erosion syndrome more commonly than are other corneal dystrophies. This dystrophy can be further subdivided into corneal dystrophy of Bowman's layer type I and type II. Type I, classic Reis-Bücklers' dystrophy, causes recurrent corneal erosions beginning in early childhood, and along with irregular corneal astigmatism can result in marked visual loss requiring corneal transplantation. Type II also causes recurrent erosions early in life, but vision loss occurs much later. Both categories are characterized by grayish "fishnet" opacities, and a network of grayish ring-like opacities in Bowman's layer and the superficial stroma.[23–25]

Stromal Dystrophies

The stromal dystrophies cause recurrent erosion less commonly than the anterior dystrophies. Because the stromal dystrophies affect the cornea more posteriorly, their usual manifestation is opacification and decreased vision resulting from deposition of foreign material in the visual axis. Nonetheless, erosive episodes do occasionally occur in stromal dystrophy patients, and the treating physician should remain aware of this possibility.

Granular dystrophy is characterized by hyaline deposits in the stroma beneath the epithelium. These deposits stain well with Masson's trichrome, and their origin is unknown. Clinically, there are discrete stromal opacities with intervening clear areas and sparing of the peripheral cornea. If vision is reduced significantly, penetrating keratoplasty is indicated, with the knowledge that recurrence in the graft can occur as early as one year.[26] Erosive episodes are rare, but occur more frequently in some family subsets.

Macular dystrophy causes recurrent erosions more often than granular dystrophy. In addition to progressive loss of vision, patients experience attacks of irritation and photophobia secondary to erosions that can be quite severe. Histologically, there is accumulation of glycosaminoglycans in every layer of the cornea, especially between the stromal lamellae. Clinically, there is diffuse opacification of the stroma with gray-white opacification. The opacities do not have intervening clear spaces and may extend from limbus to limbus. Corneal erosions can be frequent and severe.[27]

Figure 5.2. Anterior epithelial basement membrane dystrophy. Note the loose, irregular epithelium.

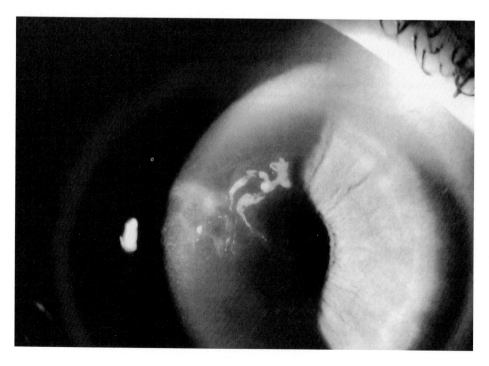

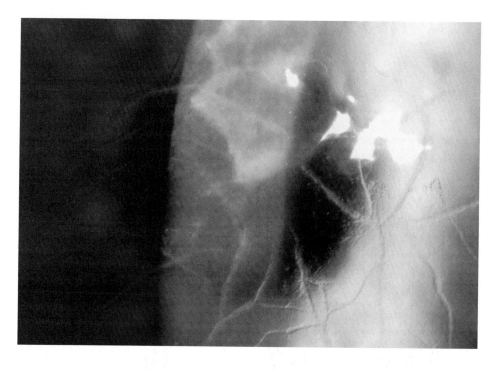

Figure 5.3. Lattice dystrophy with central subepithelial scarring in a patient who has had multiple recurrent erosions.

Lattice dystrophy is a more anteriorly occurring stromal dystrophy and, therefore, is more commonly associated with recurrent erosion syndrome (Figure 5.3). Branching linear lesions and refractile lines appear in the anterior corneal stroma during the first decade of life. This dystrophy is a form of primary localized amyloidosis. In advancing years, the deposits become more numerous and occur in deeper stroma. Management for the erosive episodes is the same as for other dystrophic causes, and will be described below.

Avellino corneal dystrophy is a hybrid of both granular and lattice dystrophy with the clinical characteristics of both, including the occurrence of recurrent erosions. In fact, the erosions occur more commonly in this dystrophy than in granular dystrophy. There are anterior stromal gray-white granular deposits with mid to posterior stromal lattice lesions.[28] Patients develop stromal haze late in the disease and foreign-body sensation, pain, and photophobia occur secondary to recurrent erosions.

Other stromal dystrophies such as Schnyder's crystalline dystrophy, fleck dystrophy, central cloudy dystrophy, and congenital hereditary stromal dystrophy do not appear to cause recurrent erosion syndrome, and the epithelium is not involved in these conditions.

Pathogenesis

Regardless of the etiology (primary or secondary) of recurrent erosion syndrome, the common fault shared by affected corneas appears to be a basic incompetence at the basement membrane level. The pathologic manifestations of individual dystrophies contribute, but probably have less primary significance.[29] Recently, studies have demonstrated that matrix metalloproteinase-2 expression is upregulated in human epithelia affected by recurrent erosion compared with that in normal control samples. Immunolocalization studies indicate that this enzyme is concentrated in basal epithelial cells, where it probably plays a pivotal role in the degradation of the epithelial anchoring system, the recurrent epithelial slippage, and the clinical erosion seen in this syndrome.[30] The source of the metalloproteinase is most likely from leucocytes and degenerated epithelial cells within the sliding epithelium.[22]

Treatment

The management of recurrent erosion syndrome is directed toward promoting re-epithelialization and maintenance of an intact corneal surface with re-establishment of a competent basement membrane complex. The healed epithelium must remain intact for sufficient time to allow the reformation of normal basement membrane complexes responsible for tight adhesions. Treatment may vary depending on the severity of disease and the underlying cause, but most cases resolve with medical therapy alone. Failing this, more elaborate techniques can be employed. These are mentioned briefly in this chapter and will be discussed more fully in later chapters.

Initial medical therapy is aimed at controlling the patient's pain and healing the epithelial defect. If the erosion is small, it will usually heal spontaneously with the aid of a pressure patch placed on the eye for 1 or 2 days. An antibiotic ointment, such as bacitracin or erythromycin can be used beneath the eye patch. The combination of these allows the epithelium to heal beneath a closed eyelid and also provides lubrication, which minimizes epithelial slippage.

However, patients with erosions associated with contact lenses should not be patched because of the increased risk of infection. Recent studies suggest that long-term use of eye ointments may actually increase the recurrence rate of recurrent erosions.[31] Sodium chloride drops (2% or 5%) have been advocated, but these drops may be no more effective than using lubricating ointment alone. The hypertonic saline exerts an osmotic effect that keeps the superficial cornea dehydrated by shifting fluid from the cells into the tear layer and ostensibly prevents lifting of the corneal epithelium on opening the eyelids in the morning. If the epithelium is not intact, however, it absorbs the salt solution, and the salt may not exert a useful effect. Lubrication may be the most important factor.[32]

Hydrophyllic therapeutic bandage contact lenses may also be helpful by protecting the healing epithelium from further lid trauma. The lenses also minimize patient discomfort. Treatment with contact lenses may not be a first-line therapy, since there is potential for infectious keratitis with long-term use, and there is need for frequent follow-up visits. The use of a therapeutic lens is usually indicated for a minimum course of 6 to 8 weeks and requires both monitoring and the use of a broad-spectrum prophylactic antibiotic.

Failing the above treatments, there are a few viable options which are very effective in treating recalcitrant cases of recurrent erosion syndrome. Briefly, anterior stromal micropuncture, superficial keratectomy, phototherapeutic keratectomy, and diamond burring of Bowman's layer after superficial keratectomy have been advocated. A more in-depth discussion of these techniques is presented in later chapters.

Neurotrophic Keratitis

Neurotrophic keratitis is a degeneration of the cornea secondary to reduced or absent corneal sensation. The corneal epithelium is affected first, and deeper layers may become involved leading to stromal melting and corneal perforation if the disease process is not arrested.

Etiology

The disorder most commonly associated with neurotrophic keratitis is infection with either Herpes zoster virus or Herpes simplex virus.[33–35] Other causes include surgeries or tumors that damage the trigeminal nerve, e.g., removal of acoustic neuroma or surgery such as rhizotomy to alleviate trigeminal neuralgia.[36,37] In addition, neurotrophic keratitis may be caused by trauma (e.g., maxillary fractures), infections (e.g., leprosy), corneal dystrophies, topical medications or toxic exposures, congenital syndromes (e.g., familial dysautonomia), and systemic diseases (e.g., diabetes, multiple sclerosis).[38,39]

Although Herpes zoster infection is a common cause

of neurotrophic keratitis, its occurrence in the cornea is fortunately rare. Patients may develop microdendritic keratitis, nummular keratitis, disciform keratitis, mucous plaque keratitis, and sclerokeratitis. If infected, eyes will develop decreased corneal sensation 21% of the time, and significant corneal hypesthesia within one year 49% of the time.[40] Of these patients, approximately 8% will develop frank signs of neurotrophic keratitis secondary to the decreased corneal sensation.

Approximately 15% of patients with anesthetic eyes develop neurotrophic disease.[41] The decreased sensation in the cornea may, however, be sectoral, and frequently the conjunctiva is uninvolved. Sensation present in either the cornea alone or the conjunctiva alone may spare the patient from disease.

Clinical Findings

The clinical findings in neurotrophic keratitis are variable, and it can be difficult to categorize the stage of the disease and customize treatment. Mackie[33] developed a useful staging system that can help guide treatment for the various stages of clinical disease: Stage I is characterized by palpebral conjunctiva staining with rose bengal, decrease in the tear film breakup time, increase in the viscosity of the tear mucous, punctate epithelial staining with fluorescein, and roughened, dry epithelium (Gaule spots). Stage II is characterized by loss of epithelium, especially from underneath the upper eyelid, a rim of loose epithelium around the epithelial defect, stromal edema, aqueous cell and flare, and smoothing of defect edges over time. Stage III corneas demonstrate stromal lysis and may run the risk of corneal perforation. The management for each stage is described later in this chapter.

The patient with neurotrophic keratitis may experience symptoms that wax and wane. A decrease in reflex tearing and a decreased blink rate are characteristic, and it has been demonstrated that aqueous tear production in patients with neurotrophic keratitis is decreased with a marked reduction in the nasal-lacrimal reflex.[42] In addition, there is an increase in mucous production and tear viscosity. The earliest sign of neurotrophic keratitis is rose bengal staining of the inferior palpebral conjunctival surface.[33,37] The loss of epithelium underneath the eyelid produces a characteristic round/oval erosion similar to that seen with recurrent erosions. Due to the loss of epithelium, the eye is susceptible to trauma and also heals poorly after injury[43] (Figure 5.4).

Pathogenesis

The molecular basis of neurotrophic keratitis was described by Cavanagh in 1989.[44] A bidirectional control process regulated by an adrenergic cAMP "off" and a cholinergic cGMP "on" is the basis for epithelial cell mitotic activity. When corneal denervation occurs, there is a decrease in intracellular acetylcholine. This decrease leads to an absent "on" response as mediated by cGMP

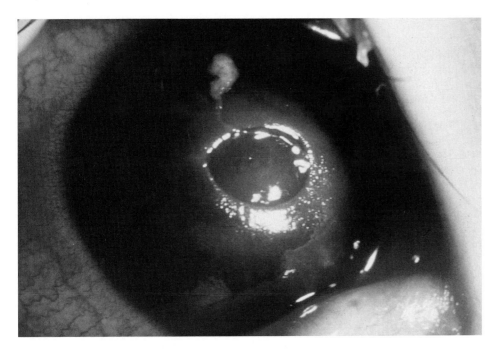

Figure 5.4. Typical nonhealing neurotrophic ulcer with raised, rolled epithelial borders. The underlying cause in this case is Herpes zoster.

and a permanent decrease in epithelial cell mitotic activity. The end result is neurotrophic keratitis.

Histopathologically, the changes are consistent with the clinical findings. The epithelium becomes thin and unhealthy. There is a decrease in epithelial cell glycogen, and the cells become swollen. There is loss of microvilli and a decrease in conjunctival goblet cells. The tear film does not adhere due to both the loss of microvilli and the disruption of normal tear composition. Although these findings are consistent with keratoconjunctivitis sicca, they are not as marked as with neurotrophic keratitis.[43-45]

Treatment

The management of neurotrophic keratitis is based on the stage of the disease. If punctate epitheliopathy is mild and only stage I disease is present, conservative treatment with frequent artificial tears is indicated. If there is no clinical response, intermittent patching of the eye may be helpful during waking hours. Oral administration of tetracycline or doxycycline may help decrease the viscosity and amount of mucous produced by anesthetic eyes, and can be used for long periods of time if there are no contraindications to their use. A therapeutic bandage contact lens may be useful to allow healing of the neurotrophic cornea. However, the eye must be closely monitored for development of infectious keratitis associated with contact lens use, since the patient may not feel pain and, therefore, will not notice problems until the infection is advanced.

In stage II disease, a contact lens is contraindicated and more aggressive measures must be taken. Protection of the cornea can be achieved either with a temporary tarsorraphy, or with the injection of Botulinum toxin into the levator palpebrae superioris to induce pto-

sis. Recently, new treatments with epidermal growth factors and nerve growth factors have been advocated, but the studies are uncontrolled and nonrandomized. The results are promising and may be helpful for patients with stage II or III disease.[46-49] The principal treatment for stage III disease is eyelid closure, as described above. Frequent topical administration of antibiotics and atropine may be indicated. Topical corticosteroids should be used with caution, since they potentiate collagenase activity, inhibit re-epithelialization, and may further thin the cornea. Other surgical procedures, such as conjunctival flaps or amniotic membrane grafts, can be helpful and are described later in this book.[50]

References

1. Binder PS, Wickham MG, Zavala EY. Corneal anatomy and wound healing. In Baraque JI: *Symposium on medical and surgical diseases of the cornea*. St. Louis, 1980, Mosby.
2. Kuwabara T, Perkins DG, Cogan DG. Sliding of the epithelium in experimental corneal wounds. *Invest Ophthalmol* 1976; 15:4–14.
3. Buck RC. Cell migration in repair of mouse corneal epithelium. *Invest Ophthalmol Vis Sci* 1979; 18:767–784.
4. Hanna C. Proliferation and migration of epithelial cells. *Am J Ophthalmol* 1966; 61:55–63.
5. Matsuda H, Smelser GK. Electron microscopy of corneal wound healing. *Exp Eye Res* 1973; 16:427–442.
6. Gipson IK. Adhesive mechanisms of the corneal epithelium. *Acta Ophthalmol Suppl* 1992; 70:13–17.
7. Khodadoust AA, Silverstein AM, Kenyon DR, Dowling JE. Adhesion of regenerating corneal epithelium: the role of basement membrane. *Am J Ophthalmol* 1968; 65:339–348.
8. Hogan MJ, Alvarado JA, Weddell JE. *Histology of the Human Eye*. Philadelphia: W.B. Saunders Company, pp. 55–84.

9. Gipson IK, Spurr-Michaud SJ, Tisdale AS. Anchoring fibrils form a complex network in human and rabbit cornea. *Invest Ophthalmol Vis Sci* 1987; 28:212–220.
10. Gipson IK, Spurr-Michaud SJ, Tisdale AS, Keough M. Reassembly of the anchoring structures of corneal epithelium during wound repair in the rabbit. *Invest Ophthalmol Vis Sci* 1989; 30:425–434.
11. Payant JA, Eggenberger LR, Wood TO. Electron microscopic findings in corneal epithelial basement membrane degeneration. *Cornea* 1991; (10)5:390–394.
12. Stepp MA, Spurr-Michaud SJ, Tisdale AS, Elwell J, Gipson IK. Alpha-6 Beta-4 Integrin heterodimer is a component of hemidesmosomes. *Proc Natl Acad Sci* 1990; 87:8970–8974.
13. Rousselle P, Lunstrum GP, Keene DR, Burgeson RE. Kalinin: an epithelium-specific basement membrane adhesion molecule that is a component of anchoring filaments. *J Cell Biol* 1991; 114:567–576.
14. Lunstrum GP, Sakai LY, Keene DR, Morris NP, Burgeson RE. Large complex globular domains of type VII procollagen contribute to the structure of anchoring fibrils. *J Biol Chem* 1986; 261:9042–9048.
15. Saka LY, Keene DR, Morris NP, Burgeson RE. Type VII collagen is a major structural component of anchoring fibrils, *J Cell Biol* 1986; 103:1577–1586.
16. Keene DR, Sakai LY, Lunstrum GP, Morris NP, Burgeson RE. Type VII collagen forms an extended network of anchoring fibrils. *J Cell Biol* 1987; 104:611–621.
17. Bron AJ, Burgess SE. Inherited recurrent corneal erosion. *Trans Ophthalmol Soc UK* 1981; 101(pt 2):239–243.
18. Williams R, Buckley RJ. Pathogenesis and treatment of recurrent erosion. *Br J Ophthalmol* 1985; 69:435–437.
19. Cogan DG, Donaldson DD, Kuwabara T, Marshall D. Microcystic dystrophy of the corneal epithelium. *Trans Am Ophthalmol Soc* 1964; 63:213.
20. Trobe JD, Laibson PR. Dystrophic changes in the anterior cornea. *Arch Ophthalmol* 1972; 87:378–382.
21. Rosenberg ME, Tervo TM, Petroll WM, Vesaluoma MH. In vivo confocal microscopy of patients with recurrent erosion syndrome or epithelial basement membrane dystrophy. *Ophthalmol* 2000; 107(3):565–573.
22. Aitken DA, Beirouty ZA, Lee WR. Ultrastructural study of the corneal epithelium in the recurrent erosion syndrome. *Br J Ophthalmol* 1995; 79(3):282–289.
23. Reis W. Familiäre, fleckige Hornhautentartung. *Dtsch Med Wochenschr* 1917; 43:575.
24. Bücklers M. Über eine weitere familiäre Hornhautdystrophie (Reis). *Klin Monatsbl Augenheilkd* 1949; 114:386–397.
25. Küchle M, Green WR, Volcker HE, Barraquer J. Reevaluation of corneal dystrophies of Bowman's layer and the anterior stroma (Reis-Bucklers' and Thiel-Behnke *typ3w*): a light and electron microscopic study of eight corneas and a review of the literature. *Cornea* 1995; 14:333–354.
26. Lyons CJ, McCartney AC, Kirkness CM, Ficker LA, Steele AD, Rice NS. Granular corneal dystrophy. Visual results and pattern of recurrence after lamellar or penetrating keratoplasty. *Ophthalmology* 1994; 101:1812.
27. Jonasson F, Johannsson JH, Garner A, Rice NS. Macular corneal dystrophy in Iceland. *Eye* 1989; 3(Pt4):446.
28. Holland EJ, Daya SM, Stone EM, Folberg R, Dobler AA, Cameron JD, Doughman DJ. Avellino corneal dystrophy: clinical manifestations and natural history. *Ophthalmology* 1992; 99:1564–1568.
29. Fogle JA, Kenyon KR, Stark WJ, Green WR. Defective epithelial adhesion in anterior corneal dystrophies. *Am J Ophthalmol* 1975; 79(6):925–940.
30. Garrana RM, Zieske JD, Assouline M, Gipson IK. Matrix metalloproteinases in epithelia from human recurrent corneal erosion. *Invest Ophthalmol Vis Sci* 1999; 40(6):1266–1270.
31. Eke T, Morrison DA, Austin DJ. Recurrent symptoms following traumatic corneal abrasion: prevalence, severity, and the effect of a simple regimen of prophylaxis. *Eye* 1999; 13(Pt3a):345–347.
32. Hykin PG, Foss AE, Pavesion C, Dart JK. The natural history and management of recurrent corneal erosion: a prospective randomized trial. *Eye* 1994; 8:35–40.
33. Mackie IA. Neuroparalytic (neurotrophic) keratitis. In *Symposium on contact lenses: transactions of the New Orleans Academy of Ophthalmology*. St. Louis, 1973, Mosby.
34. Cavanagh HD, Pihlaja D, Thoft RA, Dohlman CH. The pathogenesis and treatment of persistent epithelial defects. *Trans Am Acad Ophthalmol Otol* 1976; 81:754.
35. Cavanagh HD, Colley AM, Pihlaja DJ. Persistent corneal epithelial defects. *Int Ophthalmol Clin* 1979; 19:197.
36. Miller, NR. *Walsh and Hoyt's clinical neuro-ophthalmology*, Baltimore: 1985, Williams & Wilkins.
37. Mackie IA. Role of the corneal nerves in destructive disease of the cornea. *Trans Ophthalmol Soc UK* 1978; 93:343.
38. Schwartz DE. Corneal sensitivity in diabetics. *Arch Ophthalmol* 1974; 91:175.
39. Hyndiuk RA, Kazarian EL, Schultz RO, Seideman S. Neurotrophic corneal ulcers in diabetes mellitus. *Arch Ophthalmol* 1977; 95:2193.
40. Cobo ML. Corneal complications of herpes zoster ophthalmicus: prevention and treatment. *Cornea* 1988; 7:50.
41. Mackie IA. Neuroparalytic Keratitis (Neurotrophic Keratitis, Trigeminal Neuropathic Keratopathy). In: Fraunfelder FT, Roy H, editors. *Current Ocular Therapy 5*. Philadelphia: WB Saunders, 2000:369–371.
42. Heigle TJ, Pflugfelder SC. Aqueous tear production in patients with neurotrophic keratitis. *Cornea* 1996; 15(2):135–138.
43. Gilbard JP, Rossi SR. Tear film and ocular surface changes in a rabbit model of neurotrophic keratitis. *Ophthalmology* 1990; 97:308.
44. Cavanagh HD, Colley AM. The molecular basis of neurotrophic keratitis. *Acta Ophthalmol Suppl* 1989; 192:115–134.
45. Alper MG. The anesthetic eye: an investigation of changes in the anterior ocular segment of the monkey caused by interrupting the trigeminal nerve at various levels along its course. *Trans Am Ophthalmol Soc* 1975; 73:323.
46. Bonini S, Lambiase A, Rama P, Caprioglio G, Aloe L. Topical treatment with nerve growth factor for neurotrophic keratitis. *Ophthalmology* 2000; 107(7):1347–1351.
47. Lambiase A, Rama P, Aloe L, Bonini S. Management of neurotrophic keratopathy. *Curr Opin Ophthalmol* Aug 1999; 10(4):270–276.
48. Daniele S, Gilbard JP, Schepens CL. Treatment of persistent epithelial defects in neurotrophic keratitis with epidermal growth factor: a preliminary open study. *Graefes Arch Clin Exp Ophthalmol* 1992; 230(4):314–317.
49. Pfister RR. Clinical measures to promote corneal epithelial healing. *Acta Ophthalmol Suppl* 1992; 202:73–83.
50. Alino AM, Perry HD, Kanellopoulos AJ, Donnenfeld ED, Rahn EK. Conjunctival flaps. *Ophthalmology* 1998; 105(6):1120–1123.

6
Pterygium

Donald T.H. Tan

Introduction

A pterygium is a triangular-shaped growth consisting of bulbar conjunctival epithelium and hypertrophied subconjunctival connective tissue, occurring medially and laterally in the palpebral fissure, and encroaching onto the cornea.[1] The classic wing-like appearance (hence its name from the Greek *pterygos*, a small wing) is due to its chronic extension toward the corneal apex. Although described and recognized before 1000 B.C., the humble pterygium today remains an ophthalmic enigma, in terms of its pathogenesis.[2] Although pterygium is not generally considered to be a blinding condition in the West, in many parts of the developing world severe pterygium remains a cause of corneal blindness. In addition to being cosmetically unacceptable, symptoms of pterygium may range from mild ocular surface irritation and dryness, to decreased vision from irregular astigmatism or obscuration of the visual axis. Also frustrating is the difficulty in treating or removing this deceptively benign disease. The plethora of surgical and medical measures currently available testifies to that fact that controversies still dominate the literature. Of great import is the recognition that various treatment modalities may present with late-onset complications that may be severe and sight-threatening. This chapter explores in detail our present understanding of the causes and risk factors of pterygium, and its treatments.

Definition and Morphology

Pterygium may be defined as primary or recurrent, the latter being a generally more aggressive lesion occurring weeks to months after the excision of a primary pterygium (Figures 6.1 and 6.2). A "pseudopterygium" should be distinguished from true pterygium; it represents a conjunctival fibrovascular scar or pannus occurring secondary to mechanical or chemical trauma or peripheral degenerations such as Terrien's marginal degeneration (Figure 6.3). Although similar in histology

and believed by some to be a precursor of pterygium, a pinguecula is distinguishable from a pterygium by its conjunctival location away from the limbus and the fact that fibrovascular tissues underlying pingueculae are not radially oriented toward the corneal apex. However, a pinguecula can become a pterygium with alteration of its phenotypic appearance, and radial progression across the limbus (Figure 6.4; p. 67). Occasionally, premalignant carcinoma *in situ*, or squamous cell carcinoma of the conjunctiva, may present as an atypical pterygium (Figure 6.5; p. 67).

Primary pterygium is generally considered to be conjunctival in origin—"a triangular encroachment of the bulbar conjunctival tissue onto the cornea"—and is believed to be an acquired, chronic disorder with a distinct geographical distribution based on sunlight exposure.[1] Pterygia usually occur nasally, in the interpalpebral fissure, but may also occur temporally. Temporal pterygia, however, usually occur in the presence of a nasal pterygium ("double pterygium") (Figure 6.6; p. 68). Pterygia can also be bilateral, but are often asymmetrical in such circumstances. A pterygium consists of a "head" at the pterygium apex, usually with an avascular cap at the leading edge. Irregular, scalloped margins of the cap representing the advancing edge of pterygium may be present and are known as "Fuchs islets," or "Fuchs' islands,"[3] and commonly an epithelial iron line (Stocker's line) encircles the cap (Figure 6.7; p. 68). The neck of the pterygium lies between the head and the limbus, straddling the cornea, while the body represents the main bulk of the pterygium over the sclera and extending from the canthal region. In reality, "neck" and "head" aspects of the pterygium are morphologically indistinguishable.

Grading System

The subconjunctival or fibrovascular component of pterygium may vary considerably in appearance from a thin translucent appearance, to a thick, flesh lesion. Recurrence after excision is believed to be more ag-

Figure 6.1. Primary pterygium.

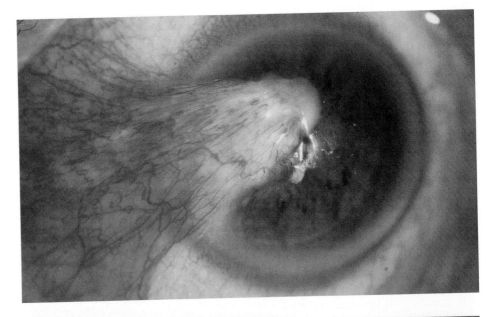

Figure 6.2. Recurrent pterygium—recurrence within 4 months of initial bare sclera surgery.

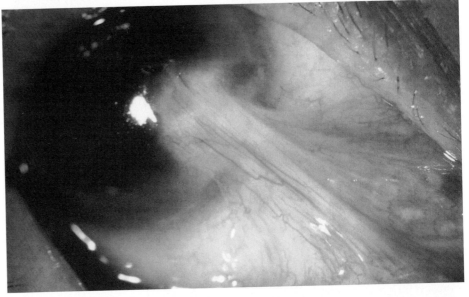

Figure 6.3. Pseudopterygium secondary to chemical burn affecting inferior limbus.

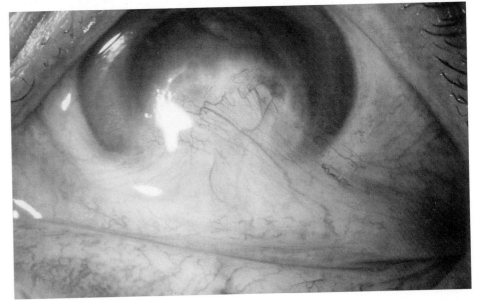

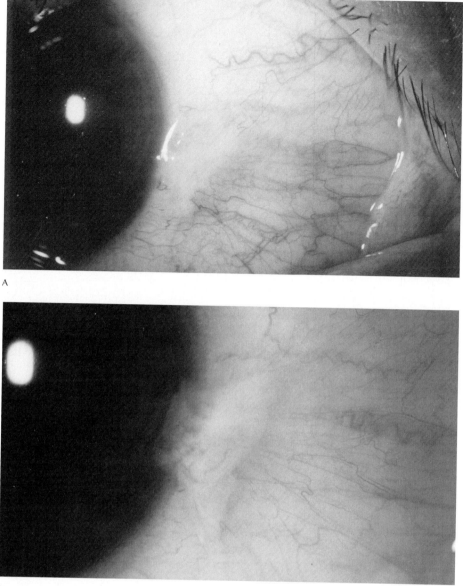

A

B

Figure 6.4. Pinguecula transforming into pterygium. A. Pre-pterygium stage. B. Progression into pterygium 21 months later—lesion has crossed the limbus and is advancing toward the corneal apex.

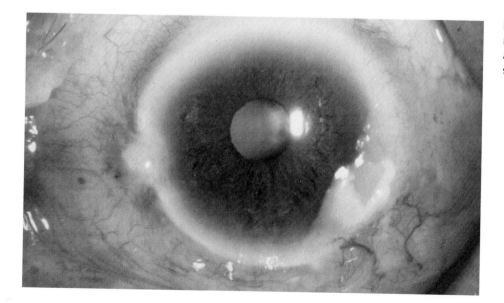

Figure 6.5. Corneal intraepithelial neoplasm (CIN) presenting with an early primary pterygium in the same eye.

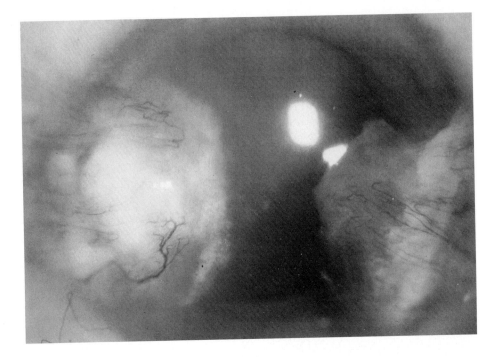

Figure 6.6. Nasal and temporal pterygium in the same eye—"double pterygium."

gressive and common in younger patients with thick, fleshy pterygia, compared with atrophic lesions in more elderly patients. We developed a simple clinical slit-lamp grading scale, based on relative translucency of the body of the pterygium, which was predictive of recurrence. In this grading, grade T1 (atrophic) denotes a pterygium in which episcleral vessels underlying the body of the pterygium were unobscured and clearly distinguished (Figure 6.8). Grade T3 (fleshy) denotes a thick pterygium in which episcleral vessels underlying the body of the pterygium are totally obscured by fibrovascular tissue (Figure 6.8). All other pterygia that do not fall into these two categories (i.e., episcleral vessel details were indistinctly seen or partially obscured) fall into grade T2 (intermediate) (Figure 6.8). Using this grading system in our randomized clinical trial comparing bare sclera excision to conjunctival autografting, we were able to show that recurrence was clearly related to the degree of fibrovascular tissue in the pterygium[4] (Figure 6.9). Surgical recurrence correlated well with translucency, with fleshy pterygium having the highest capacity for recurrence, while atrophic

Figure 6.7. Avascular pterygium cap showing scalloped extensions—"islets of Fuchs." Stocker's line is present just anterior to the cap.

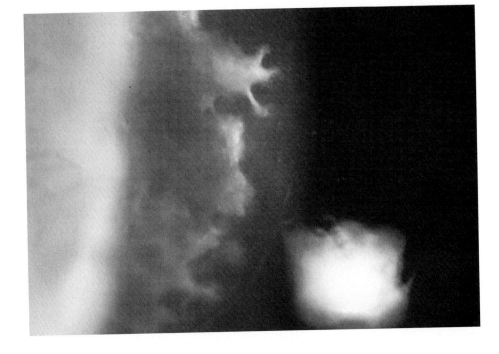

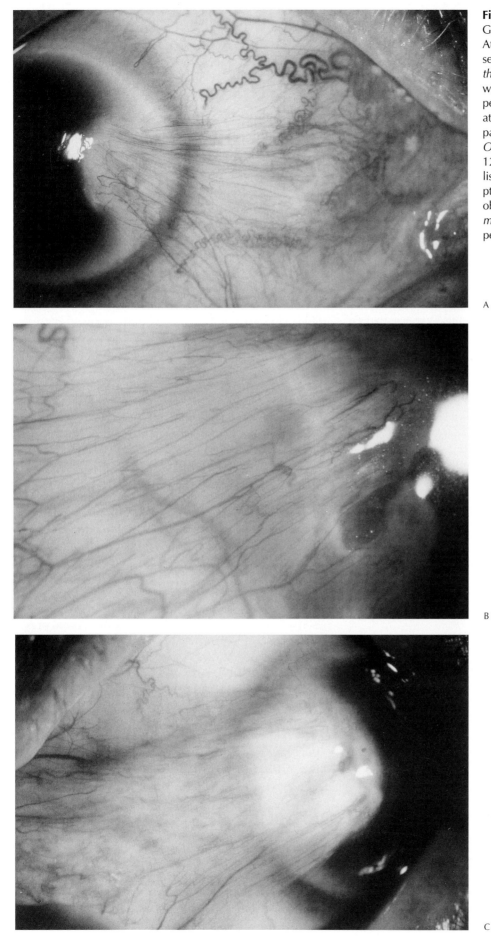

Figure 6.8. Pterygium Morphology Grading System. A. Grade T1: Atro-phic pterygium (episcleral vessels unobscured) (*Archives of Ophthalmology* 1997; 15:1235–1240, with permission from publisher pending). B. Grade T2: Intermediate pterygium (episcleral vessels partially obscured) (*Archives of Ophthalmology* 1997; 15:1235–1240, with permission from publisher pending). C. Grade T3: Fleshy pterygium (episcleral vessels totally obscured) (*Archives of Ophthalmology* 1997; 15:1235–1240, with permission).

A

B

C

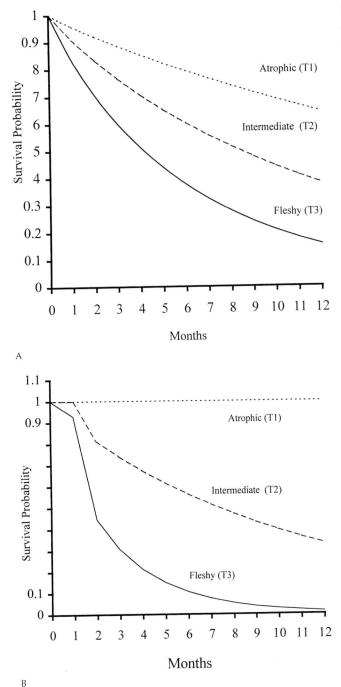

Figure 6.9. Weibull survival curve analysis according to pterygium morphologic grade. A. Primary pterygium (*Archives of Ophthalmology* 1997; 15:1235–1240, with permission from publisher pending). B. Recurrent pterygium (*Archives of Ophthalmology* 1997; 15:1235–1240, with permission).

recurrence, suggesting that pterygium morphology, and not young age is the main predictive factor for recurrence.

Epidemiology of Pterygium

One of the most striking features of pterygium is its geographical distribution. The distribution of pterygium is worldwide, but many surveys over the past half-century have consistently demonstrated that countries near the equator have higher rates of pterygia. Many of these studies have attempted to determine the prevalence of this condition, but in reality most surveys are hospital- or clinic-based studies, as opposed to randomly sampled population-based studies.[5] The potential biases from such sources include the fact that asymptomatic or mild cases may not be included; nor are those from primary health care physicians or from practice-based ophthalmologists, while hospital surveys tend to report only surgical cases. A geographical association between pterygium occurrence and variation in sunlight was first suggested by Talbot in 1948, and the ultraviolet radiation component implicated in 1961. However, it was Cameron in 1965 who surveyed the world distribution of pterygium and found that countries that are hot, dry, and dusty had a higher prevalence.[6,7] Nonetheless, other areas, neither dusty nor dry, also had high reported prevalence rates, and the common factor that emerged was latitude, with pterygium occurring primarily within the periequatorial "pterygium belt" latitudes of 37 degrees north and south of the equator. Population-based surveys have been conducted in several countries. In Australia, the prevalence rate among the aboriginal population was found to be 3.4%, as compared to non-aboriginal volunteers (1.1%).[8] Population-based surveys in the Pacific Ocean islands reveal prevalence rates ranging from 0.3% (Solomon Islands) to 29% in the Samoan islands.[9] Other surveys in selected hospitals or occupational groups have also been conducted. For example, the age-adjusted prevalence rates for male sawmill workers in Thailand was 27%, compared to 2% in white male sawmill workers in British Columbia.[10] Several studies have shown that the prevalence of pterygium increases with age.[8,11,12] The commonest age of onset appears to be in the 20s and 30s.[8,13]

Risk Factors

Many studies have attempted to correlate epidemiological and geographic features of pterygium prevalence with various etiologic risk factors. As a result, studied risk factors for pterygium development appear to be predominantly environmental in nature, such as solar and ultraviolet radiation and chronic irritation from air-

pterygium had the lowest. Differences in recurrence rates were highly significant for both primary and recurrent pterygia. Although recurrence was higher in younger patients, after controlling for pterygium morphology, age was no longer a significant factor for

borne particulate matter. Some studies implicate hereditary factors.

Ultraviolet Radiation

The major environmental risk factor for the development of pterygium is exposure to ultraviolet (UV) light. The depletion of the ozone layer in recent decades may result in increased ultraviolet radiation and a subsequent increase in sunlight-related conditions such as pterygium, cataract, and climatic droplet keratopathy.[12-16] UV light absorbed by the cornea and conjunctiva promotes cellular damage, and hence subsequent proliferation. In the mouse model, it has been demonstrated that UV radiation results in epithelial hyperplasia and Bowman's membrane degeneration.[17] "Albedo" is reflected solar radiation, which is responsible for most of the light rays striking the corneal surface and is the major factor determining focal UVB exposure of the eye. Coroneo has elegantly demonstrated the albedo effect on the eye, whereby UV light from the temporal side is focused on the nasal limbus at the exact location of a nasal pterygium.[18] Aside from local factors such as corneal curvature, anterior chamber depth, and ocular prominence determining the degree of light falling on the eye, external factors must also be important. These include latitude, reflective terrain (e.g., flat horizontal reflective surfaces, as occurs with sand, concrete pavements, and highly reflective snowfields), time spent outdoors, the use of prescription eyewear, and protective hats.[18] Several supportive studies on UV radiation as a causative factor in pterygium include occupational studies in which workers with a higher exposure to UV radiation (sawmill workers, welders, stockmen, laborers, watermen) have a higher prevalence of pterygium.[10,19,20,21,22]

Studies involving precise estimates of ultraviolet exposure are of more importance than studies in which global UV light exposure or ambient light levels of sunlight are used as crude surrogates for UV light exposure. In particular, Taylor and colleagues measured ocular exposure to a wide band of UV radiation in watermen in the Chesapeake Bay, with the use of UV-sensitive film badges placed near the eye. They compared pterygium prevalence rates with age-matched controls and found a strong association. The odds ratio for pterygium was 44.3 for patients living at latitudes less than 30 degrees and 14.1 for spending more than 50% of the time outdoors in the first five years of life.[21] Finally, in a case control study, MacKenzie and co-workers showed that study subjects who spent the first five years of their life at latitudes of less than 30 degrees were 36 times more at risk of developing pterygium compared to those at more southern latitudes, and there was a 17-fold increase in the risk of pterygium for those children spending the majority of their time outdoors, especially in the first decade of life.[23]

Genetic Factors

There is some evidence that hereditary factors may play a role in the development of pterygium. Several case reports have described clusters of family members with pterygium, and a hospital-based case control study showed family history to be significant, suggesting a possible autosomal dominant pattern.[24,25] However, in these cases, the confounding role of common exposure to UV radiation cannot be excluded. In addition, the p53 oncogene has also been suggested as a possible marker for pterygium.[21,21,21,26–29]

Other Risk Factors

Chronic irritation or inflammation occurring at the limbus or in the peripheral cornea has been suggested by many proponents of the "chronic keratitis" theory.[30–32] Actinic keratoconjunctivitis has been suggested as an irritative lesion causing chronic inflammation, scarring and vascularization, leading to pterygium progression. Studies establishing the presence of inflammatory cells and aberrant HLA-DR expression have been reported.[33,34] Interestingly, chronic inflammation is now regarded as an important cause of limbal deficiency, which is a recent theory of pterygium pathogenesis discussed later in this chapter.[21,35] Wong also suggested the presence of a "pterygium angiogenesis factor," and this theory is being reconsidered with the use of anti-angiogenetic pharmacotherapy currently undergoing clinical trials.[36,37] Dust, low humidity, and microtrauma from particulate matter such as smoke or sand have also been implicated, or suggested as confounding factors to UV light exposure, while dry eyes as a possible cause has also been investigated.[38–41] Finally, the human papilloma virus infection has also been suggested as an etiological factor in pterygium.[42]

Pathogenesis of Pterygium

In 1972, Youngson stated that "almost any respectable authority can be quoted to support the view that pterygium is a disease of corneal epithelium, basement membrane, Bowman's membrane, superficial stroma, and conjunctiva." Even today, there is no consensus as to the exact pathophysiological mechanisms underlying pterygium and its progression and recurrence.[43] Many of the classic theories of pterygium pathogenesis were reported in the 70s and 80s on the basis of histopathological studies. Today, the concept of pterygium pathogenesis has been strongly challenged, and a better understanding of the cellular and molecular processes occurring in pterygium progression and its recurrence will enable the development of specific treatment modalities.

Pinguecula and Pterygium

The histological appearance of pinguecula and pterygium is similar, and it has long been believed that most if not all pterygia arise from pinguecula. Although this theory seems to have fallen out of favor in recent years, we have certainly seen transformation of a pinguecula into a pterygium, with clear invasion of the limbus with time.

Degenerative vs. Proliferative Disorders

Pterygium has long been considered a chronic degenerative condition because of the apparently degenerative histopathological appearance. Classically described as "elastotic degeneration" by light microscopists, pterygium tissue is characterized by abnormal subepithelial tissue containing altered collagen fibers demonstrable with elastic stains, which are purely degenerative processes caused by sun exposure.[44–47] However, active or proliferative processes in pterygium have also been noted by proponents of the degenerative theory. Duke-Elder's definition of pterygium is a "triangular shaped degenerative and *hyperplastic* process."[1] Čilanova-Atanasova reviewed the histology of pterygium as compared to age-matched controls and ascertained that the degenerative or dystrophic changes in pterygium (namely elastoid and hyaline dystrophy of elastic and collagen fibers, thickening of the basement membrane, and reduction of cellular and blood vessel elements) were simply more pronounced compared with aging conjunctiva. In addition, pterygium tissue had proliferative components not present in the aging conjunctiva that included epithelial hyperplasia and the appearance of newly formed connective tissue, blood vessels and fibrous elements.[48] Cameron showed light microscopic and electron microscopic evidence of transformed, invading subconjunctival fibroblasts growing centripetally along the corneal plane, destroying Bowman's layer.[3,31] Solar or actinic degeneration of the skin has been shown to be due to radiation-activated fibroblasts that secrete elastic tissue precursors. Austin and co-workers suggested that in pterygium a similar elastodysplastic process occurred, arising from excessive production of elastin material by actinically damaged, proliferative subconjunctival fibroblasts.[44,49]

Clinically, there are also clear behavioral features of pterygium that suggest a proliferative growth disorder, not unlike properties seen in benign tumors. A primary pterygium is definitely locally invasive, growing toward the corneal apex, and pterygium epithelium exhibits varying degrees of abnormality, ranging from mild dysplasia to carcinoma *in situ*.[50] We have also seen corneal intraepithelial neoplasia (CIN) presenting together with a pterygium in the same eye. CIN should, therefore, be considered a differential diagnosis for a pterygium that is atypical in appearance. The link between pterygium and the p53 oncogene is also described in detail below, while the role of UV radiation in pterygium pathogenesis has been well elucidated above. The link between UV radiation and cancer is well known, and UV light is able to induce mutations in solar keratosis, Bowen's disease, and skin carcinomas.[51,52] Pterygia have a strong propensity for aggressive recurrence after surgical excision. Treatment modalities, therefore, mimic anticancer treatments, such as wide surgical excision to remove all possible pterygium tissue remnants, adjunctive radiotherapy with beta irradiation, and antimitotic chemotherapy with mitomycin C, an anticancer agent.

Limbal Stem Cell Deficiency and Epithelial Abnormalities in Pterygium

The concept of the ocular surface as a biological continuum was first proposed by Thoft in 1977.[53] Since then, our understanding of diseases of the ocular surface has grown significantly, stemming from the major discovery that corneal epithelial stem cells are located at the limbus and that transplantation of limbal tissue containing corneal epithelial stem cells is a viable treatment modality for ocular surface disorders with limbal stem deficiency.[54,55] Limbal stem cells are now believed to be the ultimate source of regenerating corneal epithelium via the supply of daughter transient amplifying cells that migrate centripetally onto the cornea. These cells then divide to form postmitotic suprabasal cells that ultimately migrate to the ocular surface, thus elegantly explaining Thoft's "XYZ" hypothesis of corneal epithelial cell maintenance.[56]

In the presence of limbal deficiency, conjunctivalization of the corneal surface occurs, as conjunctiva migrates across the limbus to replace the deficiency in corneal epithelial cells. The classic signs or clinical hallmarks of limbal deficiency include conjunctival ingrowth, vascularization, chronic inflammation, destruction of basement membrane, and fibrous ingrowth.[35] These signs are also the hallmark of pterygium. Accordingly, many researchers today have suggested that pterygium is a manifestation of localized, interpalpebral limbal stem cell dysfunction or deficiency, perhaps as a consequence of UV-light-related stem cell destruction.[26,35,57,58] Coroneo's hypothesis of the albedo effect of ultraviolet light localization at the nasal limbus was taken one step further by Kwok's mathematical modeling, which suggested a 20-fold peak intensity at the limbus.[18,59] They went on to propose that the initial biologic event in pterygium was an alteration of limbal stem cells due to chronic UV light exposure, resulting in concomitant breakdown of the limbal barrier and subsequent conjunctivalization of the cornea.[18,59] This theory was subsequently confirmed by Dushku and Reid, who, using specific monoclonal antibodies, demonstrated the presence of altered limbal basal cells invading normal cornea along the basement membrane in both primary and recurrent pterygium specimens.[29]

Pterygium tissues also exhibit intrinsic abnormalities in DNA repair as a result of UV radiation, as seen by a high incidence of microsatellite instability and loss of heterozygosity.[60,61] Our laboratory (and other researchers) has also shown that basal epithelial layers of both primary and recurrent pterygia exhibit overexpression of the p53 tumor-suppressor gene, an oncogene that acts as a transcription factor to activate or repress the expression of growth controlling genes, thus explaining the classic histological finding of epithelial hyperplasia[26,28,62] (Figure 6.10). Since p53 has an integral role in the transcriptional regulation of apoptosis controlling genes, it is also not surprising that we have confirmed the presence of aberrant apoptosis occurring in epithelium of primary and recurrent pterygium[63] (Figure 6.11).

The Role of the Fibrovascular Component in Corneal Invasion and Pterygium Recurrence

The hypothesized proliferative role of the fibrovascular component of pterygium has already been described above, but there is also sufficient evidence supporting intrinsic abnormalities in pterygium fibroblasts themselves. Fibroblasts isolated from pterygium tissue exhibit a transformed phenotype, growing much better in a medium containing a low concentration of serum as compared to normal conjunctival fibroblasts.[64] They can also grow in semisolid agar, which also suggests anchorage-independent growth, as occurs in neoplastic cells. We performed flow cytometry to compare DNA content and cellular proliferation rates in epithelium and fibrovascular tissues obtained from primary and recurrent pterygia, and matched superior bulbar conjunctiva[65] (Figure 6.12). The mean proliferative index (MPI) of pterygium fibrovascular tissue (13.4) was significantly higher than the MPI of superior conjunctival fibrovascular tissue (6.0, $P = 0.0001$). When we compared primary with recurrent pterygium fibrovascular tissue, an even greater difference was noted (MPI of primary fibrovascular tissue = 7.3, MPI of recurrent fibrovascular tissue = 73.75; $P = 0.003$). These results confirm that the fibrovascular layer of pterygium is the major site of excessive cellular proliferation and also suggest a clinical correlation between fibrovascular tissue upregulation and pterygium recurrence. Tseng and co-workers have recently studied pterygium fibroblasts in detail and, in particular, fibroblasts from the pterygium head. Cultured pterygium head fibroblasts exhibit a different morphological phenotype in cell culture and express collagenase (MMP-1) and stromelysin (MMP-3)—both matrix metalloproteinases that are a family of extracellular matrix-degrading enzymes responsible for tissue degradation, wound healing, and remodeling.

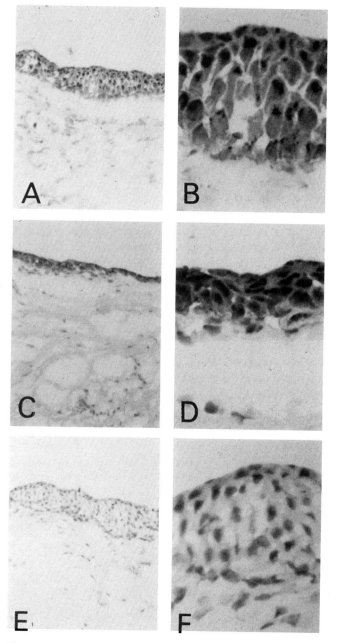

Figure 6.10. Overexpression of tumor suppressor gene p53: immunostaining with monoclonal antibody pAb 240 on sections of superior bulbar conjunctiva (A, B) and pterygium (C, D) from one eye. Also shown is negative control staining with pAb 240 on normal conjunctiva from a donor eye (E, F). (*British Journal of Ophthalmology*, 2000, Vol. 84, No. 2, p212–216, with permission from the BMJ Publishing Group). Original magnification ×100 (A, C, E) and ×400 (B, D, F). Immunoreactive p53 stains brown.

Collagenase-1 and gelatinase A have also been identified in pterygium epithelium, together with TIMP-1 and -3.[66] Tseng has also shown that pterygium-head fibroblasts respond to the TGF-β signaling differently from normal conjunctival tissues and overexpress bFGF and IGF-II. The TGF-β family contains potent cytokines in-

Figure 6.11. Aberrant apoptosis occurring in pterygium tissue: TUNEL assay of normal superior bulbar conjunctiva and pterygium from one patient. Positive cells stain brown. Original magnification ×100.

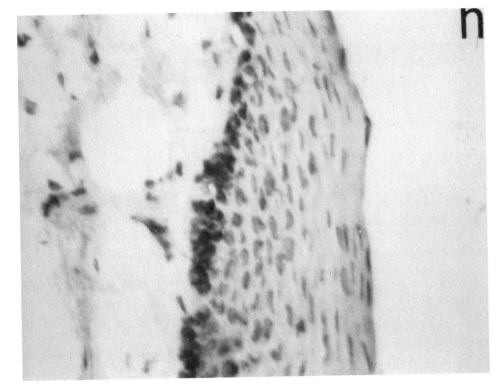

volved in scarring and fibrosis in wound healing and repair. Tseng hypothesizes that the various transformed phenotypes, overexpression of MMPs, bFGF and IGF-II are intrinsically linked with the dysregulated TGF-β signaling, which may explain the pterygium's propensity for sustained growth, invasion into the corneal stroma, and attraction of a fibrovascular and inflammatory response.[35] It is also interesting that amniotic membrane transplantation is a new treatment modality for pterygium, since evidence exists that the TGF-β signaling sys-

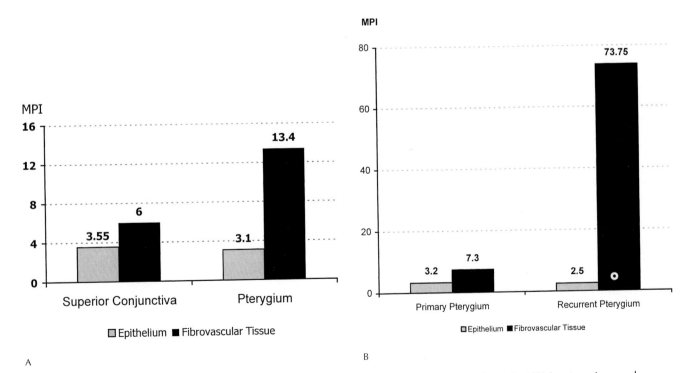

A

B

Figure 6.12. Mean proliferative indices (MPI) from flow cytometry measurements in pterygium. A. MPI in pterygium and matched superior bulbar conjunctiva from the same patients: epithelium vs. fibrovascular tissues. B. MPI in primary vs. recurrent pterygium.

tem may be downregulated by amniotic membrane stromal matrix.[27]

These new and emerging studies on molecular and cellular mechanisms occurring in pterygium will be important, since new insights into the pathophysiological mechanisms of pterygium and pterygium recurrence will alter our approach and will offer us new strategies in the medical and surgical management of pterygium.

Therapeutic Options for Pterygium

The first reported surgical excision of a pterygium dates from before 1000 B.C.[67] Susruta, the Indian physician who was the world's first surgeon-ophthalmologist, described his operative procedure, in which he combined surgical removal with adjunctive chemical therapy:

> "With the patient recumbent on an operating table, the pterygium is loosened and disturbed by sprinkling powdered salt into the eye. The pterygium is then fomented with the palm, heated by rubbing with the finger. With the patient looking laterally, a sharp hook is used to secure the growth at its loosened, upturned part, and is held up with a toothed forceps, or a threaded needle is to be passed from below the part which would be held up with the thread. The pterygium is then gotten rid of by scratching with a sharp round-topped instrument. The root of the pterygium should be pushed asunder from the black outline (cornea) of the eye to the medial canthus and then excised and removed. Any remnant of the pterygium after excision should be removed with a scarifying ointment."

Interestingly, surgical excision combined with adjunctive chemotherapy is still practiced today. The chronological inventory of pterygium surgery procedures in the historical literature is considerable, and myriad surgical and nonsurgical treatment regimens have been described. In 1953, Rosenthal reviewed surgical treatments for pterygium and reported that pterygia have been "incised, removed, split, transplanted, excised, cauterized, grafted, inverted, galvanized, heated, dissected, rotated, coagulated, repositioned and irradiated."[67] In 1950, King elegantly illustrated some of these various operations[68] (Figure 6.13). Many of the procedures are still performed today, but the emphasis on quality of pterygium surgery today perhaps requires closer scrutiny. In 1972 Cameron stated that "Many surgeons consider the humble pterygium to be unworthy of their talents and sometimes for this reason, or under pressure of work, delegate the excision to junior staff, who in turn treat the condition in cavalier fashion, with, in some cases, poor results."[3] Unfortunately this is still true in many parts of the world today, and trivialization of pterygium surgery, combined with inadequate surgical technique, are responsible for variable results and efficacy of excision procedures, leading to a general reluctance to do surgery except in severe cases of central encroachment of the visual axis. Pterygium sur-

gery today still varies from the simplest procedure of bare sclera excision to complex surgery such as lamellar keratoplasty and amniotic membrane transplantation (Figure 6.14; p. 77). These procedures have a common goal: excision of the pterygium and prevention of its subsequent recurrence. The wide variations in technique that still exist today belie the fact that unsatisfactory and inconsistent results still occur. In addition, potentially blinding complications arising from adjunctive pterygium surgery are now well recognized, and this has led to much discussion on the controversial issue of long-term complications associated with such therapies.

Recurrence of pterygium regrowth onto the cornea after surgical excision is the single most common and frustrating cause of failed pterygium surgery, but recurrence rates reported in today's literature still vary widely from 0% to 89%.[4,69–85] In the presence of a wide range in variation and success rates of pterygium surgery, some mention of appropriate indications for surgery must be made. Twelker and associates recently surveyed members of the Castroviejo Cornea Society for criteria for evaluating pterygium surgery as a potential surrogate for treatment intervention and determined that the most important factors for determining primary pterygium severity were the extent of encroachment onto the cornea, decreased visual acuity, restricted ocular motility, and increased rate of growth.[86] The study concluded that corneal specialists are in good agreement about rating pterygium severity, but a wide range of surgical techniques was reported in this U.S. study. Conjunctival autografting was the commonest procedure (58%), followed by excision and sliding conjunctival flap (19%) and simple bare sclera excision (13%), while beta irradiation and mitomycin C were not commonly used. In contrast, a 1998 survey of pterygium surgery in the Australian state of Victoria showed that excision with beta-irradiation was the most common procedure (57%), followed by simple bare sclera excision (15%) and conjunctival autografting (11%).[87] Note that bare sclera excision still features prominently in both these recent studies, while it has been clearly shown by meta-analysis methodology that bare sclera excision is clearly inferior to other procedures. The study invoked the Declaration of Helsinki, which states that in clinical trials no suboptimal treatment can be offered to a control group and concluded that "surgeons and clinical trialists should not be encouraged in the use of bare sclera resection as a surgical technique for primary pterygium."[80]

Modern pterygium surgery today can be divided into four main groups, in order of increasing complexity:

1. Bare sclera excision
2. Excision with conjunctival closure/transposition
3. Excision with antimitotic adjunctive therapies
4. Ocular surface transplantation techniques

Figure 6.13. A variety of pterygium operations illustrated in
1950 (*Archs Ophthal*, 1950,
Vol. 44, p. 856, permission
from publisher pending).

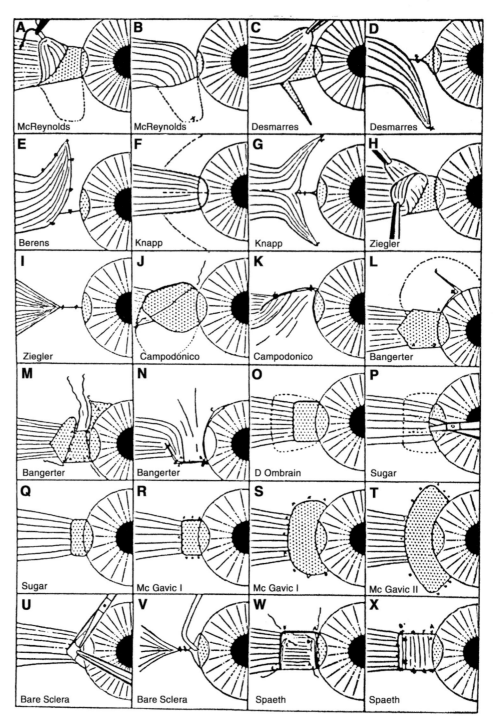

1. Bare Sclera Excision

The idea of excising the head and body of the pterygium back to the nasal canthal region, and laying the
scleral bed bare to re-epithelize, was first described in
1948 by D'Ombrain, who suggested that leaving a strip
of bare sclera allowed the cornea time to heal before the
conjunctiva grows across the limbus.[68,88] Sugar, one
year later, stated that postoperative healing was a race
between re-epithelization of the bare corneal area and

reconjunctivalization of the bare sclera area.[89] It was
presumed that, since the entire pathological tissue had
been removed, a permanent cure would be obtained if
corneal cover could be achieved before the conjunctiva
reached the limbus. Although many early studies testi-
fied to the success of this procedure, we now know today that bare sclera excision is not adequate to prevent
recurrence, and recent studies, mainly using bare sclera
excision as the surgical control for more advanced procedures, attest to high recurrence rates with simple bare

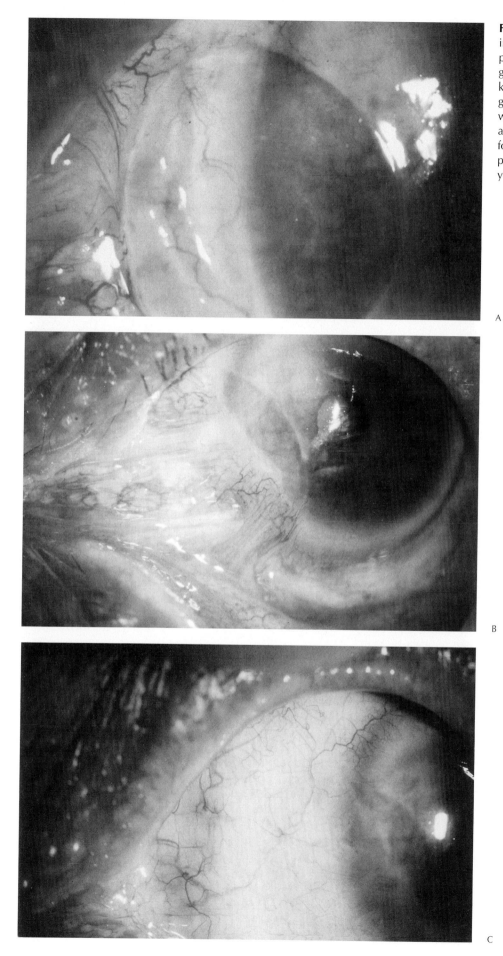

Figure 6.14. Conjunctival autografting after failure of lamellar keratoplasty for pterygium. A. Initial surgical result after lamellar keratoplasty for recurrent pterygium. B. Aggressive recurrence within 4 months. C. Conjunctival autografting successfully performed for recurrence after lamellar keratoplasty—no recurrence occurring 2 years following autografting.

A

B

C

Figure 6.15. Aggressive pterygium recurrence with symblepharon and lower eyelid adhesion to the cornea following bare sclera excision of a primary pterygium—severe ocular motility restriction with gaze dependent diplopia is present.

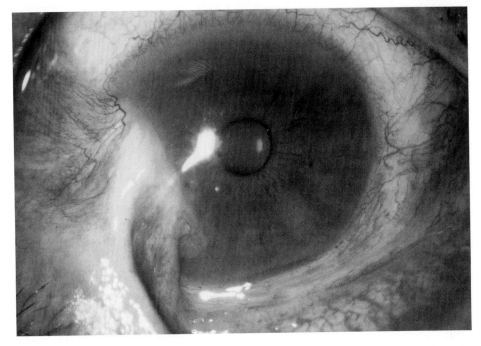

sclera excision ranging from 24% to as high as 89% (Figure 6-2).[4,71,72,77–79,82,83,90] Pterygium recurrence after bare sclera excision may also be highly aggressive, and in severe cases ocular morbidity may far exceed the primary lesion, with the development of symblepharon, restriction in ocular motility, and gaze-dependent diplopia (Figure 6.15). However, excising a pterygium is always the first step in any pterygium procedure, and an appropriate surgical technique is required to reduce the risk of complications or recurrence. The aim is to ensure complete pterygium tissue removal without excessive tissue damage or scarring. Incomplete removal of remnant pterygium tissue may result in optical degradation of the precorneal tear film, while incomplete removal at the limbus and conjunctival aspects may increase the risk of pterygium recurrence. In addition, excessive tissue removal at the time of surgery may result in irregular astigmatism at the corneal aspect or scleral thinning and dellen formation at the scleral bed. A good excision, however, may be able to reduce astigmatism related to the pterygium itself.[91] Excision of recurrent pterygium is inherently more difficult, since severe scarring obliterates tissue planes and there is, therefore, a higher risk for extraocular muscle damage and scleral or corneal tissue loss. Complete surgical details on pterygium excision technique are described in Chapter 15 on conjunctival autograft.

2. Excision with Conjunctival Closure/Transposition

In the past many surgeons have felt that laying sclera bare after excising a pterygium does not comply with general principles of wound healing and closure. Hence, many procedures describing conjunctival wound closure of the pterygium bed have been reported as far back as the 1940s. Wound closure may be simple approximation of undermined conjunctival margins, with or without relaxing incisions or may be effected by conjunctival transposition by a rotational pedicle flap from above or below. However, recurrence rates do not appear to be significantly lower than bare sclera excision. The use of antimitotic adjunctive therapy has resumed interest in wound closure procedures which, theoretically, reduce the likelihood of scleral melting after these treatments. However, two recent studies using simple closure or a superior rotational flap similarly show high recurrence rates of 37% and 29%, respectively.[73,84]

3. Excision with Adjunctive Medical Therapy

The use of chemicals or chemical cautery to treat pterygium dates back to Susruta. Powdered alum, copper sulfate, silver nitrate, zinc sulfate, and carbolic acid are among many chemicals used with or without surgical excision by surgeons over the centuries.[67] In the first half of the past century, attention focused primarily on improving surgical techniques, but adjunctive treatments included the use of thermal or electrocautery and irradiation. Radiation therapy was first advocated by Terson in 1911, who used a radium source, while Estrada advocated the use of X-rays to prevent pterygium recurrence.[67,68] In 1947, Iliff employed beta irradiation with the means of a radon applicator in 18 cases of pterygium, while Friedell in 1950 was among the first to use Strontium 90 as a source of beta radiation.[68]

Today the use of beta irradiation with Strontium 90 is considered to be a common and highly successful treatment for recurrent pterygium in many parts of the world, especially in Australia.[87,92] In 1962, emerging interest in radiomimetic antimitotic agents occurred with the report of 19 cases of pterygium successfully treated with thio-tepa (N.N.N. triethylene thiophosphamide), an alkylating agent and analog of nitrogen mustard, which is now rarely utilized due to the complication of periocular skin depigmentation.[93] One year later in 1963, Kunimoto and Mori first reported their success in reducing pterygium recurrence with postoperative instillation of 0.04% mitomycin C, then in use as an anticancer antibiotic. Today, beta irradiation and mitomycin C remain the dominant antimitotic adjunctive procedures used in pterygium surgery. Although there is universal acceptance with regard to their efficacy in reducing recurrence, the narrow therapeutic index between efficacy and safety with these agents has drawn much criticism and controversy, with numerous reports of long-term sight-threatening complications.[94–102] Controversy also stems from the fact that reported complications occurred with treatment regimens with doses that are no longer considered appropriate.[103]

a. Beta Irradiation

Ionizing radiation inhibits the mitosis of rapidly dividing cells and, therefore, actively proliferating tissues are most susceptible. Beta irradiation, therefore, has maximal effect on immature or rapidly growing tissues and both reduces fibroblast proliferation and causes an obliterative endarteritis in new vessel formation in recurrent pterygium. Strontium 90 is produced by the fission of uranium 235, with a half-life of 28 years, decaying to yttrium 90 with a half-life of 64 hours. Strontium 90 emits beta radiation without gamma emission and is the safest and most effective mode of applying radiation to the ocular surface. Opinions vary widely as to the duration of application and the optimal dose used, with total doses varying from 2000 rads to 6000 rads. Treatment periods range from a single immediate postoperative dose to weekly doses for six weeks after surgery. Although beta irradiation has been used for over half a century, studies on both efficacy and safety are generally lacking in numbers and follow-up time, and few prospective randomized trials exist.[103–105] However, most studies do show that recurrence rates are low, in the region of 10%.

The adverse events relating to beta-irradiation surgery are believed to be dose-related and include serious complications such as sectorial cataract formation, iris atrophy, scleral necrosis and melting, with or without ensuing endophthalmitis, and calcific scleral plaques[94,97,100,105–107] (Figure 6.16). Milder complications reported include conjunctivitis, conjunctival cicatrization, keratitis, photophobia, and ptosis. However, these may be evidence of early limbal stem cell dysfunction that may ultimately progress to more severe ocular surface disease. We have successfully alleviated signs and symptoms with limbal autograft transplantation in three patients with post-beta-irradiation limbal stem cell deficiency (Figure 6.17). In view of the potential seriousness of complications, the role of beta irradiation in pterygium remains controversial, while proponents of the procedure argue that reported complications relate to doses that are no longer recommended today. As such, the use of beta irradiation, while a useful adjunctive treatment, should be limited

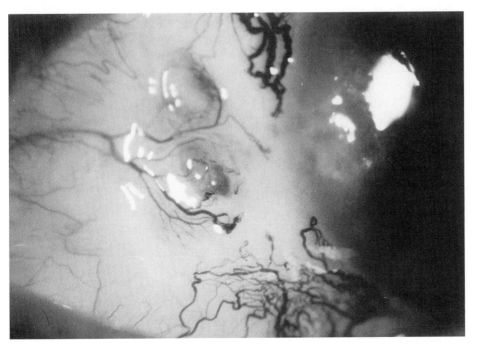

Figure 6.16. Scleral melting following pterygium excision with beta irradiation over 10 years ago—note telangiectatic conjunctival vessels, which characteristically occur after beta irradiation.

Figure 6.17. Limbal stem cell failure after beta irradiation. A. Inflamed and symptomatic pterygium recurrence after beta irradiation. B. Fluorescein staining confirms marked sectorial epithelial dysplasia corresponding to site of previous irradiation. C. Successful reconstruction of ocular surface after conjunctival limbal autograft (CLAU) with limbus and conjunctiva obtained from other eye. D. Fluorescein view shows marked improvement, with absence of epithelial staining.

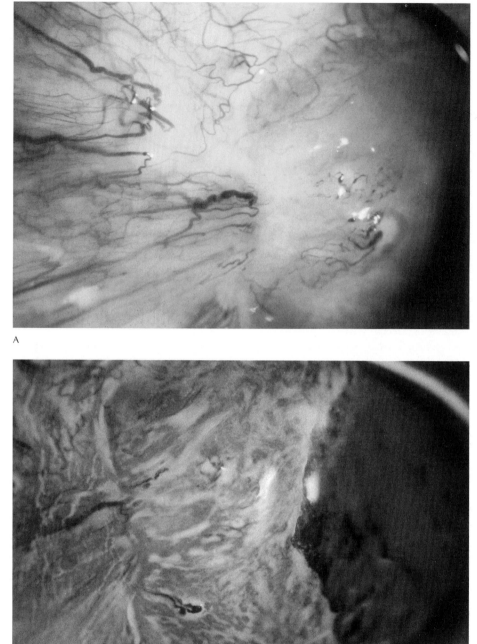

A

B

to severe or repeated pterygium recurrences with a justifiable risk-benefit ratio, and patients should be warned of the rare, but lifelong, risks of serious complications. Patients should also be followed-up for many years.

b. Mitomycin C
Mitomycin C (MMC) is an antibiotic-anticancer agent that inhibits DNA, RNA and protein synthesis. MMC causes irreversible damage to DNA in the cell and has a long-term effect on cell proliferation.[108] MMC has been

used exclusively as an adjunct to glaucoma and pterygium surgery and induces prolonged localized inhibition of Tenon's fibroblasts, thus reducing trabeculectomy bleb scarring and pterygium recurrence. Kunimoto and Mori first described the use of MMC eyedrops in Japan in 1963, while Singh in the U.S. in 1988 reported the use of 0.1% or 0.04% MMC eyedrops in a prospective randomized trial.[77,109] Singh's study reported a 2.3% recurrence rate with MMC, as compared to a 89% recurrence rate with placebo eyedrops, but reported irritative symp-

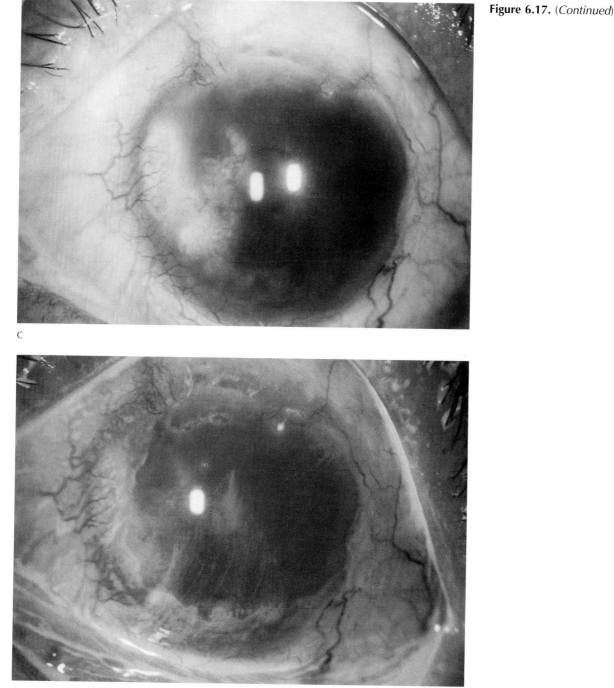

C

D

Figure 6.17. (*Continued*)

toms and punctate keratitis with the 0.1% solution. Since then, the concentration and duration of MMC eyedrop usage has dropped significantly from 0.04% four times a day for two weeks, to 0.01% twice a day for five days, with the realization of early and late complications associated with MMC.[105] Although it had originally been suggested that MMC might be a safer alternative to beta irradiation, this has not been the case, and significant sight-threatening complications with MMC remain a major issue for concern. Iritis, limbal avascularity, scle-

ral melting or calcific plaque formation, corneal decompensation, scleral or corneal perforations, secondary glaucoma and cataract have all been reported with the use or abuse of MMC eyedrops (Figures 6.18, 6.19, and 6.20).[78,95,96,99,101,102,110]

In an attempt to reduce the toxicity associated with eyedrop use, possibly related to patient overdosing, several surgeons now advocate a single intraoperative application of MMC, as was used in glaucoma filtration surgery.[76,82–85,90,111] Again, variations in dose and dura-

Figure 6.18. Severe scleral melt with partial remnant of calcific scleral plaque, following mitomycin C treatment 6 months previously, presenting as early endophthalmitis following attempted scleral plaque removal.

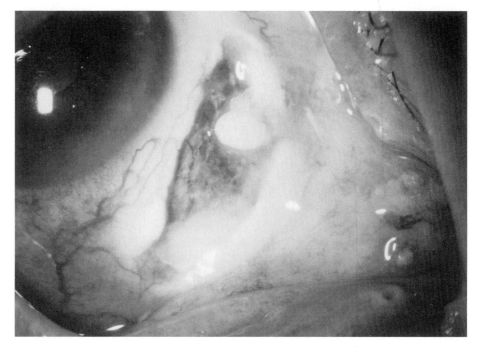

tion exist, but most studies have advocated 0.04% to 0.02% doses, and durations of 3 to 5 minutes. Recurrence rates reported with intraoperative MMC application range from 3% to 43%, and are generally comparable to MMC eyedrops. However, despite the fleeting contact with the eye, intraoperative MMC application also results in early punctate keratitis, chemosis, delayed conjunctival wound healing and conjunctival granulomas, and one case of corneal melting after intraoperative MMC application has already emerged.[82,83,112–114] It should also be noted that studies on intraoperative MMC are recent and, as such, no long-term safety data are available to date.

In view of the serious complications that are known to be associated with MMC, justification of its use in a generally nonblinding disorder like pterygium remains highly controversial. The use of MMC in pterygium surgery should probably be limited to the most severe cases, and intraoperative application of the lower dose of 0.02% would seem to be the safest method.

Figure 6.19. Acute corneal perforation with iris prolapse following mitomycin C treatment.

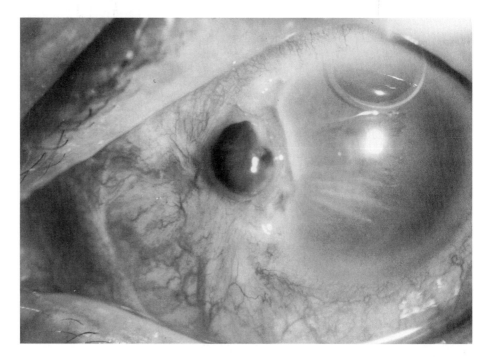

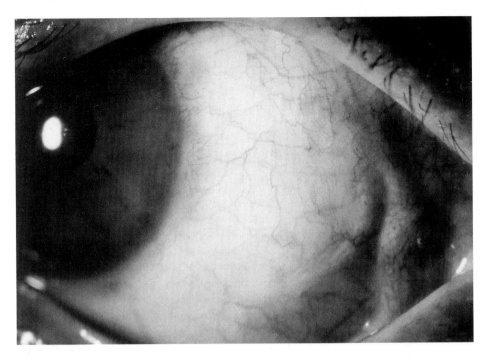

Figure 6.20. Conjunctival autograft transplantation—excellent cosmetic result with no evidence of recurrence.

4. Ocular Surface Transplantation Techniques

In recent years, the concept of ocular surface disease (OSD) has arisen, in which disorders affecting the biological continuum of the ocular surface consisting of the corneal epithelium, conjunctiva, tear film, and eyelids are grouped together as a distinct group of clinical entities.[53] New surgical techniques of ocular surface transplantation have been described in the past decade, and since pterygium is now considered by many to represent a focal form of OSD arising from chronic environmental exposure of the ocular surface, new ocular surface procedures for pterygium surgery have been developed.[115] The following ocular surface transplantation procedures are currently performed for pterygium surgery:

1. Conjunctival autograft transplantation
2. Modifications of conjunctival autografting:
    a. Conjunctival rotational autografting
    b. Annular conjunctival autografting
3. Conjunctival limbal autograft
4. Amniotic membrane transplantation

1. Conjunctival Autografting

Conjunctival autografting is today recognized by many corneal and anterior-segment surgeons to be the procedure of choice for pterygium surgery in terms of the efficacy and safety, and it represents the gold standard against which all other procedures may be benchmarked. An excellent cosmetic result is possible with this technique (Figure 6.21).[4,70] We performed a randomized controlled study comparing conjunctival autografting with bare sclera excision that showed a highly significant reduction in recurrence compared with bare sclera surgery for both primary and recurrent pterygium. The

recurrence rate for primary pterygium ($n = 123$) was 61% for bare sclera excision and 2% for conjunctival autografting (P = 0.0001), while for recurrent pterygium ($n = 17$), recurrence rate for bare sclera surgery was 82%, with no recurrences occurring in the autograft group. The recurrent pterygium study was prematurely

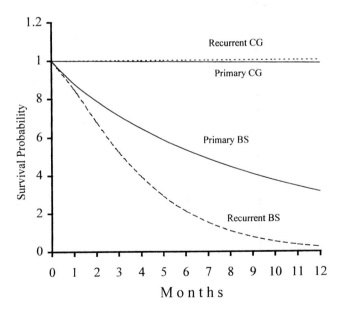

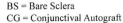

BS = Bare Sclera
CG = Conjunctival Autograft

Figure 6.21. Weibull survival curve analysis comparing success of conjunctival autografting with bare sclera excision in reducing pterygium recurrence (*Archives of Ophthalmology* 1997; 15:1235–1240, with permission from publisher pending).

terminated due to ethical considerations.[4] Conjunctival autografting has been utilized most successfully for the treatment of recurrent pterygium following failure of other procedures such as bare sclera excision and lamellar keratoplasty, but is now routinely used for primary pterygium surgery as well (Figure 6.14). Although conjunctival autografting can be highly successful, the procedure is technically demanding. Therefore, significant variation in success rates has been reported; Chapter 15 is devoted to conjunctival autografting. Along with the conjunctival autograft, newer modifications of the procedure have now been described, and these include the conjunctival rotational autograft and the annular conjunctival autograft, both described in detail in Chapter 15.[69,116]

2. Conjunctival Limbal Autograft

Recent identification of the corneal limbus as the source of limbal stem cells responsible for corneal epithelial cell maintenance has also led to the development of limbal stem cell transplantation procedures, such as limbal allograft transplantation and limbal autograft transplantation. Since focal limbal stem cell deficiency is a suggested etiological hypothesis for pterygium, limbal autografting, otherwise known as conjunctival limbal autograft (CLAU), according to Holland's classification, has also been advocated.[35,55,58,115,117] These procedures are similar to conjunctival autografting, except that the limbal edge of the donor graft is extended to include limbal epithelium either by superficial keratectomy, or by superficial lamellar dissection. This side of the graft is then placed at the limbal edge of the recipient scleral bed in order to match and reconstruct the limbus with stem-cell-containing epithelium (Figure 6.17). Despite the theoretical advantage of limbal autografting, there appears to be no significant reduction in recurrence rates compared with conventional autografting, and one large series reported a disappointing recurrence rate of 14%.[75] There also is the disadvantage of surgical trauma to an additional area of limbal stem cells.

3. Amniotic Membrane Transplantation

The use of preserved human amniotic membrane has recently been reported as an alternative basement membrane substrate for use in ocular surface transplantation procedures such as limbal allograft transplantation[118–121] pterygium surgery. Amniotic membrane transplantation (AMT) has been shown to reduce pterygium recurrence, and pterygium excision is now accepted as an indication for amniotic membrane transplantation. Amniotic membrane has also been used in conjunction with limbal autografting for severe recurrent pterygia.[73,117] Amniotic membrane is effective in reducing scarring and fibrosis in ocular surface surgery and most recently has also been shown to suppress TGF-β signaling in conjunctival and pterygium fibroblasts.[27,122–125] Although less efficient than conjunctival autografting in preventing recurrence (Prabhasawat reported a 13% recurrence rate with AMT), the procedure can provide a good cosmetic result and has advantages over conventional autografting in that the superior conjunctiva is not disturbed and the procedure is relatively simple to perform (Figure 6.22; p. 85).

Other Treatments for Pterygium

In addition to these procedures, other therapies for pterygium deserve mention. These include lamellar keratoplasty, excimer laser phototherapeutic keratectomy, and a new pharmacological treatment for pterygium utilizing an angiostatic steroid compound. Lamellar keratoplasty has been advocated on the premise that allograft corneal lamellar tissue presents a barrier limiting pterygium progression. In our personal experience, we have not found this to be so, and we have seen aggressive pterygium recurrence over a lamellar graft (Figure 6.14). Lamellar keratoplasty today is usually reserved for optical removal of pterygium scars, or as tectonic procedures for corneal or scleral melting secondary to surgical complications. Excimer laser phototherapeutic keratectomy (PTK) has also been used to smooth both the scleral bed and corneal surface after pterygium excision in order to reduce scarring and surface irregularities purported to increase the risk of recurrence, according to some studies.[126]

Finally, new pharmacological treatments are emerging, with the presence of at least one pharmacological agent to prevent pterygium recurrence currently in clinical trials. Although previous trials on compounds such as synthetic matrix metalloproteinase inhibitors have fallen by the wayside, anecortave acetate is an angiostatic steroid that has been formulated as a 1% ophthalmic suspension and is being tested in several preclinical and clinical safety trials.[37] Although the exact mechanism of action remains uncertain, angiostatic steroids are likely to inhibit angiogenesis by affecting elaboration of vascular endothelial cell proteases or their inhibitors. Since pterygium fibrovascular proliferation and recurrence is dependent on neovascularization, control of vascularization may reduce or inhibit pterygium recurrence. Santos and colleagues recently reported on a double-masked, randomized placebo-controlled trial in recurrent pterygium patients in which surgical excision was followed by anecortave acetate treatment or placebo. Treatment with anecortave acetate significantly reduced the rate of neovascularization, with a 42% recurrence rate in treated subjects, as opposed to a 70% recurrence rate in the placebo-treated group.[127] Anecortave acetate is currently undergoing further dose response and Phase III FDA clinical trials to treat pterygium recurrence.

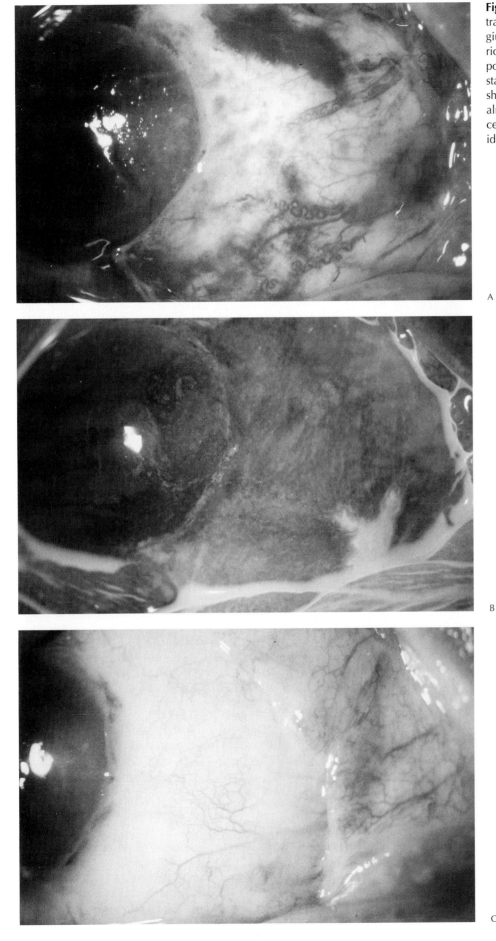

Figure 6.22. Amniotic membrane transplantation for primary pterygium. A. Early postoperative period—amniotic membrane graft in position on day 4. B. Fluorescein staining 8 days following surgery shows that amniotic membrane is almost fully epithelialized. C. Excellent cosmetic result, with no evidence of recurrence at one year.

A

B

C

References

1. Duke-Elder S. Diseases of the outer eye. *System of Ophthalmology* 1965; 8:573–585.

2. Coster D. Pterygium: an ophthalmic enigma. *British Journal of Ophthalmology* 1995; 79:304–305.

3. Cameron M. *Pterygium throughout the world*. Springfield, IL, 1965, Charles C. Thomas.

4. Tan DTH, Chee SP, Dear KBG, Lim ASM. Effect of pterygium morphology on pterygium recurrence in a controlled trial comparing conjunctival autografting with bare sclera excision. *Archives of Ophthalmology* 1997; 115: 1235–1240.

5. Saw SM, Tan D. Pterygium: prevalence, demography and risk factors. *Ophthalmic Epidemiology* 1999; Sep; 6(3):219–28.

6. Talbot G. Pterygium. *Trans Ophthalmol Soc NZ* 1948; 2: 42–45.

7. Elliott R. The aetiology of pterygium. *Trans Ophthalmol Soc NZ* 1961; 13:22–41.

8. Moran DJ, Hollows FC. Pterygium and ultraviolent radiation: a positive correlation. *British Journal of Ophthalmology* 1984; 68:343–346.

9. Verlee D. Ophthalmic survey in the Solomon Islands. *American Journal of Ophthalmology* 1968; 66:304.

10. Detels R, Dhir S. Pterygium. A geographical study. *Archives of Ophthalmology* 1967; 78:485–491.

11. Hill JC, Maske R. Pathogenesis of pterygium. *Eye* 1989; 3:218–226.

12. Coroneo M. Pterygium as an early indicator of ultraviolet insolation: a hypothesis. *British Journal of Ophthalmology* 1993; 77:734–739.

13. Hirst LW. Distribution, risk factors, and epidemiology of pterygium. In: Taylor HR, editor. *Pterygium*. The Netherlands: Kugler Publications, 2000:15–28.

14. Taylor HR. Aetiology of climatic droplet keratopathy and pterygium. *British Journal of Ophthalmology* 1980; 64:154–163.

15. Taylor HR. The environment and the lens. *British Journal of Ophthalmology* 1980; 64:303–310.

16. Cameron M. Ultra-violet radiation. *Pterygium Throughout the World* 1965; 41–54.

17. Lippincott S, Blum H. Neoplasms and other lesions of the eye induced by ultraviolet radiation in Strain A mice. *J Natl Cancer Inst* 1943; 3:545–554.

18. Coroneo M. Albedo concentration in the anterior eye: a phenomenon that locates some solar diseases. *Ophthalmic Surgery* 1990; 20:60–66.

19. Karai I, Horiguchi S. Pterygium in welders. *British Journal of Ophthalmology* 1984; 68:347–349.

20. Norn M, Franck C. Long-term changes in the outer part of the eye in welders. *Acta Ophthalmol* 1991; 69:382–386.

21. Taylor HR, West S, Muñoz B, Rosenthal FS, Bressler SB, Bressier NM. The long-term effects of visible light on the eye. *Archives of Ophthalmology* 1992; 110:99–104.

22. Khoobehi B, Saw S-M, Banerjee K, Chia S-E, Tan D. Outdoor work and the risk of pterygia: a case-control study. *International Ophthalmology* 1998; 22:293–298.

23. MacKenzie FD, Hirst LW, Battistutta D, Green A. Risk analysis in the development of pterygia. *Ophthalmology* 1992; 99:1056–1061.

24. Zhang J-D. An investigation of aetiology and heredity of pterygium. Report of 11 cases in a family. *Acta Ophthalmologica* 1987; 65:413–416.

25. Hilgers JHCh. Pterygium: Its incidence, heredity and etiology. *American Journal of Ophthalmology* 1960; 635–644.

26. Tan DTH, Lim ASM, Goh HS, Smith DR. Abnormal expression of the p53 tumor suppressor gene in the conjunctiva of patients with pterygium. *American Journal of Ophthalmology* 1997; 123.3:404–405.

27. Lee S-B, Li D-Q, Tan DTH, Meller D, Tseng SCG. Suppression of TGF-β signaling in both normal conjunctival fibroblasts and pterygial body fibroblasts by amniotic membrane. *Current Eye Research* 2000; 20:325–334.

28. Shimmura S, Ishioka M, Hanada K, Shimazaki J, Tsubota K. Telomerase activity and p53 expression in pterygia. *Investigative Ophthalmology & Visual Science* 2000; 41:1364–1369.

29. Dushku N, Reid TW. Immunohistochemical evidence that human pterygia originate from an invasion of vimentin-expressing altered limbal epithelial basal cells. *Current Eye Research* 1994; 13:473–481.

30. Pinkerton OD, Hokama Y, Shigemura LA. Immunologic basis for the pathogenesis of pterygium. *American Journal of Ophthalmology* 1984; 98:225–228.

31. Cameron ME. Histology of pterygium: an electron microscopic study. *British Journal of Ophthalmology* 1983; 67: 604–608.

32. Paton D. Pterygium management based upon a theory of pathogenesis. *Trans Am Acad Ophthalmol Otolaryngol* 1962; 79:603.

33. Nakagami T, Murakami A, Okisaka S, Ebihara N. Pterygium and mast cells—mast cell number, phenotype, and localization of stem cell factor. *J Jpn Ophthalmol Soc* 1997; 101:662–668.

34. Kadota Y. Morphological study on the pathogenesis of pterygium. *Acta Soc Ophthalmol Jpn* 1987; 91:324–334.

35. Tseng SCG, Lee S-B, Li D-Q. Limbal stem cell deficiency in the pathogenesis of pterygium. In: Taylor HR, editor. *Pterygium*. The Netherlands: Kugler Publications, 2000: 41–56.

36. Wong WW. A hypothesis on the pathogenesis of pterygiums. *Annals of Ophthalmology* 1978; 10:303–309.

37. DeFaller JM, Clark AF. A new pharmacological treatment for angiogenesis. In: Taylor HR, editor. *Pterygium*. The Netherlands: Kugler Publications, 2000:159–181.

38. Goldberg L, David R. Pterygium and its relationship to the dry eye in the Bantu. *British Journal of Ophthalmology* 1976; 60:721–731.

39. Rajiv, Mithal S, Sood A. Pterygium and dry eye—a clinical correlation. *Indian Journal of Ophthalmology* 1991; 39: 15–16.

40. Biedner B, Biger Y, Roghkoff L. Pterygium and basic tear secretion. *Annals of Ophthalmology* 1979; II:1235.

41. Dimitry T. The dust factor in the production of pterygium. *American Journal of Ophthalmology* 1937; 20:40–45.

42. Varinli S, Varinli I, Erkisi M, Doran F. Human papillomavirus in pterygium. *Central Afr J Med* 1994; 40:24–26.

43. Youngson RM. Recurrence of pterygium after excision. *British Journal of Ophthalmology* 1972; 56:120–125.

44. Austin P, Jakobiec FA, Iwamoto T. Elastodysplasia and elastodystrophy as the pathologic bases of ocular pterygia and pinguecula. *Ophthalmology* 1983; 90.1:96–109.

45. Hogan M, Alvarado J. Pterygium and pinguecula: electron microscopic study. *Archives of Ophthalmology* 1967; 78:174–186.
46. Anslari M, Rahi A, Shukla B. Pseudoelastic nature of pterygium. *British Journal of Ophthalmology* 1970; 54:473–476.
47. Vass Z, Tapaszto I. The histochemical examination of the fibers of pterygium by elastase. *Acta Ophthalmol* 1964; 42:849–854.
48. Cilanova–Atanasova B. Histological and histochemical changes of epithelium, basal membrane and Bowman's membrane in the avascular corneal part of pterygium. *Folia Medica* 1968; 23–26.
49. Ledoux-Corbusier M, Achten G. Elastosis in chronic radiodermatitis. An ultrastructural study. *Br J Dermatol* 1974; 91:287–295.
50. Clear AS, Chirambo MC, Hutt MSR. Solar keratosis, pterygium and squamous cell carcinoma of the conjunctiva in Malawi. *British Journal of Ophthalmology* 1979; 63:102–109.
51. Greenblatt MS, Bennett W, Hollstein M, Harris CC. Mutations in the p53 tumor suppressor gene: Clues to cancer etiology and molecular pathogenesis. *Cancer Research* 1994; 54:4855–4878.
52. Sim CS, Slater SD, McKee PH. Mutant p53 protein is expressed in Bowen's Disease. *American Journal of Dermatopathology* 1992; 14.3:195–199.
53. Thoft RA. Conjunctival transplantation. *Archives of Ophthalmology* 1997; 95:1425–1427.
54. Schermer A, Galvin S, Sun T-T. Differentiation-related expression of a major 64K corneal keratin in vivo and in culture suggests limbal location of corneal epithelial stem cells. *The Journal of Cell Biology* 1986; 103:49–62.
55. Tseng CG. Concept and application of limbal stem cells. *Eye* 1989; 3:141–157.
56. Thoft RA, Friend J. The X, Y, Z hypothesis of corneal epithelial maintenance. *Investigative Ophthalmology & Visual Science* 1983; 24.10:1442–1443.
57. Tan D, Tseng SCG. Pterygium and ultraviolet light-induced conjunctival disorders. In: Parrish II RK, editor. *Atlas of Ophthalmology*. Butterworth-Heinemann, 2000: 159–163.
58. Shimazaki J, Yang H-Y, Tsubota K. Limbal autograft transplantation for recurrent and advanced pterygia. *Ophthalmic Surgery and Lasers* 1996; 27.11:917–923.
59. Kwok LS, Coroneo MT. A model for pterygium formation. *Cornea* 1994; 13:219–224.
60. Detorakis ET, Sourvinos G, Tsamparlakis J, Spandidos DA. Evaluation of loss of heterozygosity and microsatellite instability in human pterygium: clinical correlations. *British Journal of Ophthalmology* 1998; 82:1324–1328.
61. Spandidos DA, Sourvinos G, Kiaris H, Tsamparlakis J. Microsatellite instability and loss of heterozygosity in human pterygium. *British Journal of Ophthalmology* 1997; 81:493–496.
62. Dushku N, Reid TW. p53 expression in altered limbal basal cells of pingueculae, pterygia, and limbal tumors. *Current Eye Research* 1997; 1179–1192.
63. Tan DTH, Tang WY, Liu YP, Goh HS, Duncan RS. Apoptosis and apoptosis related gene expression in normal conjunctiva and pterygium. *British Journal of Ophthalmology* 2000; 84:212–216.
64. Chen JK, Tsai RJF, Lin SS. Fibroblasts isolated from human pterygia exhibit transformed cell characteristics. *In Vitro Cell Dev Biol* 1994; 30A:243–248.
65. Tan DTJ, Liu YP, Sun L. Flow cytometry measurements of DNA content in primary and recurrent pterygia. *Investigative Ophthalmology & Visual Science* 2000; 41:(7) 1684–1686.
66. Girolamo ND, McCluskey P, Lloyd A, Coroneo MT, Wakefield D. Expression of MMPs and TIMPs in human pterygia and cultured pterygium epithelial cells. *Investigative Ophthalmology & Visual Science* 2000; 41:671–679.
67. Rosenthal JW. Chronology of pterygium therapy. *American Journal of Ophthalmology* 1953; 36:1601–1616.
68. King JH. The pterygium—Brief review and evaluation of certain methods of treatment. *Archives of Ophthalmology* 1950; 44:854–869.
69. Jap A, Chan C, Lim L, Tan DTH. Conjunctival rotation autograft for pterygium. *Ophthalmology* 1999;106.1:67–71.
70. Kenyon KR, Wagoner MD, Hettinger ME. Conjunctival autograft transplantation for advanced and recurrent pterygium. *Ophthalmology* 1985; 92.11:1461–1470.
71. Chen PP, Ariyasu RG, Kaza V, LaBree LD, McDonnell PJ. A randomized trial comparing mitomycin C and conjunctival autograft after excision of primary pterygium. *American Journal of Ophthalmology* 1995; 120.2:151–160.
72. Lewallen S. A randomized trial of conjunctival autografting for pterygium in the tropics. *Ophthalmology* 1989; 96.11:1612–1614.
73. Prabhasawat P, Barton K, Burkett G, Tseng SCG. Comparison of conjunctival autografts, amniotic membrane grafts, and primary closure for pterygium excision. *Ophthalmology* 1997; 104.6:974–985.
74. Wong VA, Law FCH. Use of mitomycin C with conjunctival autograft in pterygium surgery in Asian-Canadians. *Ophthalmology* 1999; 106.8:1512–1515.
75. Mutlu FM, Sobaci G, Tatar T, Yildirim E. A comparative study of recurrent pterygium surgery. *Ophthalmology* 1999; 106.4:817–821.
76. Manning CA, Kloess PM, Diaz MD, Yee RW. Intraoperative mitomycin in primary pterygium excision. *Ophthalmology* 1997; 104.5:844–848.
77. Singh G, Wilson MR, Foster CS. Mitomycin eye drops as treatment for pterygium. *Ophthalmology* 1988; 95:813–821.
78. Hayasaka S, Noda S, Yamamoto Y, Setogawa T. Postoperative instillation of low-dose mitomycin C in the treatment of primary pterygium. *American Journal of Ophthalmology* 1988; 106:715–718.
79. Mahar PS, Nwokora G. Role of mitomycin C in pterygium surgery. *British Journal of Ophthalmology* 1993; 77:433–435.
80. Sánchez–Thorin JC, Rocha G, Yelin JB. Meta-analysis on the recurrence rates after bare sclera resection with and without mitomycin C use and conjunctival autograft placement in surgery for primary pterygium. *British Journal of Ophthalmology* 1998; 82:661–665.
81. Singh G, Wilson MR, Foster CS. Long-term follow-up study of mitomycin eye drops as adjunctive treatment for pterygia and its comparison with conjunctival autograft transplantation. *Cornea* 1990; 9.4:331–334.
82. Mastropasqua L, Carpineto P, Ciancaglini M, Gallenga PE. Long-term results of intraoperative mitomycin C in

the treatment of recurrent pterygium. *British Journal of Ophthalmology* 1996; 80:288–291.

83. Caliskan S, Orhan M, Irkec M. Intraoperative and post-operative use of mitomycin-C in the treatment of primary pterygium. *Ophthalmic Surgery and Lasers* 1996; 27.7:600–604.

84. Cardillo JA, Alves MR, Ambrosio LE, Poterio MB, Jose NK. Single intraoperative application versus postoperative mitomycin C eye drops in pterygium surgery. *Ophthalmology* 1995; 102.12:1949–1952.

85. Yanyali AC, Talu H, Alp BN, Karabas L, Ay GM, Caglar Y. Intraoperative mitomycin C in the treatment of pterygium. *Cornea* 2000; 19:471–473.

86. Twelker JD, Bailey IL, Mannis MJ, Satatiano WA. Evaluating pterygium severity—a survey of corneal specialists. *Cornea* 2000; 19:292–296.

87. Snibson GR, Luu CD, Taylor HR. Pterygium surgery in Victoria: a survey of ophthalmologists. *Australian and New Zealand Journal of Ophthalmology* 1998; 26:271–276.

88. D'Ombrain A. The surgical treatment of pterygium. *British Journal of Ophthalmology* 1948; 65–71.

89. Sugar S. A surgical treatment for pterygium based on new concepts as to its nature. *American Journal of Ophthalmology* 1949; 32:912–916.

90. Frucht-Pery J, Siganos CS, Ilsar M. Intraoperative application of topical mitomycin C for pterygium surgery. *Ophthalmology* 1996; 103.4:674–677.

91. Fong KS, Balakrishnan V, Chee SP, Tan DTH. Refractive change following pterygium surgery. *CLAO Journal* 1998; 24.2:115–117.

92. Sebban A, Hirst LW. Treatment of pterygia in Queensland. *Australian and New Zealand Journal of Ophthalmology* 1991; 19.2:123–127.

93. Meacham CT. Triethylene thiophosphoramide in the prevention of pterygium recurrence. *American Journal of Ophthalmology* 1962; 54:751–753.

94. Tarr KH, Constable IJ. Pseudomonas endophthalmitis associated with scleral necrosis. *British Journal of Ophthalmology* 1980; 64:676–679.

95. Wong PK, Yeoh RLS, Lim ASM. How safe is pterygium surgery? *Asia-Pacific Journal of Ophthalmology* 1990; 2.3:102–104.

96. Rubinfield RS, Pfister RR, Stein RM, Foster CS, Martin NF, Stoleru S, et al. Serious complications of topical mitomycin-c after pterygium surgery. *Ophthalmology* 1992; 99.11:1647–1654.

97. Cameron ME. Preventable complications of pterygium excision with beta-irradiation. *British Journal of Ophthalmology* 1972; 56:52–56.

98. Margo CE, Polack FM, Mood CI. Aspergillus panophthalmitis complicating treatment of pterygium. *Cornea* 1988; 7.4:285–289.

99. Dunn JP, Seamone CD, Ostler HB, Nickel BL, Beallo A. Development of scleral ulceration and calcification after pterygium excision and mitomycin therapy. *American Journal of Ophthalmology* 1991; 343–344.

100. MacKenzie FD, Hirst LW, Kynaston B, Bain C. Recurrence rate and complications after beta irradiation for pterygia. *Ophthalmology* 1991; 98.12:1776–1781.

101. Lin C-P, Shih M-H, Tsai M-C. Clinical experiences of infectious scleral ulceration: A complication of pterygium

operation. *British Journal of Ophthalmology* 1997; 81:980–983.

102. Hsiao C-H, Chen JJY, Huang SC, Ma H-K, Chen PYF, Tsai RJF. Intrascleral dissemination of infectious scleritis following pterygium excision. *British Journal of Ophthalmology* 1998; 82:29–34.

103. Snibson GR. An evidence-based appraisal of treatment options. In: Taylor HR, editor. *Pterygium*. The Netherlands: Kugler Publications, 2000:125–140.

104. Snibson GR, Luu Chi D, Cain MS, McKenzie JD, and Taylor HR. *The surgical management of pterygium: a prospective randomised clinical trial*. In press. 2000.

105. Frucht-Pery J, Siganos CS. Adjunctive medical therapy for pterygium surgery. In: Taylor HR, editor. *Pterygium*. The Netherlands: Kugler Publications, 2000:115–124.

106. Moriarty A, Crawford G, McAllister I, Constable I. Fungal corneoscleritis complicating beta-irradiation-induced scleral necrosis following pterygium excision. *Eye* 1993; 7:525–528.

107. Moriarty AP, Crawford GJ, McAllister IL, Constable IJ. Severe corneoscleral infection: a complication of beta irradiation scleral necrosis following pterygium excision. *Archives of Ophthalmology* 1993; 111:947–951.

108. Gilman A, Rall T, Nies A, Taylor P. *Goodman and Gilman's the pharmacological basis of therapeutics*. 8th ed. New York 1990;

109. Kunimoto N, Mori S. Studies on the pterygium. Part IV. A treatment of the pterygium by mitomycin C instillation. *Nippon Ganka Gakkai Zasshi–Acta Societatis Ophthalmologicae Japonica* 1963; 67:601–607.

110. Gupta S, Basti S. Corneoscleral, ciliary body and vitreoretinal toxicity after excessive instillation of mitomycin C. *American Journal of Ophthalmology* 1992; 114:1503–1504.

111. Potério MB, Alves MR, Cardillo JA, José NK. An improved surgical technique for pterygium excision with intraoperative application of mitomycin-C. *Ophthalmic Surgery and Lasers* 1998; 29:685–687.

112. Dougherty PJ, Hardten DR, Lindstrom RL. Corneoscleral melt after pterygium surgery using a single intraoperative application of mitomycin-C. *Cornea* 1996; 15:537–540.

113. Helal M, Messiha N, Amayem A, El-Maghraby A, El-sherif Z, Dabees M. Intraoperative mitomycin C versus postoperative mitomycin C for the treatment of pterygium. *Ophthalmic Surgery and Lasers* 1996; 27:674–678.

114. Cano-Parra J, Diaz-Llopis M, Maldonado MJ, Vila E, Menezo JL. Prospective trial of intraoperative mitomycin C in the treatment of primary pterygium. *British Journal of Ophthalmology* 1995; 79:439–441.

115. Holland EJ, Schwartz GS. The evolution of epithelial transplantation for severe ocular surface disease and a proposed classification system. *Cornea* 1996; 15:549–556.

116. Yip CC, Lim L, Tan DTH. The surgical management of an advanced pterygium involving the entire cornea. *Cornea* 1997; 16.3:365–368.

117. Shimazaki J, Shinozaki N, Tsubota K. Transplantation of amniotic membrane and limbal autograft for patients with recurrent pterygium associated with symblepharon. *British Journal of Ophthalmology* 1998; 82:235–240.

118. Kim JC, Tseng SCG. Transplantation of preserved human amniotic membrane for surface reconstruction in se-

verely damaged rabbit corneas. *Cornea* 1995; 14.5:473–484.

119. Lee S, Tseng S. Amniotic membrane transplantation for persistent epithelial defects with ulceration. *American Journal of Ophthalmology* 1997; 123:303–312.

120. Pires RTF, Chokshi A, Tseng SCG. Amniotic membrane transplantation or conjunctival limbal autograft for limbal stem cell deficiency induced by 5-fluorouracil in glaucoma surgeries. *Cornea* 2000; 19:284–287.

121. Pires RTF, Tseng SCG, Prabhasawat P, Puangsricharern V, Maskin SL, Kim JC, et al. Amniotic membrane transplantation for symptomatic bullous keratopathy. *Archives of Ophthalmology* 1999; 117:1291–1297.

122. Tsubota K, Satake Y, Ohyama M. Surgical reconstruction of the ocular surface in advanced ocular cicatricial pemphigoid and Stevens–Johnson syndrome. *American Journal of Ophthalmology* 1996; 122:38–52.

123. Shimazaki J, Yang H-Y, Tsubota K. Amniotic membrane transplantation for ocular surface reconstruction in pa-tients with chemical and thermal burns. *Ophthalmology* 1997; 104.12:2068–2076.

124. Tseng SCG, Prabhasawat P, Barton K, Gray T, Meller D. Amniotic membrane transplantation with or without limbal allografts for corneal surface reconstruction in patients with limbal stem cell deficiency. *Archives of Ophthalmology* 1998; 116:431–441.

125. Tseng SCG, Prabhasawat P, Lee S-H. Amniotic membrane transplantation for conjunctival surface reconstruction. *American Journal of Ophthalmology* 1997; 124.6: 765–774.

126. Talu H, Tasindi E, Ciftci F, Yildiz TF. Excimer laser phototherapeutic keratectomy for recurrent pterygium. *J Cataract Refract Surg* 1998; 24:1326–1332.

127. Santos C, Zeiter J, Speaker M, Beasley CJ, DeFaller J, Von Tress M, et al. Efficacy and safety of topical 1.0% anecortave acetate (AL-3789) as anti-neovascular therapy for recurrent pterygium. *Investigative Ophthalmology & Visual Science* 1999; 40:S1778.

Part III

Stem Cell Deficiency Disorders

7
Congenital Stem Cell Deficiency

Joel Sugar

Although the majority of stem cell deficient states are acquired, as will be discussed in the subsequent three chapters, congenital stem cell deficiency can occur. As our understanding of stem cell function increases, deficiencies are likely to be identified in an increasing number of disorders. The best defined congenital stem cell deficient disorder is aniridia, but other disorders, including sclerocornea and some ectodermal dysplasias, also merit discussion.

Aniridia

Aniridia is generally a disorder of autosomal-dominant or sporadic occurrence. It occurs with an incidence of slightly less than 1 per 100,000 in the general population.[1] While the classic features include rudimentary development of the iris, glaucoma, foveal hypoplasia, nystagmus, and cataract, there has been increasing awareness of the presence of significant corneal disease in these patients as well. Corneal opacities have been recognized for many years,[2] but have only received significant attention relatively recently. Mackman, Brightbill, and Opitz described 19 patients with progressive corneal changes in aniridia.[3] All patients over 2½ years of age had corneal changes, while one child had no involvement at age 10 months. However, at age 22 months, peripheral corneal pannus-like changes were noted.

The corneal findings of aniridia usually begin as superficial, peripheral, gray elevated opacities extending from the limbus in patchy areas. The opacities are vascularized and "pannus-like" (Figures 7.1 and 7.2). The opacities extend to involve the entire corneal periphery and then progress to involve the cornea more centrally. The central corneal involvement may lead to visual decrease due to both opacification and irregular astigmatism. While these patients usually already have compromised vision because of their foveal hypoplasia, the corneal changes can add significant additional disability. In addition to these corneal findings, recent analysis of the ocular surface in nine aniridic patients showed

absence of the limbal palisades of Vogt in all patients, as well as the presence of goblet cells in the peripheral cornea.[4] Histopathology of eyes from aniridic children showed a fibrovascular pannus beneath the corneal epithelium with goblet cells in the epithelium, and attenuation or loss of Bowman's layer in the area of pannus.[5]

The anatomic and histopathologic findings suggest the absence of limbal stem cells. This has been further confirmed by the demonstration of the loss of corneal and increase in conjunctival phenotype markers in the cornea of a 37-year-old man with aniridia. This was shown using analysis of keratins and protein kinase C subtypes specific to cornea and conjunctiva to differentiate between the two.[6] The absence of limbal stem cells, or the presence of abnormal limbal stem cells, in aniridia explains the corneal changes seen, but does not explain the normal appearance of the cornea early in life. Nishida et al.[4] suggest the possibility that the corneal epithelium present at birth does not originate from limbal stem cells, but is replaced later by propagation of cells from the limbus. The underlying genetic defect in aniridia appears to be a mutation in the PAX6 gene. This gene is expressed in the meibomian embryogenesis and has been shown to be abnormal in both familial and sporadic aniridia.[7,8] PAX6 has been demonstrated in embryonic as well as mature corneal and conjunctival tissues, and may play a role in the maintenance and proliferation of limbal stem cells in addition to its role in embryogenesis.[9] Recent studies have shown PAX6 expression in limbal stem cells.[10]

Treatment of the keratopathy of aniridia may be of value in patients whose vision has been reduced by the corneal changes. Penetrating keratoplasty has been associated with improvement in visual acuity but, in one series of 11 eyes, all grafts developed peripheral pannus and superficial vascularization, and there was a high (64%) graft rejection rate.[11] Histopathology of corneas removed at repeat keratoplasty showed recurrence of inflammatory pannus with goblet cells.[12]

Since the underlying corneal abnormality arises in the limbal stem cell deficiency, replacement of the limbal stem cells makes the most sense. Holland[13] reported on

Figure 7.1. Cornea of a 35-year-old woman with aniridia. Note the central dense fibrous nodules and the peripheral pannus.

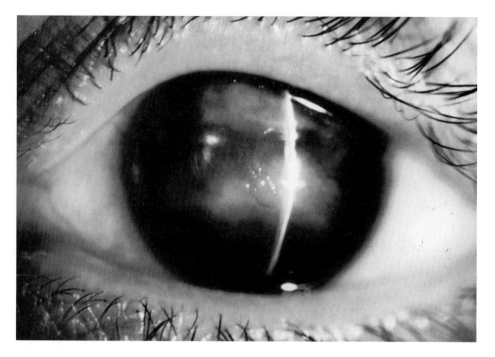

seven eyes of five patients with aniridia who underwent keratolimbal allografting, two of them with penetrating keratoplasty as well. Six (85.7%) had a stable ocular surface and 5 (71.4%) had significant improvement in vision. Tan, Ficker and Buckley[14] reported four patients with aniridia who underwent limbal allografting, one from a living related donor. All patients experienced visual improvement, although one experienced acute graft rejection when cyclosporin A was discontinued at four months postoperatively.

Dominantly Inherited Keratitis

A rare entity sharing much in common with aniridia has been described and is generally referred to as dominantly inherited keratitis, or autosomal-dominant keratitis. This disorder is characterized by symptoms of photophobia, tearing, and mucoid discharge in the first months of life and findings of progressive anterior corneal scarring and vascularization (Figure 7.3). Histopathology shows epithelial thinning and irregularity, as well as replacement

Figure 7.2. The 14-year-old daughter of patient in Figure 7.1. Note the peripheral pannus and the markedly less extensive subepithelial fibrotic nodules.

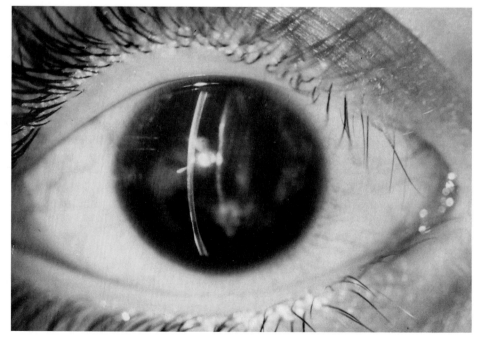

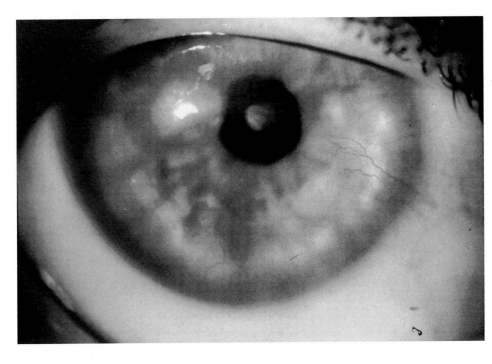

Figure 7.3. Autosomal dominant keratitis. A 27-year-old man with peripheral fibrovascular ingrowth and subepithelial fibrotic nodules. Note the mild distortion of the pupil. Courtesy of David Meisler, MD.

of Bowman's layer by fibrovascular pannus.[15] The originally reported family had no iris abnormalities, but another family demonstrated iris stromal defects and ectropion uveae, as well as macular hypoplasia, suggesting that this disorder is a variant of aniridia.[16] Another family with corneal pannus and iris changes without macular hypoplasia has been called "familial iris coloboma."[17] A PAX6 gene mutation has been found in the family with cornea, iris, and macular abnormalities.[18]

Treatment with lamellar and penetrating keratoplasty has been unsuccessful due to recurrent pannus and vascularization. Stem cell replacement has not been reported as of yet for this disorder.

Sclerocornea

Sclerocornea is an entity that is congenital and usually bilateral. Involvement ranges from peripheral corneal opacification with blunting of the limbal sulcus to total corneal opacification with corneal flattening and no evident limbus. Most cases are sporadic, although autosomal-dominant transmission is well reported.[19] Sclerocornea may be associated with other developmental anomalies including Peters' anomaly, microphthalmos, and aniridia. In peripheral sclerocornea, the changes are usually not progressive, suggesting that stem cells are present to maintain central corneal clarity.[20]

The etiology of sclerocornea is unknown. PAX6 mutations have been found rarely in Peters' anomaly and could, perhaps, occur in some sclerocornea patients.[21] Others, however, have failed to confirm PAX6 mutations in Peters' anomaly.[22] Often sclerocornea occurs in association with iris and/or lens abnormalities, suggesting Peters' anomaly. Demonstration of limbal stem

cell deficiency has not been reported, but in the more severe cases with total sclerocornea and no defined limbus, it is not unlikely that stem cell abnormalities or deficiency occur.

Treatment is often not necessary in the peripheral form of sclerocornea. With central involvement, however, keratoplasty is often necessary. Outcomes have varied, with one series reporting improved vision in 7 of 9 patients.[23] Our experience has been disappointing due to the high incidence of associated glaucoma. There is one case report of limbal transplantation for peripheral sclerocornea with regression of corneal vessels and improved visual acuity.[24]

Ectodermal Dysplasia

A number of cutaneous disorders have been associated with corneal abnormalities. Over 150 separate forms of ectodermal dysplasia exist.[25] Described here are some in which the ectodermal dysplasia appears to involve the limbal stem cells leading to keratopathy.

Ectrodactyly-Ectodermal Dysplasia-Clefting Syndrome (EEC)

This syndrome consists of ectrodactyly, or lobster-claw deformity of the hands and feet (Figure 7.4), cleft lip and palate (Figure 7.5), and ectodermal dysplasia leading to abnormal teeth and hair. Ocular findings may consist of absence of meibomian glands, nasolacrimal outflow obstruction, and keratopathy. The keratopathy includes peripheral pannus with the development of fibrous subepithelial corneal nodules (Figure 7.6).[26] Conjunctival

Figure 7.4. A 27-year-old patient with EEC showing ectrodactyly.

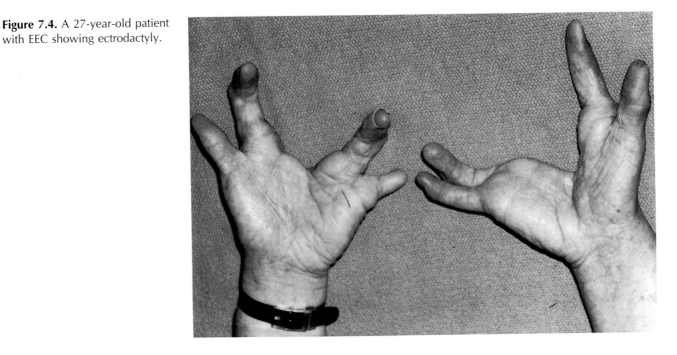

scarring and symblepharon formation also occur and may cause entropion and trichiasis.[27] Corneal scarring, opacities, and photophobia may be seen in the first few years of life.[28] Presumably the dystrophic epithelium in the limbal stem cells fails to produce normal corneal epithelium while the dysplastic conjunctival epithelium leads to the conjunctival fibrotic changes. Histopathology of the cornea shows thinning and irregularity of the epithelium with patchy absence of Bowman's layer underlying areas of pannus formation.[29]

Treatment with superficial keratectomy is not beneficial. Replacement of the dysplastic limbus with donor stem cells may prove to be beneficial in patients with severe keratopathy. Symptomatic treatment with lubrication helps provide comfort and reduces epithelial breakdown.

Other forms of ectodermal dysplasia may have corneal involvement, though this is not true of all forms. Hereditary hypohidrotic ectodermal dysplasia is usually a sex-linked recessive disorder. It presents with decreased sweating, generalized hypotrichosis, and dental abnormalities, as well as hyperkeratotic skin. Corneal punctate staining with intraepithelial cysts as well as peripheral corneal pannus has been noted. Tearing is decreased. Bowman's membrane is replaced with a fibrovascular pannus with inflammatory cells present, while the corneal epithelium demonstrates acanthosis as well as dyskeratosis.[30] Superficial keratectomy improved vision in one patient. This disorder may be a variant of the KID syndrome (see below).

An unusual variant of dyshidrotic ectodermal dysplasia has been described in two families with hair growth

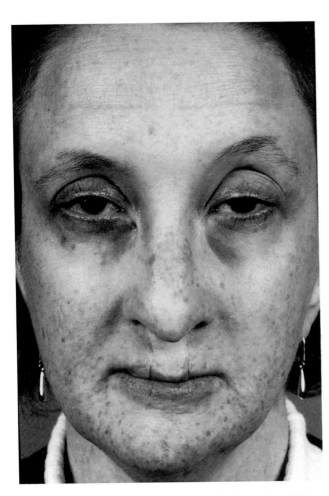

Figure 7.5. Facial appearance of patient in Figure 7.4. Note the evidence of the repaired cleft lip.

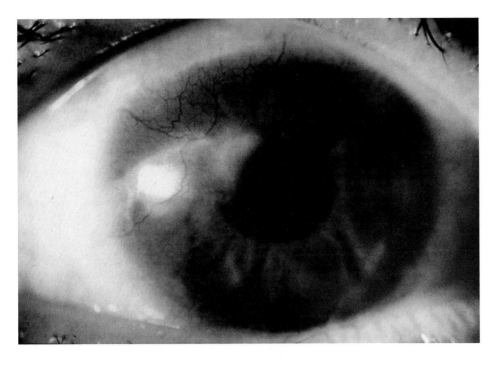

Figure 7.6. Cornea of the patient in Figure 7.4. Note the fibrovascular pannus and subepithelial fibrosis.

abnormalities, microdontia and supernumerary teeth, and excessive sweating. Meibomian glands and tear production were normal, but peripheral corneal pannus was present and limbal palisades of Vogt were not visible. Some patients had Bitot's spots with normal vitamin A levels, and one patient had hair follicles at the temporal limbus. Impression cytology showed no goblet cells. Limbal biopsy showed no stem cells. The corneal findings were attributed to limbal stem cell deficiency.[31]

Another ectodermal dysplastic syndrome with corneal involvement and presumably limbal stem cell deficiency is the keratitis-ichthyosis-deafness, or KID, syndrome, also called Senter's syndrome. This syndrome consists of congenital neurosensory hearing loss, ectodermal dysplasia with hyperkeratotic skin (not true ichthyosis),[32] and progressive corneal vascularization and pannus formation. The ocular problems are present from early in life and are associated with photophobia, tearing, and decreased vision. Chronic mycotic infection, liver disease, and mental retardation have been described as well. While occurrence is usually sporadic, dominant and recessive pedigrees have been reported.[33] Superficial keratectomy appears to be of no benefit. Systemic antifungal therapy may stabilize ocular disease in patients with associated chronic cutaneous candidiasis.[34]

A number of other dermatological disorders are associated with corneal opacities, including pannus and peripheral nebular opacities such as keratosis folicularis (Darier's disease), but the corneal changes are not progressive and probably do not reflect stem cell deficiency.[35] Various forms of epidermolysis bullosa have been associated with conjunctival and corneal scarring,

especially the dystrophic type[36] with diffuse epithelial dysfunction including limbal dysfunction. Holland[13] reported keratolimbal allografting in an eight-year-old patient with epidermolysis bullosa (type not defined) with development of a stable ocular surface and marked improvement in vision.

Other Disorders

Autoimmune Polyglandular Endocrinopathy-Candidiasis-Ectodermal Dysplasia (APECED)

Multiple endocrine deficiency, chronic mucocutaneous candidiasis, and autoimmune disease have been reported as a syndrome with some patients also developing keratitis early in life. Tear insufficiency and meibomian gland dysfunction are also present. Corneal pannus formation is characteristic.[37] This is an autosomal recessive disorder due to a defect in the AIRE (autoimmune regulator) gene.[38] Anticorneal antibodies have been demonstrated and the corneal changes may be due to both the ectodermal dysplasia and the antibody response to cornea.[39] Impression cytology shows goblet cells consistent with conjunctivalization of the cornea.[40] Whether this represents a congenital stem cell deficiency or an early acquired one it is uncertain. Stem cell grafts from living related donors have been reported in this disorder.[41]

Cryptophthalmos

Cryptophthalmos is a disorder in which the eyelids may fail to separate or the lids may be fused to the globe. Behind the abnormal lid there is no conjunctiva. When cryptophthalmos is complete, there is no ocular surface epithelium, while with partial or incomplete cryptophthalmos, some conjunctiva and limbus are present. Fraser's syndrome combines cryptophthalmos with systemic anomalies including syndactyly, urogenital abnormalities, and at times, abnormalities of the nose, ears, lips, or palate, skeleton, or mental retardation.[42] Surgical intervention has generally been directed at reforming the eyelids.[43] However, where anterior segment development is complete enough, the absence of limbal stem cells may preclude successful keratoplasty although stem cell replacement has not yet been reported in this disorder.

Conclusion

A number of disorders have so far been identified that appear to have associated congenital limbal stem cell functional deficiency. As our ability to readily identify stem cells improves, it is likely that other disorders will be recognized and our specific understanding of congenital stem cell dysfunction will increase. Hopefully, this will lead to more specific treatments that will allow better management of these presently difficult conditions.

References

1. Nelson, LB, Spaeth GL, Nowinski TS, et al. Aniridia. A review. *Surv Ophthalmol* 1984; 28:621–642.
2. Treacher Collins E. Congenital deficiency of the iris and glaucoma. *Trans Ophth Soc UK* 1893; 13:128–139.
3. Mackman G, Brightbill FS, Opitz JM. Corneal changes in aniridia. *Am J Ophthalmol* 1979; 87:497–502.
4. Nishida K, Knoshita S, Ohashi Y, et al. Ocular surface abnormalities in aniridia. *Am J Ophthalmol* 1995; 120:368–375.
5. Margo CE. Congenital aniridia: a histopathologic study of the anterior segment in children. *J Pediatr Ophthalmol Strabismus* 1983; 20:192–198.
6. Tseng SCG, Li D-Q. Comparison of protein kinase C subtype expression between normal and aniridic human ocular surfaces: implication for limbal stem cell dysfunction in aniridia. *Cornea* 1996; 15:168–178.
7. Glaser T, Walton DS, Maas RL. Genomic structure, evolutionary conservation and aniridia mutations in the human PAX6 gene. *Nat Genet* 1992; 2:232–239.
8. Jordan T, Hanson I, Zaletayev D, et al. The human PAX6 gene is mutated in two patients with aniridia. *Nat Genet* 1992; 1:328–332.
9. Koroma BM, Yang JM, Sundin OH. The Pax-6 homeobox gene is expressed throughout the corneal and conjunctival epithelia. *Invest Ophthalmol Vis Sci* 1997; 38:108–120.
10. Pan Z, Zhang W, Wu Y. Expression of Pax-6 gene in corneal epithelial cells in vitro. *Invest Ophthalmol Vis Sci* 2000; 41:S456 Abst. No. 2415.
11. Kremer I, Rajpal RK, Rapuano CJ, et al. Results of penetrating keratoplasty in aniridia. *Am J Ophth* 1993; 115: 317–320.
12. Gomes JAP, Eagle RC, Gomez AKGDP, et al. Recurrent keratopathy after penetrating keratoplasty in aniridia. *Cornea* 1996; 15:457–462.
13. Holland EJ. Epithelial transplantation for the management of severe ocular surface disease. *Trans Am Ophth Soc* 1996; 94:677–743.
14. Tan DTH, Ficker LA, Buckley RJ. Limbal transplantation. *Ophthalmology* 1996; 103:29–36.
15. Kivlin JD, Apple DJ, Olson RJ, et al. Dominantly inherited keratitis. *Arch Ophthalmol* 1986; 104:1621–1623.
16. Pearce WG, Mielke BW, Hassard DTR, et al. Autosomal dominant keratitis: a possible aniridia variant. *Can J Ophthalmol* 1995; 30:131–137.
17. Soong HK, Raizman MB. Corneal changes in familial iris coloboma. *Ophthalmology* 1986; 93:335–339.
18. Mirzayans F, Pearce WG, MacDonald IM, et al. Mutation of the PAX6 gene in patients with autosomal dominant keratitis. *Am J Hum Genet* 1995; 57:539–548.
19. Elliott JH, Feman SS, O'Day DM, et al. Hereditary sclerocornea. *Arch Ophthalmol* 1985; 103:676–679.
20. Waizenegger UR, Kohnen T, Weidle EG, et al. Kongenitale familiäre cornea plana mit Ptosis, peripherer Sklerokornea und Bindehaut-Xerose. *Klin Monatsbl Augenheilk* 1995; 206:111–116.
21. Hanson IM, Fletcher JM, Jordan T, et al. Mutations at the PAX6 locus are found in heterogenous anterior segment malformations including Peters' anomaly. *Nat Genet* 1994; 6:168–173.
22. Churchill AJ, Booth AP, Anwar R, et al. PAX 6 is normal in most cases of Peters' anomaly. *Eye* 1998; 12:299–303.
23. Zingirian M. Keratoplasty for sclerocornea in early infancy. *Fortschr Ophthalmol* 1987; 84:429–431.
24. Tsai R J-F, Tseng SCG. Human allograft limbal transplantation for corneal surface reconstruction. *Cornea* 1994; 13:389–400.
25. Freire-Maia N, Pinheiro M. Ectodermal dysplasias: a review of the conditions described after 1984 with an overall analysis of all the conditions belonging to this nosologic group. *Rev Brasil Genet* 1988; 10:403–414.
26. Mawhorter LG, Ruttum MS, Koenig SB. Keratopathy in a family with the ectrodactyly-ectodermal dysplasia-clefting syndrome. *Ophthalmology* 1985; 92:1427–1431.
27. Ireland IA, Meyer DR. Ophthalmic manifestations of ectrodacytyly-ectodermal dysplasia-clefting syndrome. *Ophthal Plast Reconstr Surg* 1998; 14:295–297.
28. Mondino BJ, Bath PE, Foos RY, et al. Absent meibomian glands in the ectrodactyly, ectodermal dysplasia, cleft lip-palate syndrome. *Am J Ophthalmol* 1984; 97:496–500.
29. Baum JL, Bull MJ. Ocular manifestations of the ectrodactyly, ectodermal dysplasia, cleft lip-palate syndrome. *Am J Ophthalmol* 1974; 78:211–216.
30. Wilson FM, Grayson M, Pieroni D. Corneal changes in ectodermal dysplasia. *Am J Ophthalmol* 1973; 75:17–27.
31. Tijmes NT, Zaal MJW, DeJong PTVM, et al. Two families with dyshidrotic ectodermal dysplasia associated with ingrowth of corneal vessels, limbal hair growth, and Bitot-like conjunctival anomalies. *Ophthalmic Genet* 1997; 18: 185–192.

32. Caceres-Rios H, Tamayo-Sanchez L, Duran-McKinster C, et al. Keratitis, ichthyosis, and deafness (KID) syndrome: A review of the literature and proposal of a new terminology. *Pediatr Dermatol* 1996; 13:105–113.

33. Wilson GN, Squires RH, Weinberg AG. Keratitis, hepatitis, ichthyosis, and deafness: report and review of KID syndrome. *Amer J Med Genet* 1991; 40:255–259.

34. Hazen PG, Walker AE, Stewart JJ, et al. Keratitis, ichthyosis, and deafness (KID) syndrome: management with chronic oral ketoconazole therapy. *Int J Dermatol* 1992; 31:58–59.

35. Blackman HJ, Rodrigues MM, Peck GL. Corneal epithelial lesions in keratosis follicularis (Darier's disease). *Ophthalmology* 1980; 87:931–943.

36. Granek H, Baden HP. Corneal involvement in epidermolysis bullosa simplex. *Arch Ophthalmol* 1980; 98:469–472.

37. Wagman RD, Kazdan JJ, Kooh SW, et al. Keratitis associated with multiple endocrine deficiency, autoimmune disease, and candidiasis syndrome. *Am J Ophthalmol* 1987; 103:569–575.

38. Bjorses P, Halonen M, Palvimo JJ, et al. Mutations in the AIRE gene: effect on subcellular location and transactivation function of the autoimmune polyendocrinopathy-candidiasis-ectodermal dystrophy protein. *Am J Hum Genet* 2000; 66:378–392.

39. Kaye SB, Willoughby CE, Haslett R, et al. Keratopathy in autoimmune polyglandular endocrinopathy-candidiasis-ectodermal dystrophy (APECED). *Invest Ophthalmol Vis Sci* 2000; 41:S266, Abst No. 1396.

40. Puangsricharern V, Tseng SCG. Cytologic evidence of corneal diseases with limbal stem cell deficiency. *Ophthalmology* 1995; 102:1476–1485.

41. Tseng SCG, Meller D, Pires RTF, et al. Corneal surface reconstruction by limbal epithelial cells ex vivo expanded in amniotic membrane. *Investigative Ophthalmol Vis Sci* 2000; 41:S756 Abst No. 4016.

42. Walton WT, Enzenauer RW, Cornell FM. Abortive cryptophthalmos: a case report and a review of cryptophthalmos. *J Pediatr Ophthalmol Strabismus* 1990; 27:129–132.

43. Ferri M, Harvey JT. Surgical correction for complete cryptophthalmos: case report and review of the literature. *Can J Ophthalmol* 1999; 34:233–236.

8
Chemical and Thermal Injuries to the Ocular Surface

Terry Kim and B. Alyse Khosla-Gupta

Epidemiology

Chemical burns to the eye can result in mild injury, or severe ocular damage. Most chemical injuries are due to alkali or acid compounds. The extent of ocular injury depends on several factors: the strength of the chemical agent, concentration, volume of solution, and duration of exposure.[1,2] Most injuries are accidental and occur in the workplace, particularly in an industrial setting. A large retrospective study including 171 patients and 236 injured eyes reviewed in Germany from 1990–1991 demonstrated that 121 of the patients were male (70%) and 39 patients (23%) were female. The majority of the patients were between 16 and 45 years of age. Sixty-one percent of these injuries occurred in an industrial workplace, 37% were due to household injuries, and 2% were of unknown origin.[3,4] Another large retrospective study performed in the United Kingdom also showed that the majority of victims in chemical-related ocular injuries were young males. Morgan demonstrated that in a study of 180 patients from 1985–1986, 136 patients (75.6%) were male and only 44 (24.4%) were female. In this series, the majority of the cases occurred in the workplace (63%), 33% occurred at home, and 3% occurred at school. Alkali injuries were twice as common as acid injuries.[4,5]

Alkali Injuries

Alkaline Chemicals

The most severe alkali injuries are usually due to ammonia or lye. Ammonia is found in fertilizers and household cleaners. It has the potential to cause the most severe eye damage because of its characteristic of both lipid and water solubility. It penetrates the eye very quickly and can reach the anterior chamber in one minute.[6,7] Lye, or sodium hydroxide, is commonly found in drain cleaners and can also penetrate the eye quickly, although not as rapidly as ammonia. It can reach the anterior chamber in three minutes.[6] Magne-

sium hydroxide is an alkali that in itself does not cause severe chemical injuries, but it is often a component of fireworks and flares. The thermal injuries associated with magnesium hydroxide may, therefore, be quite severe.[8] Lime, or calcium hydroxide, is the most common cause of alkaline injury but fortunately, does not penetrate as well as ammonia or lye. Calcium hydroxide is found in cement, mortar, and plaster. This compound saponifies the epithelial cell membrane and forms calcium soaps that precipitate and limit its further penetration into tissue.[9] For this reason, it causes early opacification, but superficial injury. Precipitates of lime may remain in the fornices or on tissue despite irrigation and continue to serve as a source of alkali.[2] Table 8.1 lists the common chemical substances causing ocular injuries.

Pathogenesis

Alkali injury results in ocular damage due to the saponification and disruption of fatty acids in cell membranes, leading to cell death. The lipid saponification associated with alkali injuries allows rapid penetration of the alkali substance into tissue, in contrast to most acidic compounds. A pH of 11.5 or higher is associated with severe ocular damage. The hydroxyl ions cause collagen fiber edema with subsequent thickening and shortening.[10] Injury by a similar mechanism occurs to other tissues in the eye such as conjunctiva, blood vessels, nerves, endothelium and keratocytes.[2] Intense pain caused by an alkali agent is secondary to stimulation of the nerve endings in the conjunctiva and cornea.[11] The effect on goblet cells is unclear; some studies have shown that the goblet cell population decreases, while other studies have demonstrated an increase in cell population.[12,13] Intraocular structures such as iris, ciliary body, and trabecular meshwork may also be affected, depending upon the degree of penetration and the pH of the aqueous. Aqueous pH can remain elevated from thirty minutes to three hours despite external irrigation.[6,14] Glucose and ascorbic acid levels decrease after an alkaline

Table 8.1. Common chemicals causing ocular injury.

Compound	Sources	Associated Facts
Alkaline Substances		
Sodium Hydroxide	Drain Cleaners	Rapid penetration
Ammonium Hydroxide	Fertilizers, refrigerants, Cleaning agents	Very rapid penetration Lipid and water soluble
Magnesium Hydroxide	Fireworks, sparklers	Often combined chemical and thermal injury
Calcium Hydroxide	Plaster, cement, mortar	Poor penetration, most common alkali injury
Acidic Substances		
Sulfuric Acid	Car batteries	Most common acid injury
Sulfurous Acid	Exposure of sulfur dioxide to water	Rapid penetration, lipid and water soluble
Hydrofluoric Acid	Glass frosting, etching, rust removal	Rapid penetration
Hydrochloric Acid	Industrial uses	Hydrogen chloride gas released—irritating to eye; severe injury associated with concentrated acids
Chromic Acid	Chrome plating	Causes brown discoloration of superficial cornea
Silver Nitrate	Neonatal ocular prophylaxis, conjunctival cauterization	High concentrations may lead to permanent corneal opacification

injury and may remain at low levels for prolonged periods of time.[15,16] Ascorbate is required for collagen and glycosaminoglycan synthesis and is normally twenty times higher in aqueous than in plasma. The low levels of ascorbate in alkali burns are due to a decreased active transport mechanism in the damaged ciliary body.[2]

Stromal corneal ulceration may also occur (Figure 8.1). Factors affecting ulceration include defects in the corneal epithelium, inflammation, release of proteolytic enzymes,

anesthesia, tear deficiency, and impaired collagen synthesis.[2] Type I collagenase plays an instrumental role in corneal ulceration and is released by keratocytes and polymorphonuclear leukocytes (PMNs).[17,18] Type I collagenase has been detected as early as nine hours after injury,[19] but peaks 14 to 21 days after the primary insult.[20,21] Type I collagenase is normally inhibited by epithelial cytokines,[22] which highlights the importance of an intact epithelium in ulcer prevention.

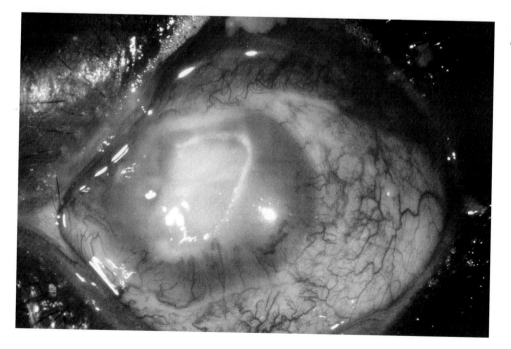

Figure 8.1. Central corneal ulceration after an alkali injury.

It has been shown that an epithelial injury is repaired by centripetal movement of the proximal epithelium.[23] A complete epithelial defect requires repair from limbal stem cells.[24,25] If limbal stem cells are not available due to extensive injury, then the conjunctiva must re-epithelize the corneal surface. This pathologic re-epithelialization is a prolonged process and does not produce a normal phenotypic corneal epithelium.[23] Regardless of the source of epithelium, the re-epithelialization process in chemical injury may be slower than normal due to inflammation and basement membrane damage.[26] Epithelialization is enhanced by adequate lubrication and control of inflammation.[4]

Inflammation also plays a key role in the pathogenesis of alkaline burns. Infiltration of PMNs and mononuclear leukocytes occurs within 12 to 24 hours after initial alkaline exposure. These cells undergo chemotactic attraction by cellular and extracellular proteins released from necrotic tissue and injured blood vessels.[21,27] In addition to type I collagenase released by neutrophils, superoxide free radicals are created by the oxidative respiratory bursts of these neutrophils and result in further tissue damage.[1]

Fibroblasts that repair stromal damage in the cornea are immature, and the collagen produced from these cells is underhydroxylated, resulting in an abnormal winding pattern that does not follow the triple helical structure of normal collagen. In addition, this new collagen is vulnerable to enzymatic lysis.[1]

Clinical Manifestations and Classification

Acute Phase
Chemical injuries must be treated immediately with irrigation and removal of chemical debris. Other aspects of the examination such as history and vision checks should be postponed until emergency treatment is under way or complete. Injury to cellular structures in the conjunctiva, cornea, nerves, and vessels occurs almost immediately after the injury. The conjunctiva may be injected, chemotic, or necrotic. Partial or complete epithelial defects may occur over the cornea and conjunctiva. Epithelial defects may be extensive or complete. In addition, there may be perilimbal ischemia (Figure 8.2). The corneal stroma may vary from being clear to completely opacified (Figure 8.3). Inflammatory membranes may also form in the anterior chamber. Immediately after injury, the collagen fibers in the cornea and trabecular meshwork shrink, causing an increase in intraocular pressure. Within a few hours, prostaglandins are released from damaged intraocular structures, and the trabecular meshwork may become occluded with inflammatory debris. Later, the ciliary body may shut down from damage, resulting in hypotony. For these reasons, intraocular pressures may vary widely in the first few days and should be closely monitored.[2] Burns to the periocular skin and eyelids, cataract formation, scleral thinning and necrosis, and damage to the retina may also occur. A useful classification of chemical injuries was first proposed by Hughes[28] and then modified by Roper-Hall.[29] This classification divides the clinical manifestations into four categories which help to guide prognosis and treatment. Pfister has further adapted the Hughes–Roper-Hall classification into another helpful classification as well (Table 8.2 and Figure 8.4).

Early Repair Phase
During the early repair phase, epithelial migration and regeneration occurs in grade I and II injuries. Grade III

Figure 8.2. Opacified cornea secondary to an alkali injury.

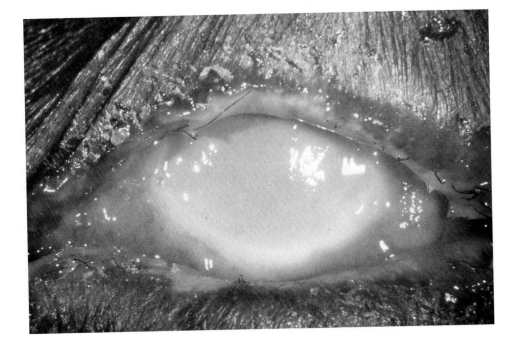

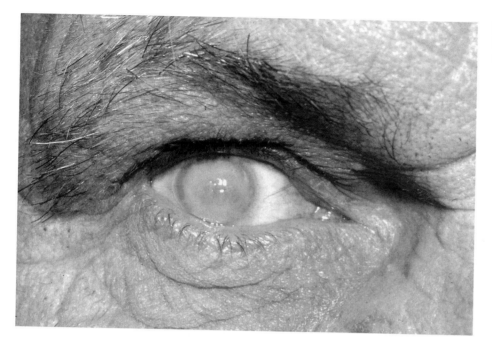

Figure 8.3. Severe acute alkali injury resulting in a thin, opacified cornea with limbal ischemia.

injury retards re-epithelialization loss of limbal stem cells. Little if any change occurs in grade IV cases.[4] Fibrovascular pannus and an influx of inflammatory components may develop during this early stage also. Symblephara can develop between denuded surfaces of the palpebral and bulbar conjunctiva.[2] Keratocyte proliferation, collagen synthesis, and collagenase synthesis peak during this period, and the stroma begins to clear gradually.[4] Stromal ulceration may develop between seven to ten days, although it most typically occurs between two to three weeks.[2]

Late Repair Phase

Conjunctival scarring, trichiasis, cicatricial entropion, and corneal scarring can progress during the later period of repair (Figure 8.5). The patient may also develop tear deficiency abnormalities secondary to loss of goblet cells, or decreased aqueous production. Corneal nerve sensation may also be decreased, depending upon the extent of injury. Intraocular pressure problems of hypotonia or elevated pressure may persist as well.[2]

Table 8.2. Hughes–Roper-Hall classification of chemical burns

Grade	Findings	Prognosis
I	Corneal epithelial damage; no limbal ischemia	Good
II	Cornea hazy but iris detail seen; ischemia less than one third of limbus	Good
III	Total loss of corneal epithelium; stromal haze blurring iris details; ischemia at one third to one half of limbus	Guarded
IV	Cornea opaque, obscuring view of iris or pupil; ischemia at more than one half of limbus	Poor

Treatment

Treatment can be divided into acute and chronic management strategies. Acute treatment is primarily medical, and chronic management may require surgical therapy. The acute management can be subdivided into three phases: immediate, intermediate, and long term. Immediate treatment includes management of pH, pressure control, and anti-inflammatory therapy. Intermediate goals include promoting re-epithelialization, preventing infections, and restoration of the ocular surface. Long-term goals involve prevention and management of scarring of the ocular surface.

Acute Treatment

An alkali injury constitutes a true eye emergency and immediate ocular irrigation is necessary. Irrigation should occur prior to taking a history, or completing the rest of the ocular exam. Although an isotonic solution with a neutral pH is preferable, such as normal saline or Ringer's lactate, any nontoxic solution is acceptable in an emergency. Irrigation is usually performed with an ocular device attached to intravenous tubing such as a Morgan lens.[30] If such a device is not available, irrigation can be performed with intravenous tubing and a lid speculum, and should continue for a minimum of thirty minutes, or until the pH becomes neutral. The fornices should be tested with litmus paper 5 to 10 minutes after irrigation. Studies have demonstrated that external irrigation of the eye for ninety minutes lowers the pH in the aqueous humor by 1.5 pH units.[14] Removal of aqueous humor by paracentesis decreases pH by 1.5 units. If possible, the aqueous humor should be replaced by balanced salt solution, or a buffered phosphate solution.[30] However, some authorities do not advocate an-

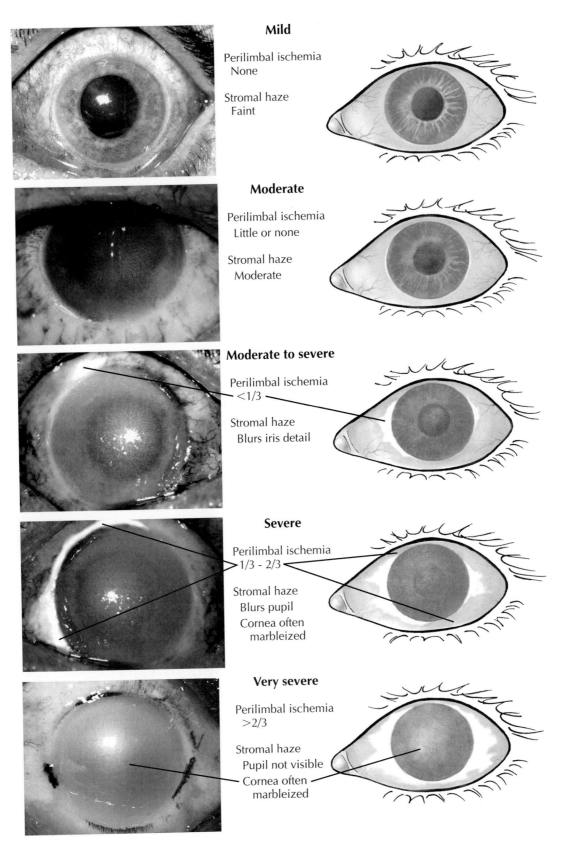

Mild

Perilimbal ischemia
None

Stromal haze
Faint

Moderate

Perilimbal ischemia
Little or none

Stromal haze
Moderate

Moderate to severe

Perilimbal ischemia
<1/3

Stromal haze
Blurs iris detail

Severe

Perilimbal ischemia
1/3 - 2/3

Stromal haze
Blurs pupil
Cornea often
marbleized

Very severe

Perilimbal ischemia
>2/3

Stromal haze
Pupil not visible
Cornea often
marbleized

Figure 8.4. Classification of alkali-burned eyes (from the Pfister classification of chemical injury). **Normal eye: Mild**: corneal epithelial erosion, faint anterior stromal haziness, no ischemic necrosis of perilimbal conjunctiva and sclera. Prognosis: healing with little or no corneal scarring; visual loss usually no greater than 1 to 2 lines. **Moderate**: Moderate corneal opacity, little or no significant ischemic necrosis of perilimbal conjunctiva. Prognosis: slow healing of epithelium with moderate scarring, peripheral corneal vascularization, and visual loss of 2 to 7 lines. **Moderate to severe**: Corneal opacity blurring iris details, ischemic necrosis of conjunctiva limited to less than one-third of perilimbal conjunctiva. Prognosis: prolonged corneal healing with significant corneal vascularization and scarring; vision usually limited to 20/200 or less. **Severe**: Blurring of pupillary outline, ischemia of approximately one-third to two-thirds of perilimbal conjunctiva, cornea often marbleized. Prognosis: very prolonged corneal healing with inflammation and high incidence of corneal ulceration and perforation. In the best cases, severe corneal vascularization and scarring with counting-fingers vision. **Very severe**: Pupil not visible, greater than two-thirds ischemia of perilimbal conjunctiva, cornea often marbleized. Prognosis: very prolonged corneal healing with inflammation and high incidence of corneal ulceration and perforation. In the best cases, severe corneal vascularization and scarring with counting-fingers vision. (Adapted from *Cornea and External Disease: Diagnosis and Management*, editors, J Krachmer, M Mannis, E Holland, 1997.)

terior chamber paracentesis, and the practice remains controversial.[22] The lid should be double-everted to remove any remaining solid material that could act as a reservoir for alkali. Particulate matter can be removed with forceps, scraping, or a cotton-tipped applicator. If calcium hydroxide is the culprit, sodium EDTA (0.01 M) can be used to loosen the sticky paste that it can form.[31] Once the pH is neutralized, a complete history should be taken, including the mechanism of the injury, the chemicals involved, and whether eye protection was used. A thorough ocular exam should also be performed.

Any necrotic tissue should be removed carefully, since it can act as a stimulus for inflammatory components, such as neutrophils that can incite an enzymatic cascade causing further damage.[32] A cycloplegic drop such as scopolamine should be administered for comfort. Vasoconstrictors such as phenylephrine should be avoided, especially in cases of perilimbal ischemia, since they may potentially worsen the ischemia. Medications should be kept at a minimum, because the preservatives they contain can cause epithelial toxicity, and thus hinder epithelial repair. A broad-spectrum topical antibiotic such as ciprofloxacin would be prudent to avoid a microbial keratitis. Increases in intraocular pressure should be controlled with beta-blockers (timolol maleate 0.5%), topical carbonic anhydrase inhibitors (dorzolamide 2.0%), alpha adrenergic agents (bromonidine tartrate 0.2%), or oral carbonic anhydrase inhibitors (arcelazatamide).

Frequent lubrication with preservative-free drops should be utilized to enhance epithelialization. A hydrophilic bandage contact lens can also be used to promote epithelial repair. Usually the bandage contact lens is not removed until the epithelium is healed; this process may take several days to months. The use of bandage contact lenses is controversial because of the increased risk of infection. Thus, careful follow-up is crucial. If the healing is not adequate by these more conservative measures, then patching, tarsorrhaphy, or an amniotic patch can also be considered.[33] If a descene-

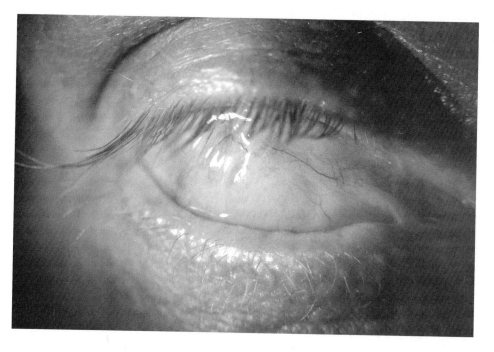

Figure 8.5. Symblephara resulting from a severe alkali injury.

tocele or small perforation takes place, cyanoacrylate glue is helpful as a temporary measure until a more permanent treatment such as a penetrating keratoplasty is scheduled.[30]

Topical corticosteroids can be utilized to decrease inflammation in the first 7 to 10 days of treatment because their effect on collagenase activity is minimal. After 10 days, however, the risk/benefit ratio shifts, and corticosteroids then increase the risk of ulceration and stromal melting.[34] Topical NSAIDS such as ketoralac are inflammatory inhibitors that have proved useful in controlling ocular inflammation in several settings. Although their effect on stromal ulceration and collagenase activity has not been fully evaluated,[35] this class of compounds may be useful as a substitute for topical steroids after the first week. Topical, subconjunctival, or systemic medroxyprogesterone (Provera) has also demonstrated an anticollagenase effect and has been shown to inhibit neovascularization.[36,37] Medroxyprogesterone may be a useful adjunct in early treatment as well. Finally, moderate to severe burns in which stromal ulceration is expected, tetracycline (250 mg four times a day), doxycycline (100 mg twice a day), or minocycline (100 mg twice a day) may be added for anticollagenolytic effect. Topical tetracycline preparations (1% solution or 3% ointment) have also been effective in addition to oral tetracycline.[30] Tetracycline and its derivatives do not work in an antimicrobial fashion, but rather by chelating zinc at the active site of the collagenase enzyme.[38] It may also reduce neutrophil activity by decreasing its ability to produce collagenase.[39]

Ascorbate is another useful agent in stromal ulcer prophylaxis. It is a water-soluble vitamin that is necessary for collagen synthesis. Low levels of ascorbic acid are found in the aqueous humor after damage to the ciliary body and its active transport mechanisms. Topical or systemic administration of ascorbate has demonstrated efficacy in preventing the incidence of ulceration in experimental chemical injuries if an aqueous humor concentration of 15 mg/dl can be achieved.[40,41] A 10% solution of sodium ascorbate applied hourly or 1000 mg of oral ascorbic acid given four times a day will help to increase ascorbate to therapeutic levels.[30] Topical application has proved superior to systemic administration in severe cases.[40] However, studies have not demonstrated any efficacy in preventing progression of established ulcers in chemical injuries.[42]

Citrate is a calcium chelator that inhibits intracellular and membrane levels of calcium, thus decreasing leukocyte phagocytosis, adherence, mediator release, and lysosomal enzyme release.[43] It has been shown to reduce neutrophil infiltration by 63% in the early phase and 92% in the late phase of experimental chemical injury studies.[44] It has also been demonstrated that topical administration is more effective than systemic administration.[45] A 10% solution of sodium citrate can be applied hourly. Citrate has been proven more effective than ascorbate in corneal ulcer prophylaxis.[44] It has also been shown to help retard ulcer progression in established stromal ulcers, unlike ascorbate.[46] Citrate and ascorbate act to reduce the incidence of ulceration through different mechanisms and, therefore, work well in combination. When used together in experimental alkali injuries, the incidence of corneal ulceration fell to only 4.6%, compared to 80% in the untreated eye.[47] A study of patients with alkali burns revealed that intensive therapy with topical steroids, ascorbate, citrate, and antibiotics was most helpful in grade 3 injuries in the Roper-Hall classification with regard to time of re-epithelialization and visual acuity. Intensive therapy actually delayed re-epithelialization in grade 1 and 2 injuries, probably due to epithelial toxicity.[48]

Acetylcysteine was one of the earliest collagenase inhibitors discovered and is still available. Acetylcysteine (Mucomyst) 10% solution can be applied every hour and has little toxic effect beyond a mild, temporary stromal haze.[30] It must be refrigerated, kept in a dark bottle because of its instability to light, replaced weekly, and does not penetrate the stroma well.[4,44] However, it is widely available. It is not recommended in severe injuries. Agents such as tetracycline are far more effective than acetylcysteine in severe injuries. Synthetic collagenase inhibitors such as thiol peptides are powerful new agents that are 10,000 times more potent than acetylcysteine and have also been shown to reduce corneal ulceration and thinning in experimental studies.[4,6,49] Recombinant metalloproteinase tissue inhibitors are anticollagenolytics with an efficacy similar to that of thiol peptides.[50] Neither of these compounds is available for clinical use at this time.

Attention should also be given to symblephara that may form during the early phase of treatment. Damage to the conjunctiva from the alkali, in addition to the subsequent inflammatory reaction, causes fibrin adhesions to form between conjunctival surfaces. Subconjunctival fibrosis can cause shortening of the conjunctiva and symblepharon formation.[1] A glass rod can be used to break developing symblephara on a daily basis, and helps to prevent shortening of the fornices. A symblepharon ring in combination with a bandage contact lens is also a favored method for separating the bulbar and palpebral conjunctiva.[2] Another alternative method is to apply a thin plastic wrap, such as food wrap, to the palpebral conjunctiva and secure it with sutures through the upper and lower fornices.[1]

Chronic Treatment

A method that can re-establish limbal vascularity is the conjunctival/Tenon's advancement procedure. This technique, as described by Teping and Reim, involves excising all necrotic or ischemic tissue from the limbal area and then separating Tenon's capsule from the equator of the globe and the extraocular muscles with blunt dissection. Tenon's flap and its vascular supply are then advanced to the limbus and secured to the sclera.[4,47] This method works well in arresting corneal ulceration and re-establishing a limbal vascular supply. In a study of 24 eyes with severe chemical injuries, Tenon's advancement alone was performed. In 100% of these cases, stromal ulceration was either halted or prevented.[51] However, this technique has not worked as well in establishing appropriate phenotypic re-epithelialization of the cornea.[51,52]

In severe injuries such as grade 4 chemical burns, in which there is a great deal of perilimbal ischemia, anterior segment necrosis may occur due to the loss of blood vessels and failure to re-epithelialize the cornea. Techniques involving transplantation of a source of epithelium to the damaged ocular surface are necessary in these cases. The nomenclature classification proposed by Holland and Schwartz has simplified the terminology used for these procedures. This nomenclature is based on the donor source, the carrier tissue used, and the location of the epithelium harvested. A donor source may be the fellow eye (autograft), a cadaveric source (allograft), or a living relative (allograft). The source of epithelium may be the conjunctiva or limbal stem cells. If limbal stem cells are used, the carrier tissue may be cornea or conjunctiva. A conjunctival autograft (CAU) uses conjunctiva from a fellow eye, whereas a conjunctival allograft (CAL) uses conjunctiva from a living relative (Lr-CAL) or a cadaveric donor (c-CAL). A conjunctival limbal autograft (CLAU) refers to conjunctival tissue from a fellow eye, whereas cadaveric conjunctival limbal allograft (c-CLAL) designates a cadaveric source for the limbal graft. If a living relative donates conjunctiva and limbal tissue, the transplant is termed a living related conjunctival limbal allograft (lr-CLAL). Keratolimbal allograft (KLAL) refers to a cadaveric source of corneal and limbal tissue.[53]

Limbal stem cell transplantation should be considered in cases with severe partial or total damage to the limbal area. Limbal stem cell transplantation is the only technique currently known that promotes proper phenotypic differentiation of the corneal epithelium. This technique, first described by Kenyon and Tseng,[54] involves the transplantation of sectorial crescents of healthy limbal tissue from the uninjured or minimally injured eye to the injured contralateral eye. Each tissue section should be approximately three clock hours or greater in diameter.[55] This technique can be applied for acute (less than one month) or chronic (greater than one year) cases. If the chemical injury is chronic, then fibrovascular pannus may have developed and would need to be removed with a superficial keratectomy prior to limbal stem cell autografting. If a limbal stem cell transplant is performed early, complications such as corneal fibrovascular pannus, ulceration, and scarring

may be prevented.[55] To perform an autograft early in the course of injury, ocular inflammation must be controlled with appropriate medical therapy. In all cases, a sufficient vascular supply must be established to support the graft.

In a unilateral injury, a CAU or CLAU could be considered. If extensive bilateral injury is present and precludes limbal stem cell autografting, a KLAL or lr-CLAL may be indicated. Appropriate HLA typing is necessary in choosing the living related donor to prevent stem cell rejection, and postoperative immunosuppression is required to avoid allograft rejection.[55]

In a primate study reported by Weise involving 12 eyes with limbal allografts, all 12 eyes re-epithelialized well, and the donor tissue survived.[56] Pfister also reported on two anectodal human cases involving limbal allografts and subsequent penetrating keratoplasties. In both cases, the patients did well over one year after penetrating keratoplasty with improved visual acuity.[57]

Amniotic membrane transplants are also helpful in reconstructing the corneal epithelium and suppressing fibrovascular membrane formation, particularly in cases with extensive conjunctival damage. In an experimental study, Kim and Tseng examined rabbit corneas with total limbal stem cell deficiency and significant conjunctival damage after penetrating keratoplasties alone, or in conjunction with amniotic membrane transplants. Control corneas all revascularized to the center of the cornea with conjunctivalization. In contrast, 5 of the 13 corneas in the experimental group were clear with minimal or no vascularization. Five experimental corneas showed mid-peripheral vascularization, and 3 corneas were completely vascularized with a cloudy stroma.[58]

Other treatment options include combined amniotic membrane and stem cell transplants. A small series by Shimazaki et al. involving patients with severe chemical and thermal burns were treated with amniotic-membrane transplants and limbal stem cell autografts ($n = 4$) or allografts ($n = 2$) if necessary. In all 7 eyes, the corneal epithelium was successfully reconstructed, and visual acuity improved dramatically.[59] However, long-term clinical trials involving limbal stem cell allografts must still be examined to discern the potential value of the technique. Another possibility described by Tsai et al. employs cultured human limbal stem cells that are harvested, grown in vitro, and then transplanted back to the original host on amniotic-membrane grafts.[60,61] Current studies in this area of research appear promising and would create treatment options for severely injured individuals.

If corneal thinning progresses to the level of a descemetocele, then an impending corneal perforation must be prevented. A lamellar keratoplasty may be the procedure of choice to re-establish structural integrity to the cornea.[30] For a perforation greater than 1 millimeter in diameter, in which cyanoacrylate glue cannot be used, a penetrating keratoplasty may be necessary. Penetrating keratoplasty is indicated in cases of severe scarring to improve visual potential as long as the ocular surface can support a graft. The eye should be quiet prior to proceeding with surgery. Ideally, it is best to wait two years after the initial injury before performing a penetrating keratoplasty. These patients have a better prognosis than patients who undergo early penetrating keratoplasty.[62] Care must be taken intraoperatively and postoperatively to protect the epithelium of the donor graft to prevent future epithelial healing defects. Bandage contact lens wear, patching, or a partial tarsorrhaphy should be considered for 4 to 6 weeks after surgery to protect the graft surface and promote healing. Lubrication is critical.

The ocular environment is critical to the success of the penetrating keratoplasty as well. Glaucoma or any other intraocular abnormality that may affect visual potential should be controlled prior to the procedure. Any lid abnormality such as an ectropion, entropion, or trichiasis needs to be addressed prior to the penetrating keratoplasty in order to create as normal an ocular environment as possible with an appropriate lid-globe relation. Conjunctival transplantation can be helpful in this regard, if shortening of the fornix, cicatricial entropion, symblepharon formation, or conjunctival keratinization and scarring hinders normal anatomic relationships. Conjunctiva can be taken from the contralateral eye if it contains healthy tissue. If bilateral injury exists and it is not possible to use conjunctiva, a mucous membrane, or an amniotic membrane graft, can act as a substitute for conjunctiva. Some authorities recommend the use of nasal mucosal grafts rather than buccal mucosa because it contains goblet cells that may restore some mucous-secreting ability to the eye and improve tear film stability.[63,64] Finally, if these surgical options fail, a permanent keratoprosthesis can be utilized as a last resort to obtaining visual function. However, these devices are fraught with complications.[65]

Acid Injuries

Acidic Chemicals

Acid injuries to the eye are common due to the frequency of acidic compounds found in household chemicals such as cleaners, rust removers, and car batteries.[66] Acids are commonly used in various industrial applications under high pressure, which can exacerbate the nature of the ocular insult. Although acid injuries are generally considered less severe to the eye than alkali injuries, this is not necessarily the case. Strong acids in high concentration can cause devastating ocular injuries. As with alkaline compounds, acid injury to the eye depends on several factors: strength of the acid, concentration, volume of solution, and duration of exposure.[2,4] The extent of ocular injury is also dependent upon the ability of the acidic compound to adhere to and penetrate the tissue. The acid's ability to penetrate tissue is affected by its lipid solubility.[67]

Sulfuric acid is the most common cause of acidic chemical injury to the eye. Although it is widely used in industry, most ocular chemical burns result from car battery accidents. Lead batteries contain up to 25% sulfuric acid. During the recharging of a battery, hydrogen and oxygen are produced by electrolysis and form an explosive mixture.[68] This mixture can be easily ignited when a match or lighter are used to inspect the battery in the dark, or when jumper cables are improperly attached to the battery. These injuries may be compounded by contusions or lacerations to the eye from the explosion itself. Sulfurous acid is formed when sulfur dioxide combines with water in the tears or cornea. It is highly soluble in both hydrophobic and hydrophilic substances and, therefore, penetrates rapidly.[2] Sulfurous acid penetrates more quickly into tissue than hydrochloric, sulfuric, or phosphoric acids.[30]

Hydrofluoric acid also penetrates tissue easily. Although it is a weak acid, its fluoride anion can dissolve cellular membranes. In addition, its small molecular size and weight also enhance its ability to penetrate tissue very easily.[2] It is commonly used in cleaning, etching, and rust removal in industrial settings.[30] Hydrochloric acid is usually not damaging to the eye except in high concentrations. Regardless of concentration, this acid releases hydrogen chloride gas, which is irritating to the eye even at low levels. Chromic acid is used in the chrome-plating industry and in washing laboratory equipment. It can cause a chronic conjunctivitis and a brown discoloration of the corneal epithelium.[7] Silver nitrate burns can occur in neonatal ocular prophylaxis if a solution greater than one percent is used. It can also occur if silver nitrate sticks are used to cauterize conjunctiva. In addition to acid burns, silver deposition can occur with silver nitrate injury.[2] High concentrations of silver nitrate can result in corneal opacification that may be permanent.[69] Table 8.1 lists the common acids and their sources.

There are many similarities between alkali and acid injuries to the eye. Only differences between the two types of injuries will be highlighted in the following sections.

Pathogenesis

Acids dissociate to form hydrogen ions in solution. These free hydrogen ions cause cellular necrosis. The acid anion causes protein denaturation and precipitation. As these proteins precipitate, they form a barrier to prevent further acid penetration, thus protecting the eye. This precipitation gives the eye its "ground glass" appearance after injury.[67] This barrier may protect against weaker acids, but strong acids may continue to penetrate deeply. The cornea itself can act as a partial buffer to acids. Corneal pH begins to neutralize within fifteen minutes and can normalize within an hour.[70,71,72] Although hydrofluoric acid is a weak acid, its anion is highly reactive and acts as an alkali. It is very toxic and penetrates tissue easily.

After acid penetration into the corneal stroma, extracellular glycosaminoglycans precipitate, epithelial cells coagulate causing corneal opacification, and hydration and shortening of collagen fibrils occur.[67,72] The intraocular pressure rises due to the collagen shrinkage and distortion in the trabecular meshwork. The rise in intraocular pressure is then maintained for at least 3 hours by prostaglandin release.[73,74] Ascorbate levels are also decreased with acid injuries, as they are with alkali injuries. Low ascorbate levels are probably due to dual mechanism of damage to the ciliary body causing decreased active transport of ascorbate and to a disrupted blood-aqueous barrier.[70,75]

Clinical Manifestations and Classification

Although there is no separate classification for ocular acid injuries, the Hughes–Roper-Hall classification is applicable. Evidence of intraocular injury and perilimbal ischemia are important prognostic factors. Corneal opacification is less important in acid injuries because epithelial and anterior stromal opacification may cover a clear underlying cornea. A delay of 1 to 2 days may be necessary in order to appropriately classify the injury. Pfister has also adapted the Hughes–Roper-Hall classification into a separate classification for acid injuries to the eye.[66] This classification is based on the extent of damage to the epithelium, extent of stromal edema, degree of conjunctival involvement, and degree of limbal ischemia. As with alkali injuries, clinical presentations

vary depending upon the severity of injury. Complications such as glaucoma, corneal neovascularization, stromal ulceration, conjunctival scarring, or inflammatory responses can occur (Figure 8.6). Unlike alkali injuries, certain compounds such as nitric or chromic acids can turn the corneal epithelium or conjunctiva yellow-brown.[2]

Treatment

Treatment of ocular acid injuries is similar to ocular alkali injuries. Immediate irrigation is critical with any nontoxic solution available until transfer to an appropriate medical center. Irrigation should never be performed with a base in an effort to neutralize the effects of the acid, since this may produce further thermal injury from an exothermic reaction.[66] Other treatment guidelines have been discussed under the subtitle of alkali injury treatment.

Thermal Injuries

Epidemiology

Most thermal injuries can be divided into two main categories: flame and contact burns.[76] Flame burns are secondary to fire and contact burns are from direct exposure to hot liquids or hot objects. In a large series involving 552 burn patients, 20% of the victims suffered from ocular burns. In this study, the leading cause of ocular burns was from house fires.[77] Another large series conducted over a three-year period at a burn center revealed that 47% of the patients had facial burns, 27% had burns involving the eyelids or eyes, and 11% required an ophthalmic consult. Of the 54 patients with eye injuries, 50 patients had lid burns and 17 patients had corneal involvement.[78] The low incidence of corneal involvement was probably due to the rapid blink reflex

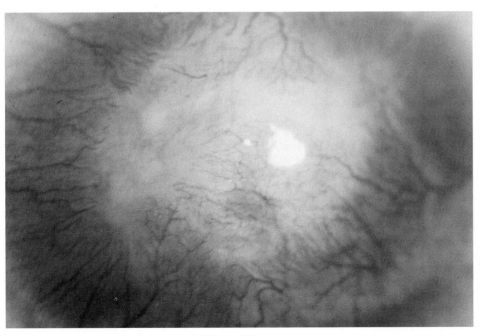

Figure 8.6. Previous acid injury with subsequent fibrovascular pannus secondary to chronic inflammation.

and Bell's phenomenon. The most common cause of ocular injury in this study was from gas explosions. Another large study of ocular thermal contact burns conducted in India revealed that splashes from boiling fluid were the most prominent causes of contact burns. An overwhelming majority of these cases (90%) occurred at home.[76] Another leading cause of contact thermal burns in the United States is from curling iron injuries, which occur almost exclusively to young women.[79]

Pathogenesis
Early work by Shahan demonstrated that cautery applied to rabbit corneas resulted in epithelial loss and stromal edema. If the insult was applied near the limbus, sectorial pannus would develop.[80] In a study by Goldblatt et al. defined heat doses were applied to rabbit corneas, and they determined that the cornea could tolerate a temperature of 45°C for up to fifteen minutes without any detectable damage grossly or histologically. Mild stromal edema was first noted grossly one day after injury was induced at a temperature of 45°C applied for 45 minutes. At one week follow-up, no tissue damage was noticed. A temperature of 52°C for 5 minutes induced stromal edema at one week follow-up. When this level of heat was applied for 45 minutes, nuclear degeneration of keratocytes and partial destruction of Bowman's membrane occurred by one week. Higher thermal doses produced a spectrum of damage, with complete destruction of keratocytes and endothelial cells at a temperature of 59°C for 45 minutes. This degree of thermal damage resulted in total necrosis of the cornea at one week.[81] However, Shahan demonstrated that deep corneal damage could occur at high temperatures for shorter periods of time. Coagulation necrosis of the deep stroma with corneal neovascularization was achieved with a temperature of 130°F for 10 minutes.[80]

Clinical Manifestations and Management
The severity of a thermal ocular injury depends on three factors: the temperature of the agent, the area over which the heat is applied, and the duration of contact.[79] Most thermal injuries to the ocular surface are superficial burns to the corneal epithelium or conjunctiva. Superficial burns tend to produce a gray to white elevated burn on the cornea, usually limited to the epithelium.[82] Any necrotic tissue should be gently debrided, and a cycloplegic drop such as homatropine should be administered. An antibiotic drop should also be given if there is a corneal abrasion, and pressure patching should be employed. Most superficial burns heal within 24 to 48 hours without sequelae. Treatment of deeper burns affecting the stroma should also include control of inflammation and neovascularization. Deeper tissue injuries induce a characteristic "ground glass" appearance and usually result in a stromal scar. The eschar eventually sloughs, leaving thin tissue that may be ectatic or staphylomatous.[82] Severe injuries may cause corneal necrosis and perforation. Appropriate surgical intervention, such as a lamellar keratoplasty, penetrating keratoplasty, or a limbal stem cell transplant procedure, may be necessary in these cases.

References

1. Pfister R, Pfister D. Alkali-Injuries of the eye. In: Krachmer M, Mannis M, Holland E, editors. *Cornea and External Disease: Clinical Diagnosis and Management.* St. Louis: Mosby-Year Book, 1997: 1443–1451.
2. Arffa R. Chemical injuries. In: *Grayson's diseases of the cornea.* St. Louis: Mosby-Year Book, 1991: 649–665.
3. Kuckelkorn R, Luft I, Kottek AA. Chemical and thermal eye burns in the residential area of RWTH Aachen. Analysis of accidents in 1 year using a new automated documentation of findings. *Klin Monatsbl Augenheilkd* 1993; 203:397–402.
4. Wagoner M. Chemical Injuries of the Eye: current concepts in pathophysiology and therapy. *Surv Ophthalmol* 1997; 41:276–313.
5. Morgan S. Chemical burns of the eye: causes and management. *Br J Ophthalmol* 1987; 71:854–857.
6. Pfister R. Collagenase activity of intact corneal epithelium in peripheral alkaline burns. *Arch Ophthalmol* 1971; 86: 308–310.
7. Grant W, Schuman J. *Toxicology of the Eye*, 4th ed. Springfield: Charles C. Thomas, 1993.
8. Harris L, Cohn K, Galin M. Alkali injury in fireworks. *Ann Ophthalmol* 1971; 3:849–851.
9. McCulley J. Chemical injuries. In: Smolin G and Thoft R, editors. *The Cornea: Scientific Foundation and Clinical Practice.* Boston, Little, Brown, and Co, 1987: 527–542.
10. Cejkova J. Alkali burns of the rabbit cornea. A histochemical study of glycosaminoglycans. *Histochemistry* 1975; 45:71–75.
11. Pfister R. Chemical injuries of the eye. *Ophthalmology* 1983; 90:1246–1253.
12. Nelson J, Wright J. Conjunctival goblet cell densities in ocular surface disease. *Arch Ophthalmol* 1984; 102:1049–1051.
13. Ohji M. Goblet cell density in thermal and chemical injuries. *Arch Ophthalmol* 1987; 105:1686–1688.
14. Paterson C, Pfister R, Levinson R. Aqueous humor pH changes after experimental alkali burns. *Am J Ophthalmol* 1975; 79:414–419.
15. Pfister R, Paterson C. Ascorbic acid in the treatment of alkali burns of the eye. *Ophthalmology* 1980; 87:1050–1057.
16. Levinson R, Paterson C, Pfister R. Ascorbic acid prevents corneal ulceration and perforation following experimental alkali burns. *Invest Ophthalmol* 1976; 15:986–988.
17. Fujisawa K, Katakami C, Yamamoto M. Keratocyte activity during wound healing of alkali-burned cornea. *Nippon ganka Gakkai Zasshi* 1991; 95:59–66.
18. Kao W, Ebert J, Kao C. Development of monoclonal antibodies recognizing collagenase from rabbit PMN: the presence of this enzyme in ulcerating corneas. *Curr Eye Res* 1986; 5:801–05.
19. Gordon J, Bauer E, Eisen A. Collagenase in the human cornea: immunologic localization. *Arch Ophthalmol* 1980; 98:341–45.

20. Berman M, Dohlman C, Davison F. Characterization of collagenolytic activity in the ulcerating cornea. *Exp Eye Res* 1971; 11:225–27.

21. Brown S, Weller C. The pathogenesis and treatment of collagenase-induced diseases of the cornea. *Trans Am Acad Ophthalmol Otolaryngol* 1970; 74:375–83.

22. Johnson-Wint B. Regulation of stromal cell collagenase production in adult rabbit cornea: in vitro stimulation and inhibition by epithelial cell products. *Proc Natl Acad Sci USA* 1980; 77:5531–5535.

23. Shapiro M, Friend J, Thoft R. Corneal re-epithelialization from the conjunctiva. *Invest Ophthalmol Vis Sci* 1981; 46:135–142.

24. Huang A, Tseng S. Corneal epithelial wound healing in the absence of limbal epithelium. *Invest Ophthalmol Vis Sci* 1991; 32:96–105.

25. Thoft R, Wiley L, Sundarraj N. The multipotential cells of the limbus. *Eye* 1989; 3:109–113.

26. Gartaganis S, Margaritis L, Koliopoulous J. The corneal epithelium basement membrane complexes after alkali burns: an ultrastructural study. *Ann Ophthalmol* 1987; 19: 263–268.

27. Burnett J, Smith L, Prauss J. Acute inflammatory cells and collagenase in tears of human melting corneas. *Invest Ophthalmol Vis Sci* 1990; 31:107–114.

28. Hughes W. Alkali burns of the eye. Review of the literature and summary of present knowledge. *Arch Ophthalmol* 1946; 35:423–428.

29. Roper-Hall M. Thermal and chemical burns. *Trans Ophthalmol Soc UK* 1965; 85:631–633.

30. Ralph R. Chemical Injuries of the eye. In: Tasman W, Jaeger E. *Duane's Clinical Ophthalmology*. Vol. 4. Philadelphia: Lippincott Williams & Wilkins, 1998: 1–23.

31. Grant W, Kern H. Action of alkalies on the corneal stroma. *Arch Ophthalmol* 1955; 54:931–933.

32. Pfister R. Identification and synthesis of chemotactic tripeptides from alkali-degraded whole cornea: A study of N-acetyl-Proline-Glycine-Proline and N-methyl-Proline-Glycine-Proline. *Invest Ophthalmol Vis Sci* 1995; 36:1306–1316.

33. Kim J, Kim J, Na B. Amniotic membrane patching promotes healing and inhibits proteinase activity on wound healing following acute corneal alkali burn. *Experiment Eye Res* 2000; 70:329–37.

34. Donshik P, Berman M, Dohlman C. Effect of topical corticosteroids on ulceration in alkali-burned corneas. *Arch Ophthalmol* 1978; 96:2117–2120.

35. Hersch P, Rice B, Baer J. Topical nonsteroidal agents and corneal wound healing. *Arch Ophthalmol* 1990; 68:577–583.

36. Newsome D, Gross J. Prevention by medroxyprogesterone of perforation of the alkali-burned rabbit cornea: inhibition of collagenolytic activity. *Invest Oophthalmol Vis Sci* 1988; 16:21–31.

37. Gross J, Azizkhan R, Biswas C. Inhibition of tumor growth, vascularization, and collagenolysis in the rabbit cornea by medroxyprogesterone. *Proc Natl Acad Sci USA* 1981; 78: 1176–1180.

38. Brion M, Lambs L, Berthon G. Metal ion-tetracycline interactions in biological fluids: Part 5. Formation of zinc complexes with tetracycline and some of its derivatives and assessment of their biological significance. *Agents Actions* 1985; 17:229–242.

39. Lauhio A, Sorsa T, Lindy O. The anticollagenolytic potential of lymecycline in the long-term treatment of reactive arthritis. *Arthritis Rheum* 1992; 35:195–198.

40. Pfister R, Paterson C, Spiers J. The efficacy of ascorbate treatment after severe experimental alkali-burns depends upon the route of administration. *Invest Ophthalmol Vis Sci* 1980; 19:1526–1529.

41. Pfister R, Paterson C. Additional clinical and morphological observations on the favorable effect of ascorbate in experimental ocular burns. *Invest Ophthalmol Vis Sci* 1977; 16:478–487.

42. Pfister R, Paterson C, Hayes S. Effects of topical 10% ascorbate solution on established corneal ulcers after severe alkali burns. *Invest Ophthalmol Vis Sci* 1982; 22:382–395.

43. Pfister R, Haddox J, Dodson R. Polymorphonuclear leukocyte inhibition by citrate, other heavy metal chelators, and trifluoperazine: evidence to support calcium binding protein involvement. *Invest Ophthalmol Vis Sci* 1984; 25:955–970.

44. Pfister R, Nicolaro M, Paterson C. Sodium citrate reduces the incidence of corneal ulcerations and perforations in extreme alkali-burned eyes—acetylcysteine and ascorbate have no favorable effect. *Invest Ophthalmol Vis Sci* 1980; 21:486–490.

45. Pfister R, Haddox J, Paterson C. The efficacy of sodium citrate in the treatment of severe alkali burns of the eye is influenced by the route of administration. *Cornea* 1982; 1:205–211.

46. Burns F, Gray R, Paterson C. Inhibition of alkali-induced corneal ulceration and perforation by a thiol peptide. *Invest Ophthalmol Vis Sci* 1990; 31:107–114.

47. Teping C, Reim M. Tenoplasty as a new surgical principle in the early treatment of the most severe chemical eye burns. *Klin Monatsbl Augenheilkd* 1989; 194:1–5.

48. Brodovsky S, McCarty C, Snibson G. Management of Alkali Burns. *Ophthalmol* 2000; 10:1829–1835.

49. Darlak K, Miller R, Stack M. Thiol-based inhibitors of mammalian collagenase. *J Biol Chem* 1990; 265:5199–5205.

50. Paterson C, Wells J, Koklitis P. Recombinant tissue inhibitor of metalloproteinase type-1 suppresses alkali-burn-induced corneal ulceration in rabbits. *Invest Ophthalmol Vis Sci* 1994; 35:677–684.

51. Reim M, Overkamping B, Kuckelkorn R. 2 years experience with Tenon-plasty. *Ophthalmologe* 1992; 89:524–30.

52. Kuckelkorn R, Wschrage N, Reim M. Treatment of severe eye burns by tenoplasty. *Lancet* 1995; 345:657–658.

53. Holland E, Schwartz G. The evolution of epithelial transplantation for severe ocular surface disease and a proposed classification system. *Cornea* 1996; 15:549–556.

54. Kenyon K, Tseng S. Limbal autograft transplantation for ocular surface disorders. *Ophthalmology* 1989; 96:709–722.

55. Gangadhar D, Kenyon K, Wagoner M. The surgical management of chemical ocular injuries: present and future strategies. *Inter Ophthalmol Clinics* 1995; 35:63–69.

56. Weise R, Mannis M, Vastine D. Conjunctival transplantation. Autologous and homologous grafts. *Arch Ophthalmol* 1985; 103:1736–1740.

57. Pfister R. Corneal stem cell disease: concepts, categorization, and treatment by auto- and homotransplantation of limbal stem cells. *CLAO J* 1994; 20:64–72.

58. Kim J, Tseng S. Transplantation of preserved human am-

niotic membrane for surface reconstruction in severely damaged rabbit corneas. *Cornea* 1995; 14:473–484.

59. Shimazaki J, Yang H, Kazuo T. Amniotic membrane transplantation for ocular surface reconstruction in patients with chemical and thermal burns. *Ophthalmol* 1997; 104: 2068–2076.

60. Tsai R, Li L, Chen J. Reconstruction of damaged corneas by transplantation of autologous limbal epithelial cells. *New Engl J Med* 2000; 343:86–93.

61. Schwab IR, Reyes M, Isseroff RR. Successful transplantation of bioengineered tissue replacements in patients with ocular surface disease. *Cornea* 2000; 19(4):421–426.

62. Kramer S. Late numerical grading of alkali burns to determine keratoplasty prognosis. *Trans Am Opthalmol Soc* 1983; 81:97–100.

63. Kuckelkorn R, Wenzel M, Lamprecht J. Autologous transplantation of nasal mucosa after severe chemical and thermal eye burns. *Klin Monatsbl Augenheilkd* 1994; 204:155–161.

64. Naumann G, Lang G, Rummelt V. Autologous nasal mucosa transplantation in severe bilateral conjunctival mucous deficiency syndrome. *Ophthalmology* 1990; 97:1011–1017.

65. Yaghouti F, Dohlman C. Innovations in keratoprosthesis: proved and unproved. *Int Ophthalmol Clin* 1999; 39:27–36.

66. Pfister D, Pfister R. Acid injuries of the eye. In: Krachmer J, Mannis M, Holland E, editors. *Cornea and External Disease: Diagnosis and Management*. St. Louis: Mosby-Year Book, 1997; 1437–1442.

67. Friedenwald J, Hughes W, Herman H. Acid injuries of the eye. *Arch Ophthalmol* 1946; 35:98–108.

68. Holekamp T, Becker B. Ocular injuries from automobile batteries. *Trans Am Acad Ophthalmol Otolaryngol* 1977; 83: 805–807.

69. Grayson M, Peroni D. Severe silver nitrate injury to the eye. *Am J Ophthalmol* 1970; 70:227–229.

70. Guidry M, Allen J, Kelly J. Some biochemical characteristics of acid injury of the cornea. *Am J Ophthalmol* 1955; 40: 111–119.

71. Friedenwald J, Hughes W, Herrmann H. Acid-base tolerance of the cornea. *Arch Ophthalmol* 1944; 31:279–283.

72. Schultz G, Henkind P, Gross E. Acid injuries of the eye. *Am J Ophthalmol* 1968; 66:654–657.

73. Chinag T, Moorman L, Thomas R. Ocular hypertensive response following acid and alkali burns in rabbits. *Invest Ophthalmol* 1971; 10:270–273.

74. Paterson C, Eakins K, Paterson R. The ocular hypertensive response following experimental acid burns in the rabbit eye. *Invest Ophthalmol Vis Sci* 1979; 18:67–74.

75. Friedenwald J. Discussion. *Am J Ophthalmol* 1955; 40:119–120.

76. Vajpayee R, Gupta N, Angra S. Contact thermal burns of the cornea. *Can J Ophthalmol* 1991; 26:215–218.

77. Linhart R. Burns of the eyes and eyelids. *Ann Ophthalmol* 1978; 10:999–1001.

78. Guy R, Baldwin J, Kwedar S. Three years' experience in a regional burn center with burns of the eyes and eyelids. *Ophthal Surg* 1982; 13:383–386.

79. Mannis M, Miller R, Krachmer J. Contact thermal burns of the cornea from electric curling irons. *Am J Ophthalmol* 1984; 98:336–339.

80. Shahan W, Lamb H. Histologic effect of heat on the eye. *Am J Ophthalmol* 1916; 33:225–227.

81. Goldblatt W, Finger P, Perry H. Hyperthermic treatment of rabbit corneas. *Invest Ophthalmol Vis Sci* 1989; 30: 1778–1783.

82. Hamill B. Corneal Injury. In: Krachmer J, Mannis M, Holland E, editors. *Cornea and External Disease: Diagnosis and Management*. St. Louis: Mosby-Year Book, 1997; 1403–1422.

9

Autoimmune Diseases Affecting the Ocular Surface

Joseph Tauber

Introduction

Autoimmune diseases are extremely diverse in origin, pathogenesis and clinical ocular manifestations. As a group, these diseases are the ones that clinicians think of as the most destructive to the ocular surface. No matter whether the pathologic mechanism is neutrophil-mediated, immune-complex-mediated, or T-cell-mediated, the end result is scarring or destruction of ocular tissues and interference with the physiologic processes necessary to maintaining ocular surface homeostasis. Understanding the management of patients with this group of diseases requires a comprehensive understanding of how all of the components of the ocular surface work together. The clinician responsible for caring for patients who suffer from these diseases must simultaneously manage eyelid and meibomian gland disease, conjunctival and episcleral inflammatory disease, tear film disorders and keratitis, which may be exposure-related, infectious, inflammatory, toxic, or combinations of all these categories. While the details of treating autoimmune diseases vary with each specific disease entity, it is critical that the treating clinician remain constantly aware of the interactions between all of the components of the ocular surface and direct appropriate treatment toward each abnormality simultaneously. Just as it is impossible to provide comfort to the dry eye patient with blepharitis by using ocular lubricants alone, the severe pathologies involved in autoimmune diseases require a multi-armed therapeutic approach. This chapter will discuss the ocular aspects of three different conditions as examples of the category of autoimmune disease.

Cicatricial Pemphigoid

Cicatricial pemphigoid is an autoimmune, cicatrizing disease of mucosal epithelium and, less often, skin. Cicatricial pemphigoid (CP) was first defined as a disease entity separate from pemphigus by Thost in 1911.[1] It has been termed "chronic pemphigus," "essential shrinkage of the conjunctiva," "ocular pemphigoid" and has been widely described as "benign mucous membrane pemphigoid" in dermatologic literature.[2–7] Since this disease is often anything but benign with regard to its ophthalmic consequences, the term cicatricial pemphigoid is suggested as the preferred terminology and will be used herein.

Presentation

Patients with CP may first present to their ophthalmologist, dermatologist, dentist, gastroenterologist, otolaryngologist or primary care physician (Table 9.1). To the ophthalmologist, the usual presentation is chronic conjunctivitis with an insidious onset.[3,8,9] The course of the disease is usually slow but may be punctuated by periods of explosive inflammatory activity.[10] Ten to thirty years or more may be required for the disease to run its full course, with bilateral blindness as the result. Unilateral presentation is not rare, but eventually most patients develop bilateral ocular involvement[11]; slowly progressive subconjunctival cicatrization is the hallmark of this disease. Sixty-five to ninety percent of CP patients have ocular involvement,[2,3,7,12,13] while approximately 25% have lesions on non-mucosal skin.[3,8,9,14] Oral disease occurs in 70–90% of CP patients, and the mouth may be the sole site of involvement. Desquamative gingivitis is the most common oral manifestation, although non-healing ulcers of buccal mucosa are not rare.[8,14,15] Commonly, bullae develop after local trauma during chewing, and last several days. Once the bullae rupture, nonhealing erosions may last for weeks. Involvement of nasal, pharyngeal, laryngeal, esophageal, urethral, vaginal or anal mucosal surfaces may manifest as chronic ulcerations or strictures.[3,7,9,12,16–18] The average age of onset of CP is reported to be 65 years, but this does not take into account the observation that most cases of CP are relatively advanced at the time of diagnosis.[3,9,19]

Table 9.1. Distribution of tissue involvement in cicatricial pemphigoid.

Reference	# of cases	Skin	Mouth	Eye	Larynx	Nose	Genitalia	Esophagus
Hardy 1971 (10)	81	23%	84%	77%	30%	38%	30%	7%
Person 1977 (35)	65	34%	89%	52%	11%	28%	23%	5%
Mondino 1981 (11)	78	21%	50%	100%	—	—	—	—
Foster 1986 (5)	130	9%	15%	100%	4%	12%	7%	9%
Hanson 1988 (83)	142	21%	88%	61%	9%	23%	—	4%
Total	496	22%	65%	78%	14%	25%	20%	6%

Many childhood cases of CP have been reported, as early as 5 years.[3,20,21]

Incidence and Prevalence

Published reports of the incidence of CP have varied between 1 : 12,000 to 1 : 20,000 in the general population and 1 : 20,000 to 1 : 46,000 in ophthalmic practices[3,8,22]; however, significant underreporting is likely, since early stages of disease are often missed, several different subspecialties may be involved and many elderly patients do not report their symptoms at all.

Ophthalmic Clinical Features

Early ocular symptoms in patients with CP include burning or foreign-body sensation, excess tearing and mucous production. Early ocular findings include conjunctival injection or suffusion, vascular dilatation, mucous threads in the inferior fornix and patchy conjunctival epitheliopathy and conjunctival thickening.[3,9] Subconjunctival fibrosis, very subtle and difficult to detect, may be visible as fine, fibrillar white lines beneath the palpebral or tarsal conjunctiva.[3,8,9] The cicatrizing process results in progressive subconjunctival fibrosis and fornix foreshortening (inferior > superior). Later,

fibrous bands, or symblepharon, form between the lid and globe, best visualized by everting the lower lid with the patient gazing upward. Sequelae of the primary cicatrizing process include squamous metaplasia with keratinization of the ocular surface, eyelid deformation with resultant entropion or ectropion, trichiasis, distichiasis, meibomian gland obstruction, lacrimal duct destruction, corneal epitheliopathy, scarring and neovascularization. Secondary microbial keratitis and blepharitis are common.[23] Progressive corneal opacification, due to all of the above processes, results in eventual loss of useful vision. Corneal perforation may result in complete loss of the eye.

Several grading systems have been used for describing patients with CP.[3,8,24] Many centers now use the more sensitive modified-Foster system (see Figure 9.1).[25] Subepithelial fibrosis without foreshortening of the fornix characterizes stage I, while the development of fornix foreshortening defines stage II. The extent of foreshortening is graded either A (0–25%), B (25–50%), C (50–75%), or D (>75%). The presence of symblepharon characterizes stage III, with the extent of horizontal involvement graded as above, between A and D. Stage IV, end stage disease, is characterized by ankyloblepharon and ocular surface keratinization. Thus, a patient with

Figure 9.1. A. Stage I cicatricial pemphigoid of the conjunctiva. Note the tarsal subepithelial white stria and formation of a "feltwork" of subepithelial fibrosis.

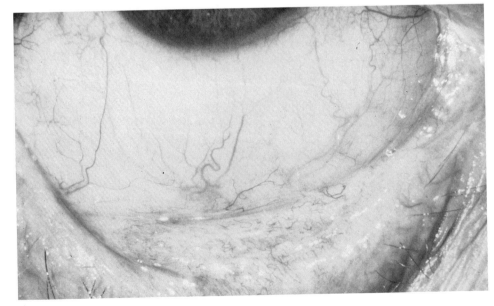

A

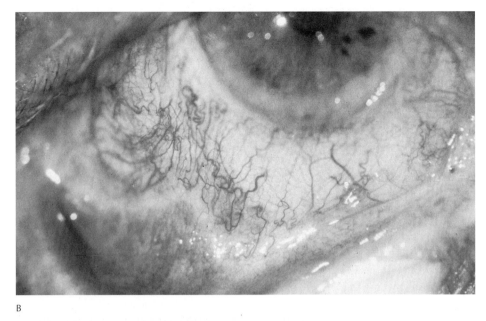

B

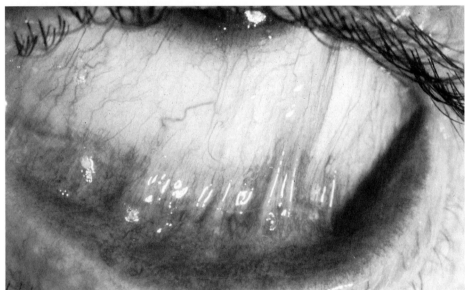

C

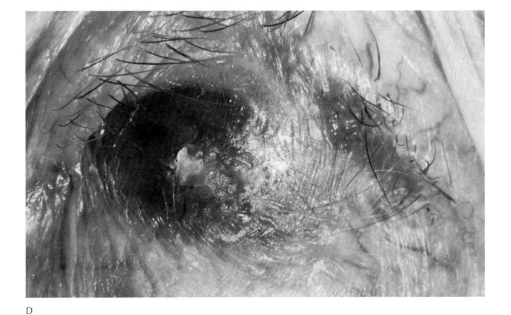

D

Figure 9.1. (*Continued*) B. Stage II cicatricial pemphigoid of the conjunctiva. In addition to white fibrotic stria, note the loss of deep fornix and the blunting of the angle of reflection of the fornix conjunctiva onto the globe (fornix foreshortening). C. Stage III cicatricial pemphigoid of the conjunctiva. In addition to subepithelial stria and fornix foreshortening, there is formation of symblephara, especially temporally, best demonstrated with the lower lid retracted and the patient gazing upward. D. Stage IV cicatricial pemphigoid affecting the eyes. Ankyloblepharon has developed. Complete keratinization of the ocular surface epithelium is apparent.

30% fornix foreshortening and a single thin symblepharon would be graded IIBIIIA. It is important to grade both the fornix and symblepharon carefully at each evaluation because progressive cicatrization is as likely to manifest as increased fornix foreshortening as the development of new symblepharon, or as an increase in the horizontal extent of symblepharon.[25] Progression in subconjunctival cicatrization does not occur in all CP patients, but the likelihood of progression increases with disease stage.[8] As many as 75% of patients who have stage III CP can be expected to have progressive disease without treatment within 2 years. However, such estimates may be skewed by the limited number of patients followed with stage I or stage II disease.[3,8,25–32]

Subconjunctival cicatrization is not the only process threatening the eyes of the CP patient; complications of the primary disease process are themselves serious problems. Secondary keratitis sicca is common and extremely difficult to manage due to the multifactorial compromise of all three layers of the tear film by scarring and obstruction of lacrimal ductules and meibomian ductules and loss of conjunctival goblet cells.[3,9,33,34] Entropion and trichiasis are the common sequelae of scarring beneath palpebral conjunctiva and commonly become chronic, unremitting sources of ocular morbidity. Surgical correction of the eyelid often induces progressive scarring.[8] Trichiasis is difficult to eradicate, often necessitating multiple treatments by lid cryotherapy, diathermy, or electrolysis and repeated epilations. Glaucoma has been reported to be present in up to 26% of patients with CP, and it is very difficult to accurately evaluate or control.[35]

Diagnosis

Histologic findings are not, by themselves, diagnostic for CP. Similar findings occur in bullous pemphigoid (BP), herpes gestations, linear IgA disease, dermatitis herpetiformis, lupus erythematosus, epidermolysis bullosa aquisita, erythema multiforme and hereditary epidermolysis bullosa.[36,37] Nonetheless, in most cases, an accurate diagnosis is possible when the clinical presentation and histologic and immunologic findings are brought together.

Histologic findings in CP vary, depending on the biopsied tissue and the timing of biopsy relative to disease duration. In early disease, skin biopsy specimens may demonstrate vacuolization beneath basal epithelial cells with minimal inflammatory cell infiltration, while later in the disease course subepidermal bullae formation without acantholysis is often seen.[38–40] While intact bullae are extremely rare in biopsies from mucosal or conjunctival lesions,[3] biopsies from oral lesions may demonstrate separation of epithelium from underlying connective tissue at the level of the basement membrane. Conjunctival biopsies often show submucosal scarring

and fibrosis. Other typical findings on light microscopy in CP include a marked chronic inflammatory infiltrate with prominent plasma cell and mast cell involvement, perivasculitis and squamous metaplasia of the epithelium with loss or absence of goblet cells.[3,33,34,41,42] In earlier stages of disease, and in ocular specimens from acutely inflamed conjunctiva, a variable neutrophil infiltrate may be seen.[10] Immunopathologic studies in CP biopsy specimens have further described the types of inflammatory cells found in involved tissues. Increases in T helper/T suppressor cell ratio, Langerhans cells, macrophages and mast cells have been demonstrated[43–46] and, while B lymphocytes are rarely seen, more mature plasma cells are plentiful.

Direct immunofluorescence microscopy of biopsied tissue demonstrates linear deposition of immunoglobulins and/or complement components at the basement membrane zone, the *sine qua non* for the diagnosis of CP. The sensitivity of this technique has been reported as between 80 and 100%.[3,47–51] Deposited immunoreactants are most often C3 and IgG, with up to 25% being IgA, 20% IgM, and less often, IgD and other complement components.[3,48–51] Linear immunoreactant deposition may be seen in other diseases,[36,37] and thus by itself is not pathognomonic of CP. It is critical for the managing physician to work with a laboratory experienced in immunofluorescence microscopy, and also necessary for the opthalmologist to work with a laboratory expert in the handling of tiny conjunctival specimens for an accurate diagnosis of CP. In cases of high clinical suspicion, it may be necessary to process tissue using the far more sensitive, but labor intensive, avidin-biotin immunoperoxidase staining technique, as 10–15% of CP specimens only demonstrate immunoreactant deposition with this method.[3]

A negative biopsy does not rule out the diagnosis of CP. In some cases, the diagnosis is made on the clinical findings and course of disease despite a negative biopsy.

Management

The management of CP is difficult because of the broad spectrum of disease involvement that different practitioners face. Treatment must be individualized according to the location of lesions, the course of progression, patient age, underlying medical problems, and response to medications. Disease limited to the upper aerodigestive tract is often controllable with topical corticosteroid ointments or sprays and intralesional injections of corticosteroids.[16–18] Severe cutaneous disease is most often treated with dapsone, a sulfone derivative used primarily to treat leprosy and dermatitis herpetiformis. It was an evolution of clinical success using dapsone and other sulfonamides for the treatment of pemphigus, BP, and dermatitis herpetiformis that led dermatologists to the first trials in CP patients.[52,53] Dapsone is now widely considered to be the first drug in a stepladder approach to treating CP unresponsive to initial treatment with corticosteroids, provided the patient is not glucose-6-phosphate dehydrogenase deficient, or allergic to sulfa.[3,26-29] Success rates as high as 83% have been reported for cutaneous and oral disease.[27,31,54] The mechanism of action of dapsone remains poorly understood, though it is known to interfere with the peroxide system of neutrophil cytotoxicity.[3,52,53] Side effects are not uncommon, including hemolytic anemia in as many as 95% of patients in some series.[3]

Gingivitis and oral ulcerations are often controllable with topical corticosteroid ointments or sprays,[16-18] and some anecdotal success has been reported in treating oral lesions with swishes of cyclosporin solution.[55] Esophageal or laryngeal involvement may be severe and become life-threatening as a result of stricture formation and asphyxiation or aspiration[3,16-18]; surgery may be required for the management of strictures, webs or large scars.[18]

Management of ocular involvement in CP is complex, requiring the managing ophthalmologist to consider separately treatment for the underlying disease process and the management of its sequelae. Differentiating these is difficult, but is of critical importance in achieving control of ocular inflammation and minimizing scarring while avoiding iatrogenic complications.

It cannot be overemphasized that one must methodically eliminate all external aggravants in CP patients with ocular inflammation. Aggressive treatment of keratitis sicca is imperative and often requires frequent application of preservative-free ophthalmic eyedrops and ointments. If it has not occurred as a result of lid scarring, punctal closure is valuable, as are eyeglass side shields and moisture chambers. Compulsive management of eyelid disease is also critical, including frequent and vigorous lid hygiene for blepharitis and systemic tetracycline or doxycycline for meibomianitis. Nightly application of antibiotic ointment is commonly required, as the incidence of bacterial superinfection of the lids is high.[23] Keratinization of the eyelid margin, or of the conjunctival surface, may also produce reactive conjunctival inflammation. In selected patients, specially prepared topical all-trans vitamin A ointment or eyedrops may be effective for this vexing problem.[56]

Trichiasis is an extremely common cause of sight-threatening corneal epithelial defects, scarring and secondary bacterial keratitis. Treatment approaches have included cryotherapy, electrocautery (hyfrecation), diathermy, laser destruction of follicles, surgical excision and repeated epilation of the aberrant lashes, but no one method is entirely successful. Cryotherapy is the most widely used treatment, though repeated treatments are often necessary to completely eliminate conjunctival and corneal trauma from cilia as an etiology for persistent conjunctival inflammation.

Treatment of entropion is difficult, as surgery may accelerate conjunctival shrinkage.[10] Eyelid rotation procedures may be effective early in the course of disease. Once inflammation is controlled, mucous membrane grafting of the inferior cul-de-sac may be effective, but the technical difficulties of this procedure, together with a high complication rate, limits its widespread use.[57] While not clearly a sequela of CP, glaucoma is a serious problem occurring in up to 26% of patients with CP.[35] All aspects of glaucoma management in the patient with CP are difficult. Diagnosis is hampered by the limited accuracy of tonometry due to corneal scarring, by difficulties in adequate examination of the optic nerve head, and by the frequent inability to obtain an accurate visual field assessment in these patients. Treatment options are limited by the potentially causative role of commonly used antiglaucomatous drugs in pseudopemphigoid[3,58-65] and by the impossibility of filtration surgery in eyes with inflamed, scarred conjunctiva.

Once the treating physician is certain that external aggravants are not responsible for the presence of conjunctival inflammation, treatment must address the primary disease process. Decades of unfortunate patient outcomes have made it clear that topical anti-inflammatory treatments are ineffective in halting progressive conjunctival scarring. Systemic corticosteroids, such as prednisone, are extremely valuable in the treatment of acute inflammation in CP, but long-term administration carries unacceptable risk of serious side effects.[3,10] Many studies, including several randomized, controlled clinical trials have unequivocally demonstrated that systemic immunosuppressive chemotherapy is capable of halting the progression of conjunctival scarring in CP and in eliminating disease-driven conjunctival inflammation.[3,7,27,30,32,66,67] It is important to remember that not all cases of ocular CP are progressive, and therefore, not all patients with CP require systemic therapy. It is of the utmost importance to limit the institution of systemic chemotherapy to those CP patients with immunologically driven inflammation. It is impossible to eliminate conjunctival inflammation due to sicca, trichiasis or meibomitis with systemic chemotherapy, but it is possible to produce life-threatening pancytopenia, or a fatal infectious complication, by injudicious treatment. While there are some ophthalmologists with specific training in ocular immunologic disease, including chemotherapeutic management, most ophthalmologists will benefit from working together with an oncologist or rheumatologist experienced in the use of cytotoxic agents. Long-term follow-up of patients treated with systemic chemotherapy has shown success rates as high as 94% in preventing progression of conjunctival scarring.[26,27]

Over time, a stepwise approach to immunosuppression for CP has evolved. Mildly active disease is treated first with dapsone (provided the patient is not glucose-

6-phosphate-dehydrogenase-deficient, or allergic to sulfa), which is effective in up to 70% of patients as a single drug treatment.[27] Azathioprine may be effective in cases of dapsone intolerance or side effect, but only a small group of patients will experience disease remission with this drug.[27,30] Methotrexate, 7.5–25 mg once a week, can sometimes control CP inflammation. For resistant cases, and for patients who have extreme conjunctival inflammation at initial presentation, cyclophosphamide is the drug of choice. Commonly, treatment is initiated at 2.0 mg/kg/day together with prednisone at 1 mg/kg/day. Prednisone is tapered over 6 weeks as the chemotherapeutic agent reaches an effective therapeutic level. Treatment is usually continued for a year after elimination of conjunctival inflammation. Relapse may occur in up to 27% of patients following discontinuation of chemotherapy and may occur as long as 17 months following treatment.[26,28] Lifetime follow-up is mandatory in this frequently relentless disease.

There may be a role for local subconjunctival or intrasymblepharon injections of mitomycin-C in selected patients with CP.[68,69] This local therapy may be highly effective in reducing inflammation and slowing subconjunctival cicatrization. This local therapy may be used for selective patients at higher risk for complications with systemic immunosuppressive therapies, or as adjunct treatment for patients on maximum systemic therapy who are still inflamed.

Ocular surgery in patients with cicatricial pemphigoid should be considered only in limited situations. Cataract surgery may be safely performed in patients who have had all conjunctival inflammation thoroughly eliminated, usually requiring systemic chemotherapy for not less than several months.[70] Corneal grafting should be reserved for relatively desperate scenarios, such as impending or actual perforation or bilateral blindness. Although tectonic stabilization may be achieved, in one study, clear grafts were maintained in only 50% of patients, and only 18% of patients achieved vision greater than 20/200.[71] Unless the local ocular environment is successfully rehabilitated, with abolition of keratinization and trichiasis, replacement of adequate lubrication, and restoration of epithelial integrity, corneal transplantation is highly likely to result in chronic nonhealing epithelial defects, stromal melting and perforation.[71,72] Amniotic membrane grafting may have a role in establishing a healthy substrate for ocular surface epithelium and also as a protective "blanket," beneath which healing of the epithelium can occur. Studies in recent years have demonstrated that limbal stem cell deficiency from CP or other causes manifests as corneal epithelial conjunctivalization, vascularization and chronic inflammation.[73] Stem cell transplantation may be necessary and effective in allowing restoration of a healthy epithelial surface in such eyes.[74]

Correction of eyelid abnormalities may be successfully performed once conjunctival inflammation has been abolished.[57] Keratoprosthesis may be effective in providing limited vision to patients with extreme degrees of corneal scarring.[74] Overall, cicatricial pemphigoid is among the most difficult conditions ophthalmologists treat. Optimal care requires differentiation between many possible causes of ocular inflammation, making difficult treatment decisions and maintaining adequate control of the diverse complications of this chronic and frequently blinding disease.

Stevens–Johnson Syndrome

Stevens–Johnson syndrome (SJS), also known as erythema multiforme major, is an immune-mediated, acute blistering disease affecting skin and mucous membranes. First described by Hebra in 1866, it was the 1922 report by Stevens and Johnson that led to the widespread recognition of this disorder. Excellent reviews of this disease have been published, detailing the differences of erythema multiforme minor and major from related diseases such as toxic epidermal necrolysis and staphylococcal scalded skin syndrome (SSSS).[75]

Incidence

SJS is an uncommon disease. Studies from Italy and France have reported incidence figures ranging from 0.6 to 1.3 per million per year, while a Swedish study reported an incidence of 5 cases per million per year. Peak incidence appears to be during the second and third decades of life, with males affected three times as often as females.[75]

Clinical Presentation

While erythema multiforme minor may last from 1 to 4 weeks and erythema multiforme major may last up to 6 weeks, the acute phase of ocular disease generally lasts only 2 to 3 weeks.[76] Most patients hospitalized with SJS develop ocular involvement. The acute stage of SJS may involve the entire ocular surface, including the eyelids, conjunctiva and cornea (see Figure 9.2). Eyelids are typically edematous and erythematous, with crusting and ulceration of the lid margin and tarsal conjunctiva. Bilateral purulent or pseudomembranous conjunctivitis occurs in 15–80% of patients.[77–79] Secondary infectious conjunctivitis is common. Conjunctival vesicles have only rarely been reported.[79,80] The acute inflammation in SJS may produce rapid symblepharon formation. Keratitis of some kind occurs in most patients, and may be toxic or infectious in nature. Bacterial keratitis may progress to corneal perforation and, more rarely, endophthalmitis.[81,82] Acute uveitis is uncommon, but has

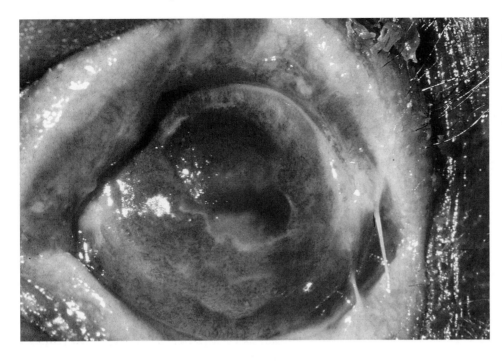

Figure 9.2. Stevens–Johnson syndrome, 3 weeks following onset. Abnormal findings include severe eyelid inflammation with lid margin keratinization, marked conjunctival inflammation, corneal epithelial disruption, and pannus formation.

been reported. In its chronic stage, many of the ocular features reported in patients with SJS are the same as those seen in patients with CP.[76,82,83] Eyelid involvement may include cicatricial entropion or ectropion, recurrent trichiasis, and meibomian gland dysfunction. Conjunctival cicatrization with shortening of the inferior fornix, symblepharon and subconjunctival scarring may be indistinguishable from that seen in CP, though it is generally not as advanced. Dry eye disease secondary to goblet cell destruction, meibomian gland dysfunction and lacrimal gland ductule scarring may be ex-

tremely difficult to manage.[34,83] Corneal involvement is much more severe later in the course of SJS, and may include chronic epitheliopathy, nonhealing epithelial defects, fibrovascular pannus formation, subepithelial scarring and stromal neovascularization, scarring or thinning (see Figure 9.3). Many of the corneal manifestations in chronic SJS are secondary to abnormal eyelid anatomy and/or lid margin keratinization and severe dry eye disease. In a small subset of patients, recurrent episodes of immunologically driven inflammation may occur.[84]

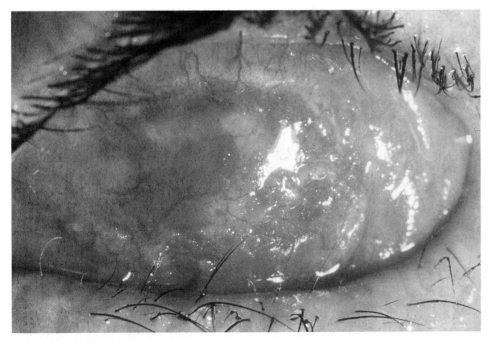

Figure 9.3. Stevens–Johnson syndrome, chronic stage. Findings include trichiasis, distichiasis, secondary conjunctival inflammation produced by misdirected lashes, vascularized corneal scarring and a near-absent tear film.

Diagnosis—Clinical Criteria

Differential diagnosis of acute SJS is usually not difficult. Thorough history taking generally reveals the characteristic sudden onset with classic skin lesions. It is critical to differentiate SJS from staphylococcal scalded skin syndrome, which requires proper antibiotic therapy to arrest release of the staphylococcal exotoxins responsible for the cutaneous disease. While it can be difficult or impossible to ascribe a precise cause to the onset of SJS, a number of etiologic factors have been implicated as triggers of the disease.[85–87] These include the administration of certain systemic medications (especially sulfonamides and phenytoin) and immunologic processes following certain infections (especially Herpes simplex or mycoplasma pneumonia). Topical ocular administration of scopolamine, sulfonamide, or tropicamide has been associated with SJS.[88,89]

The differential diagnosis of chronic SJS includes those diseases that produce cicatricial scarring of the eyelid and conjunctiva, including CP, atopic keratoconjunctivitis, ocular rosacea, linear IgA disease, chemical burns, radiation exposure, avitaminosis A, and trachoma. Careful history taking generally establishes the diagnosis, though biopsy is needed in some cases.

Management

The clinician managing a patient with SJS must simultaneously optimize treatment of all involved tissues. Organizing the approach to treatment into some general guiding principles can be helpful in avoiding complications. These include: (1) good hygiene is important; (2) do no harm; (3) prevention is easier than treatment; (4) timing is everything.

Good hygiene of the ocular surface is imperative, including frequent lid soaks to remove adherent discharge, mucous and crusts. Likewise, frequent conjunctival irrigation is helpful to wash away mucoid discharge, which tends to accumulate in the fornices. Inadequate attention to lid hygiene will result in significant keratitis. Another critical treatment principle in these patients is the seemingly simple aphorism "do no harm." Keratitis medicamentosa secondary to unnecessary or inappropriately dosed topical medications with toxicity to corneal epithelium must be avoided. This may occur with topical nonsteroidal anti-inflammatory agents, beta blockers, aminoglycoside antibiotics, antiviral agents, preserved artificial lubricants, or cycloplegics. A minimalist approach to the use of topical medications will avoid unnecessary complications.

Prevention of the complications of the inflammatory process in SJS is far more efficiently accomplished than treatment of these complications. Prophylactic topical antibiotics, optimal dry eye management with nonpreserved artificial tears and punctal occlusion, and prompt treatment of intraocular inflammation should be considered. Early correction of abnormal eyelid anatomy is important. Trichiasis may be managed by epilation, electrolysis, diathermy, or cryotherapy. Lid margin keratinization is often responsive to topical all-transretinoic acid.[56,90] Often, aggressive lubrication regimens are needed to prevent breakdown of the corneal epithelium, including administration of topical growth factors, use of serum tears and moisture chambers, and control of ocular surface inflammation with topical steroids, tetracycline or cyclosporine. Once corneal epithelial defects have developed, efforts must be directed to preventing stromal loss, including administration of systemic and topical and systemic anticollagenolytics. Judicious use of topical corticosteroids may be necessary but must be carefully followed due to the risk of accelerated stromal lysis. Tectonic grafting with amniotic membrane, lamellar corneal or scleral tissue may be required once significant stromal lysis has developed.

Efforts may be necessary to maintain normal ocular anatomy and limit cicatrization, including lysis of early symblepharon and use of the sutured symblepharon ring. On occasion, Saran wrap sutured to ocular[91,92] or amniotic membrane grafting may be valuable in the acute stage of SJS. The timing of surgical intervention in patients with SJS is important in achieving good outcomes. Keratoplasty should only be considered in selected settings. Often, the treating clinician has no choice, as in impending or actual corneal perforation. The success of surgical intervention is less related to the control of the underlying inflammatory processes than to the degree of tissue destruction during the acute phase of SJS.[75] The most common postoperative complication is recurrent, nonhealing corneal epithelial defect, which often requires regrafting.[71,72,93] Graft rejection is less likely to cause graft failure than ocular surface failure.[71]

The recent increased interest in amniotic membrane grafting and stem cell transplantation has helped improve outcomes in patients with SJS. Stem cell grafts may be necessary to facilitate healing of chronic epithelial defects or to achieve a smooth corneal surface, which allows for useful vision. The importance of timing this surgery properly cannot be overstated. In the setting of active inflammation, inadequate lubrication, active blepharitis and trichiasis, delicate stem cell grafts cannot survive. Amniotic membrane grafting may have a role in both the acute and chronic stages of SJS.[94–100] The anti-inflammatory qualities of amniotic membrane provide reduction of inflammation in acute SJS while simultaneously providing a better substrate for subsequent stem cell grafting. Superior results appear to be achieved by performing these two procedures separately, rather than simultaneously.[94–96] In chronic SJS, amniotic membrane transplantation and stem cell transplantation are often necessary procedures to optimize the ocular surface before contemplating keratoplasty. In some cases, keratoplasty will not be necessary after restoration of a noninflamed, smooth epithelial surface.[94]

Rheumatoid Arthritis

Rheumatoid arthritis (RA) is a systemic autoimmune disease far more commonly encountered than CP or SJS. Reported to affect from 1–2% of the world's population with an incidence of 1 per thousand persons per year,[101,102] RA has no racial predilection, affects women three times as often as men and increases in prevalence with increasing age.[103] Extra-articular manifestations are commonly observed with RA, including vasculitis, subcutaneous nodules, pulmonary, neurologic and ocular involvement. Ocular manifestations may include keratitis sicca, scleral inflammation, corneal ulcerations and, more rarely, retinal vasculitis.[104]

Keratoconjunctivitis sicca (KCS) is the most common ocular manifestation of RA. Symptoms are indistinguishable from other types of chronic dry eye disease, including complaints of scratchiness, grittiness, foreign-body sensation, burning, stinging, mucous accumulation, photophobia, itching and numerous functional limitations. Since many autoimmune disorders occur simultaneously, some RA patients have coexistent Sjögren's syndrome and extremely severe dry eye disease. Punctate corneal epitheliopathy is the most common finding, easily visualized with vital dyes such as fluorescein sodium, lissamine green or rose bengal. Other findings suggestive of KCS include diminished tear meniscus height, conjunctival staining, decreased Schirmer test scores and rapid tear breakup time. Extensive recent research into the pathophysiology of KCS has given a better under-

standing of the role of ocular surface inflammation in producing lacrimal gland dysfunction.[105,106] Management of KCS is the same as in non-RA patients, including tear film replacement and tear film conservation strategies. Aggressive tear film supplementation with nonpreserved drops, gels or ointments together with punctal occlusion using cautery or silicone plugs is needed in most patients. Severe cases may require newer approaches to control ocular surface inflammation, such as tetracycline, judicious topical steroids or cyclosporin.[107–110]

Scleral involvement in RA may vary greatly among patients. Manifestations may include focal, diffuse or nodular episcleritis or scleritis (see Figure 9.4). Less commonly seen are forms of necrotizing scleritis, either without (scleromalacia perforans) or with associated inflammation (see Figure 9.5). Therapeutic approaches for scleral involvement include systemic nonsteroidal drugs, steroids and immunosuppressive drugs. Methotrexate has increased in popularity as a first choice for immunosuppression in these patients because of its anti-inflammatory properties. Treatment options for scleritis have been extensively reviewed elsewhere[111,112] and are beyond the scope of this chapter.

Corneal involvement in RA tends to involve patients with advanced systemic disease, often with vasculitis.[104] Corneal involvement may occur with or without coexistent scleral inflammation, and may be inflammatory or noninflammatory. Sclerosing keratitis is the most common corneal abnormality reported to occur in association with scleritis.[112] This grayish, crystalline thickening and opacification of stroma generally progresses centrally, before neovascularization and lipid exudation are seen. Acute stromal keratitis is a more rare finding that may progress to significant ulceration.[104]

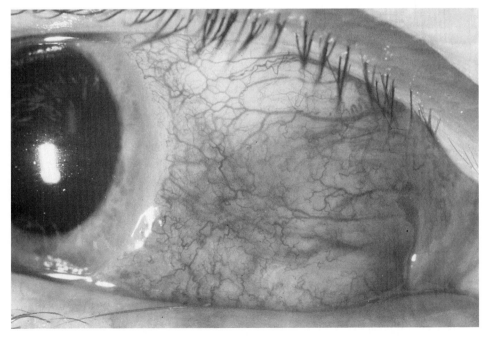

Figure 9.4. Episcleritis in a patient with rheumatoid arthritis. The dilated episcleral blood vessels demonstrate the typical fine tortuosity.

Figure 9.5. Necrotizing scleritis in a patient with rheumatoid arthritis. Diffuse inflammation with large, dilated scleral vessels is apparent. Inferiorly, an area of whitening corresponds to scleral necrosis. Though the white area appears limited to the inferior bulbar region, the process of necrosis extends well beyond, beneath the inflamed superficial scleral tissue.

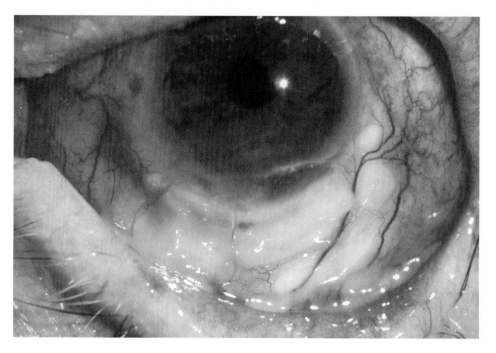

Central or paracentral ulceration is generally related to severe KCS, which may not be symptomatic prior to detection of corneal ulceration.[112–114] As in other forms of KCS, severe disease may produce remarkably rapid stromal lysis, with descemetocele formation or perforation. These types of corneal ulcers generally respond well to aggressive treatment of KCS, though nonresponsive ulcers may benefit from topical cyclosporin eyedrops.[114]

Peripheral corneal stromal thinning may occur with or without associated inflammation. Noninflammatory

limbal guttering or furrows are a well-described complication of RA.[115–119] Usually located inferiorly, furrows may become quite large circumferentially and deep, eventually developing vascularization or lipid deposition. Typically, the epithelium remains intact over the area of stromal loss (see Figure 9.6).[104] Vision may be greatly compromised by irregular astigmatism, but perforation rarely occurs in the absence of trauma.

In contrast, peripheral ulcerative keratitis (PUK) is a necrotizing process that may be rapidly destructive. Stromal loss may occur within hours or days, with active

Figure 9.6. Marginal furrow in a patient with rheumatoid arthritis. Note the absence of significant inflammation.

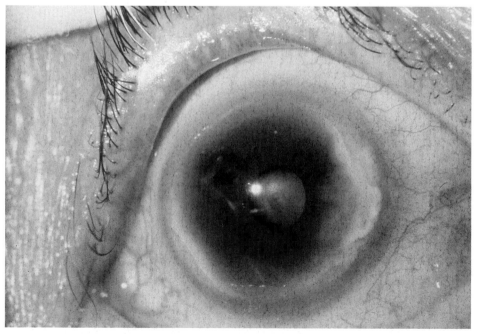

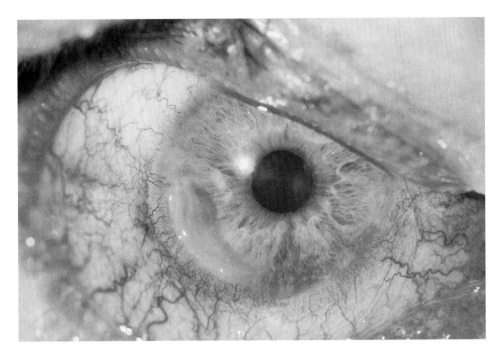

Figure 9.7. Peripheral ulcerative keratitis in a patient with rheumatoid arthritis. Findings include ciliary flush, contiguous episcleral inflammation and crescentic corneal stromal ulceration.

proteolysis by gelatinases, collagenases and matrix metalloproteinases.[104,120,121] Clinical findings include epithelial loss with stromal ulceration and active keratitis. Scleritis may occur in adjacent areas (see Figure 9.7). Rapid progression may require emergency application of tissue adhesives or lamellar tectonic grafts. Most importantly, PUK in RA is an important marker of systemic vasculitis involvement. Five-year mortality of RA patients with PUK may be as high as 50% in the absence of systemic immunosuppressive chemotherapy.[122] Extensive reviews have been published, but there is no consensus on the proper therapeutic approach for corneal ulceration associated with RA.[123–126] As a rule, management must first focus on treating the systemic disease, usually with immunosuppressive agents.[122,127–129] Treatment plans must include aggressive management of KCS, which may be sufficient in central ulceration. Management of rapidly progressive peripheral ulcers is more complex. In small ulcers without associated inflammation, application of tissue adhesive and a bandage contact lens may be sufficient.[127,130] In more rapidly progressive cases of PUK, conjunctival resection performed together with the application of tissue adhesive and bandage contact lens has been shown effective in temporizing the inflammatory process,[131] presumably by reducing the access of activated neutrophils to the exposed stromal surface. Tectonic corneal grafting may be necessary to stabilize globe integrity prior to later penetrating keratoplasty for visual rehabilitation.[114,127] Results of emergency corneal surgery are often poor, with recurrent keratolysis and descemetocele formation.[127] In experienced hands, anatomic success has been reported in 87% of patients, though recovery of vision was less impressive.[132] Surgical success is significantly increased if the clinical course permits the institution of systemic immunosuppressive therapy prior to surgery.[127,132,133]

Summary

The three autoimmune diseases discussed herein present a range of pathogenic mechanisms, and each produces devastating multifactorial ocular surface disease. Clinicians who care for such patients must remain mindful of the need to comprehensively treat all aspects of the disease processes in order to optimize rehabilitation of the ocular surface. Great strides have been made in our ability to intervene surgically to achieve a healthier ocular surface. Stem cell transplantation and amniotic-membrane grafting offer hope that many eyes previously considered lost may be rehabilitated. However, in treating ocular surface disease related to autoimmune systemic disease, timing is everything. In most patients, the primary immunologic process must be controlled before surgical intervention may be reasonably attempted. There are few experiences more disheartening than watching an excellent surgical outcome following a delicate stem cell graft destroyed within days in the face of uncontrolled inflammation. Future advances in our ability to modulate the immunopathophysiologic process will facilitate better success in the restoration of vision to these severely diseased eyes.

References

1. Thost A. Der chronische Schleimhautpemphigus der oberen luftwege. *Arch Laryng Rhinol* (Berlin) 1911; 25:459–478.

2. Person JR, Rogers RS. Bullous and cicatricial pemphigoid: clinical histopathological and immunopathological correlations. *Mayo Clin Proc* 1977; 52:54–66.

3. Foster CS. Cicatricial pemphigoid. *Tr Am Ophthalmol Soc* 1986; 84:527–663.

4. Jones BR. The ocular diagnosis of benign mucous membrane pemphigoid. *Proc R Soc Med* 1961; 54:109–110.

5. Wright P. Cicatrising conjunctivitis. *Trans Ophthalmol Soc UK* 1979; 99:663–670.

6. Wright P. The enigma of ocular cicatricial pemphigoid. *Trans Ophthalmol Soc UK* 1979; 99:141–145.

7. Hardy KM, Perry KO, Pingree GC, Kirby TJ. Benign mucous membrane pemphigoid. *Arch Dermatol* 1971; 104:467–475.

8. Modino BJ, Brown SI. Ocular cicatricial pemphigoid. *Ophthalmology* 1981; 88:95–100.

9. Mondino BJ. Cicatricial pemphigoid and erythema multiforme. *Ophthalmology* 1990; 97:939–952.

10. Mondino BJ, Brown SI, Lempert S, Jenkins MS. The acute manifestations of ocular cicatricial pemphigoid: diagnosis and treatment. *Ophthalmology* 1979; 86:543–555.

11. Duke-Elder S, Leigh AG. Diseases of the outer eye, In: *System of Ophthalmology*, Vol. 8 (Part 1), London, Henry Kimpton, 1965, pp. 502–512.

12. Shklar G, McCarthy PL. Oral lesions of mucous membrane pemphigus, a study of 85 cases. *Arch Otolaryngol* 1971; 93:354–364.

13. Lever WF. *Pemphigus and Pemphigoid*. Springfield IL, Charles C. Thomas, 1965. 9–23.

14. Lever WF. Pemphigus and Pemphigoid: a review of the advances made since 1964. *J Amer Acad Dermatol* 1979; 1:2–31.

15. Moschella SL, Pillsbury DM, Hurley HJ. In: *Dermatology*. Philadelphia: WB Saunders, 1975; 460–476.

16. Ahmed AR, Hombal SM. Cicatricial pemphigoid. *Int J Dermatol*, 1986; 25:90–96.

17. Ellison DE, Ward PH, Ahmed AR. Pemphigus and pemphigoid of the upper aerodigestive tract. *Trans Am Laryngol Assoc* 1984; 105:132–139.

18. Hanson RD, Olsen KD, Rogers RS. Upper aerodigestive tract manifestations of cicatricial pemphigoid. *Ann Otol Rhinol Laryngol* 1988; 97:493–499.

19. Laskaris G, Sklavounou A, Stratigos J. Bullous pemphigoid, cicatricial pemphigoid and pemphigus vulgaris. A comparative clinical survey of 278 cases. *Oral Surg* 1982; 54:656–662.

20. Sklavounou A, Laskaris G. Childhood cicatricial pemphigoid with exclusive gingival involvement. *J Oral Maxillofac Surg* 1990; 19:197–199.

21. Moy W, Kumar V, Friedman RP, Schaeffer ML, Beutner E, Helm F. Cicatricial pemphigoid. A case of onset at age 5. *J Periodont* 1986; 57:39–43.

22. Smith RC, Myers EA, Lamb HD. Ocular and oral pemphigus: Report of a case with anatomic findings in the eyeball. *Arch Ophthalmol* 1934; 11:635–640.

23. Ormerod LD, Fong LP, Foster CS. Corneal infections in mucosal scarring disorders and Sjögrens syndrome. *Am J Ophthalmol* 1988; 105:512–518.

24. Mondino BJ, Brown SI. Immunosuppressive therapy in ocular cicatricial pemphigoid. *Am J Ophthalmol* 1983; 96:453–459.

25. Tauber J, Jabbur N, Foster CS. Improved detection of disease progression in ocular cicatricial pemphigoid. *Cornea* 1992; 11:446–451.

26. Neumann R, Tauber J, Foster CS. Ocular cicatricial pemphigoid (OCP)—The potential for cure. *Ophthalmology* 1990; 97(9)Suppl:132.

27. Tauber J, Sainz de la Maza M, Foster CS. Systemic chemotherapy for ocular cicatricial pemphigoid. *Cornea* 1991; 10:185–195.

28. Neumann R, Tauber J, Foster CS. Remission and recurrence after withdrawal of therapy for ocular cicatricial pemphigoid, *Ophthalmology* 1991; 98:858–862.

29. Foster CS, Neumann R, Tauber J. Long-term results of systemic chemotherapy for ocular cicatricial pemphigoid. *Doc Ophthalmol* 1992; 82:223–229.

30. Dave VK, Vickers CFH. Azathioprine in the treatment of muco-cutaneous pemphigoid. *Br J Dermatol* 1974; 90:183–186.

31. Person JR, Rogers RS. Bullous pemphigoid responding to sulfapyridine and the sulfones. *Arch Dermatol* 1977; 113:610–615.

32. Foster CS, Wilson LA, Ekins MB. Immunosuppressive therapy for progressive ocular cicatricial pemphigoid. *Ophthalmology* 1982; 89:340–353.

33. Kinoshita S, Kiorpes TC, Friend J, Thoft RA. Goblet cell density in ocular surface disease. *Arch Ophthalmol* 1983; 101:1284–1287.

34. Ralph RA. Conjunctival goblet cell density in normal subjects and dry eye syndromes. *Inves Ophthal Vis Sci* 1975; 14:299–302.

35. Tauber J, Melamed S, Foster CS. Glaucoma in patients with ocular cicatricial pemphigoid. *Ophthalmology* 1989; 96:33–37.

36. Frith PA, Venning VA, Wojnarowski F, Millard PR, Bron AJ. Conjunctival involvement in cicatricial and bullous pemphigoid: a clinical and immunopathologic study. *Br J Ophthalmol* 1989; 73:52–56.

37. Leonard JN, Hobday CM, Haffenden GP, Griffiths CEM, Powles AV, Wright P, Fry L. Immunofluorescence studies in ocular cicatricial pemphigoid. *Br J Dermatol* 1988; 118:209–217.

38. Williams DM. Vesiculo-bullous mucocutaneous disease: Benign mucous membrane and bullous pemphigoid. *J Oral Path Med* 1990; 19:16–23.

39. Labahn R. A review of cicatricial pemphigoid. *Periodontal Abstracts* 1992; 40:5–9.

40. Norn MS, Kristensen EB. Benign mucous membrane pemphigoid. II. Cytology. *Acta Ophthalmol* 1974; 52:282–290.

41. Hoang-Xuan T, Foster CS, Raizman MB, Greenwood B. Mast cells in conjunctiva affected by cicatricial pemphigoid. *Ophthalmology* 1989; 96:1110–1114.

42. Thoft RA, Friend J, Kinoshita MA, Nikolic L, Foster CS. Ocular cicatricial pemphigoid associated with hyperproliferation of the conjunctival epithelium. *Am J Opthalmol* 1984; 98:37–42.

43. Rice BA, Foster CS. Immunopathology of cicatricial pemphigoid affecting the conjunctiva. *Ophthalmology* 1990; 97:1476–1483.

44. Bahn AK, Fujikawa LS, Foster CS. T cell subsets and Langerhans cells in normal and diseased conjunctiva. *Am J Ophthalmol* 1982; 94:205–212.

45. Sacks EH, Jacobiec FA, Wieczorek R, Donnenfeld E, Pery H, Knowles DM. Immunophenotypic analysis of the inflammatory infiltrate in ocular cicatricial pemphigoid: further evidence for a T cell mediated disease. *Ophthalmology* 1989; 96:236–243.

46. Sacks EH, Wieczorek R, Jacobiec FA, Knowles DM. Lymphocytic subpopulations in the normal human conjunctiva: a monoclonal antibody study. *Ophthalmology* 1986; 93:1276–1283.

47. Fine J-D. Epidermolysis Bullosa: Variability of expression of cicatricial pemphigoid, bullous pemphigoid, and epidermolysis bullosa acquisita antigens in clinically uninvolved skin. *J Inves Dermatol* 1985; 85:47–49.

48. Laskaris G, Angelopolous A. Cicatricial pemphigoid: Direct and indirect immunofluorescent studies. *Oral Surg, Oral Med, Oral Pathol* 1981; 51:48–54.

49. Griffith MR, Fukuyama K, Tuffanelli D, Silverman S. Immunofluorescence studies in mucous membrane pemphigoid. *Arch Dermatol,* 1974; 109:195–199.

50. Proia AD, Foulks GN, Sanfilippo FP. Ocular cicatricial pemphigoid with granular IgA and complement deposition. *Arch Ophthalmol* 1985; 103:1669–1672.

51. Rogers R, Perry HO, Bean SF, Jordan RE. Immunopathology of cicatricial pemphigoid: Studies of complement deposition. *J Inves Dermatol* 1977; 68:39–43.

52. Rogers RS, Seehafer JR, Perry HO. Treatment for cicatricial (benign mucous membrane) pemphigoid with dapsone. *J Am Acad Dermatol* 1982; 6:215–223.

53. Rogers RS, Mehregan DA. Dapsone therapy of cicatricial pemphigoid. *Seminars in Dermatol* 1988; 7:201–205.

54. Aultbrinker EA, Starr MB, Donnenfeld ED. Linear IgA disease. The ocular manifestations. *Ophthalmology* 1988; 95:340–343.

55. Azana JM, de Misa RF, Boixeda JP, Ledo A. Topical cyclosporine for cicatricial pemphigoid. *J Am Acad Dermatol* 1993; 28:134–135.

56. Wright P. Topical retinoic acid therapy for disorders of the outer eye. *Trans Ophth Soc UK* 1985; 104:869–874.

57. Shore JW, Foster CS, Westfall CT, Rubin PAD. Results of buccal mucosal grafting for patients with medically controlled ocular cicatricial pemphigoid. *Ophthalmology* 1992; 99:383–395.

58. Patten JT, Cavanagh HD, Allansmith MR. Induced ocular pseudopemphigoid. *Am J Ophthalmol* 1976; 82:272–276.

59. Hirst LW, Werblin T, Novak M. Drug induced cicatrizing conjunctivitis simulating ocular pemphigoid. *Cornea* 1982; 1:121–128.

60. Lass JH, Thoft RA, Dohlman CH. Idoxuridine induced conjunctival cicatrization. *Arch Ophthalmol* 1983; 101:747–750.

61. Pouliquen V, Patey A, Foster CS, Goichot L, Savoldelli M. Drug induced cicatricial pemphigoid affecting the conjunctiva; light and electron microscopic features. *Ophthalmology* 1986; 93:775–783.

62. Fiore PM, Jacobs IH, Goldberg DB. Drug induced ocular pemphigoid: a spectrum of diseases. *Arch Ophthalmol* 1987; 105:1660–1663.

63. Tseng SC, Maumenee AE, Stark WJ, Maumenee IH, Jensen AD, Green WR, Kenyon KR. Topical retinoid treatment for various dry eye disorders. *Ophthalmology* 1985; 92:717–727.

64. Udell IJ. Trifluridine associated conjunctival cicatrization. *Am J Ophthalmol* 1985; 99:363–364.

65. Kristensen EB, Norn MS. Benign mucous membrane pemphigoid. I. Secretion of mucous and tears. *Acta Ophthalmol* (Copenh) 1974; 52:266–281.

66. Foster CS. Immunosuppressive therapy for external ocular inflammatory diseases. *Ophthalmology* 1980; 87:140–150.

67. Brody HJ, Pirozzi DJ. Benign mucous membrane pemphigoid. *Arch Dermatol* 1977; 113:1598–1599.

68. Donnenfeld ED, Perry HD, Wallerstein A, et al. Subconjunctival mitomycin C for the treatment of ocular cicatricial pemphigoid. *Ophthalmology* 1999; 106:72–79.

69. Secchi AG, Tognon MS. Intraoperative Mitomycin C in the Treatment of Cicatricial Obliterations of Conjunctival Fornices. *Am J Ophthalmol* 1996; 122:728–730.

70. Sainz de la Maza M, Tauber J, Foster CS. Cataract surgery in ocular cicatricial pemphigoid. *Ophthalmology* 1988; 95:481–486.

71. Tugal-Tutkun I, Akova YA, Foster CS. Penetrating Keratoplasty in Cicatrizing Conjunctival Diseases. *Ophthalmology* 1995; 102:576–585.

72. Nobe JR, Moura BT, Robin JB, et al. Results of penetrating keratoplasty for the treatment of corneal perforations. *Arch Ophthalmol* 1990; 108:939–941.

73. Basti S, Mathur U. Unusual intermediate term outcome in three cases of limbal autograft transplantation. *Ophthalmology* 1999; 106:958–963.

74. Rao GN, Blatt HL, Aquavella JV. Results of keratoprostheses. *Am J Ophthalmol* 1979; 88:190–196.

75. Holland EJ, Palmon FE, Webster GF. Erythema multiforme, Stevens Johnson Syndrome and Toxic Epidermal Necrolysis. In: Mannis MJ, Macsai MS, Huntley AC, eds. *Eye and Skin Disease.* Lippincott-Raven Publishers, Philadelphia, 1996. pp. 273–284.

76. Dohlman CH, Doughman DJ. The Stevens Johnson syndrome. In: Symposium on the Cornea. *Transactions of the New Orleans Academy of Ophthalmologists.* St. Louis: Mosby, 1965. pp. 236–252.

77. Power WJ, Ghoraishi M, Merayo-Lloves J, et al. Analysis of the acute ophthalmic manifestations of the erythema multiforme/Stevens Johnson syndrome/toxic epidermal necrolysis disease spectrum. *Ophthalmology* 1995; 102: 1669–1676.

78. Nelson JD, Wright JC. Conjunctival goblet cell densities in ocular surface disease. *Arch Ophthalmol* 1984; 102:1049–1051.

79. Patz A. Ocular involvement in erythema multiforme. *Arch Dermatol* 1950; 43:244–256.

80. Howard GM. The Stevens Johnson Syndrome. Ocular prognosis and treatment. *Am J Ophthalmol* 1963; 55:893–900.

81. Beyer C. The management of special problems associated with Stevens Johnson syndrome and ocular pemphigoid. *Trans Am Acad Ophthalmol Otolaryngol* 1977; 83:701–707.

82. Wright P, Collin JR. The ocular complications of erythema multiforme (Stevens Johnson syndrome) and their management. *Trans Ophthalmol Soc UK* 1983; 103:338–341.

83. Arstikaitis MJ. Ocular aftermath of Stevens Johnson syndrome. Review of 33 cases. *Arch Ophthalmol* 1973; 90: 376–379.

84. Foster CS, Fong LP, Azar D, et al. Episodic conjunctival inflammation after Stevens Johnson syndrome. *Ophthalmology* 1988; 95:453–462.

85. Huff JC, Weston WL, Tonnesen MG. Erythema multiforme: A critical review of characteristics, diagnostic criteria, and causes. *J Am Acad Dermatol* 1983; 8:763–775.

86. Major PP, Morriset R, Kustak C. Isolation of herpes simplex virus type 1 from lesions of erythema multiforme. *Can Med J* 1978; 118:821–822.

87. Yetiv JZ, Bianchine JR, Owens JA. Etiologic factors of the Stevens Johnson syndrome. *South Med J* 1980; 73:599–602.

88. Genvert GI, Cohen EJ, Donnenfeld ED, et al. Erythema multiforme after use of topical sulfacetamide. *Am J Ophthalmol* 1985; 99:465–468.

89. Guill MA, Goette DK, Knight CG, et al. Erythema multiforme and urticaria. *Arch Dermatol* 1979; 115:742–743.

90. Tseng SCG, Maumenee AE, Stark WJ, et al. Topical retinoid treatment for various dry eye disorders. *Ophthalmology* 1985; 92:717–727.

91. Revuz J, Roujeau J-C, Guillaume J-C, et al. Treatment of toxic epidermal necrolysis. Creteil's experience. *Arch Dermatol* 1987; 123:1156–1158.

92. Robin JB, Dugel R. Immunologic disorders of the cornea and conjunctiva. In: Kaufman HE, Barron BA, McDonald MV, Waltman SR, eds. *The Cornea*. New York: Churchill-Livingstone, 1988; 511–561.

93. Killingsworth DW, Stern GA, Driebe WT, et al. Results of therapeutic penetrating keratoplasty. *Ophthalmology* 1993; 100:534–541.

94. Tsubota K, Satake Y, Ohyama M, et al. Surgical reconstruction of the ocular surface in advanced ocular cicatricial pemphigoid and Stevens-Johnson Syndrome. *Am J Ophthalmol* 1996; 122:38–52.

95. Honavar SG, Bansal AK, Sangwan VS, et al. Amniotic membrane transplantation for ocular surface reconstruction in Stevens Johnson Syndrome. *Ophthalmology* 2000; 107:975–979.

96. Shimmura S, Ando M, Shimazaki J, et al. Complications with one-piece lamellar keratolimbal grafts for simultaneous limbal and corneal pathologies. *Cornea* 2000; 19:439–442.

97. Tseng SCG, Prabhaswat P, Barton K, et al. Amniotic membrane transplantation with or without limbal allografts for corneal surface reconstruction in patients with limbal stem cell deficiency. *Arch Ophthalmol* 1998; 116:431–441.

98. Lee S, Tseng SCG. Amniotic membrane transplantation for persistent epithelial defects with ulceration. *Am J Ophthalmol* 1997; 123:303–312.

99. Tsubota K, Shimazaki J. Surgical treatment of children blinded by Stevens Johnson Syndrome. *Am J Ophthalmol* 1999; 128:573–581.

100. Shimazaki J, Shimmura S, Fujishima H, et al. Association of preoperative tear function with surgical outcome in severe Stevens Johnson Syndrome. *Ophthalmology* 2000; 107:1518–1523.

101. Wolfe AM. The epidemiology of rheumatoid arthritis: a review: Part I. Surveys Part II. Incidence and Diagnostic Criteria. *Bull Rheum Dis* 1968; 19:518–529.

102. Harris ED Jr. Mechanism of disease: rheumatoid arthritis—pathophysiology and implications for therapy. *NEJM* 1990; 322:1277–1289.

103. Dubord P, Ho V, Shojania K, Chalmers A. *Rheumatoid Arthritis in Eye and Skin Disease*, ed. MJ Mannis, MS Macsai and AC Huntley. Lippincott-Raven Publishers, Philadelphia 1996, pp. 191–198.

104. Robin JR, Schanzlin DJ, Verity SM, et al. Peripheral corneal disorders. *Survey Ophthalmol* 1986; 31:1–36.

105. Stern ME, Beuerman RW, Fox RI, et al. The pathology of dry eye: The interaction between the ocular surface and lacrimal glands. *Cornea* 1998; 17:584–589.

106. Turner K, Pflugfelder SC, Zhanghua J, et al. Interleukin 6 levels in the conjunctival epithelium of patients with dry eye disease treated with cyclosporine ophthalmic emulsion. *Cornea* 2000; 19:492–496.

107. Marsh P, Pflugfelder SC. Topical nonpreserved methylprednisolone therapy for keratoconjunctivitis sicca in Sjogren syndrome. *Ophthalmology* 1999; 106:811–816.

108. Tishler M, Yaron I, Geter O, et al. Elevated tear interleukin-6 levels in patients with Sjogren syndrome. *Ophthalmology* 1998; 105:2327–2329.

109. Solomon A, Rosenblatt M, Li D, et al. Doxycycline inhibition of interleukin-1 in the corneal epithelium. *Invest Ophthalmol Vis Sci* 2000; 41:2544–2557.

110. Stevenson D, Tauber J, Reis BL, et al. Efficacy and safety of cyclosporin A ophthalmic emulsion in the treatment of moderate-to-severe dry eye disease. *Ophthalmology* 2000; 107:967–974.

111. Foster CS, Sainz de la Maza M. *The Sclera*. (pp. 299–307.) Springer-Verlag, 1993.

112. Watson PG, Hayreh SS. Scleritis and episcleritis. *Br J Ophthalmol* 1976; 60:163–191.

113. Pfister RR, Murphy GE. Corneal ulceration and perforation associated with Sjogrens syndrome. *Arch Ophthalmol* 1980; 98:89–94.

114. Kervick GN, Pflugfelder SC, Haimovici R, et al. Paracentral rheumatoid corneal ulceration. Clinical features and cyclosporine therapy. *Ophthalmology* 1992; 99:80–88.

115. Brown SI, Grayson M. Marginal furrows: A characteristic corneal lesion of rheumatoid arthritis. *Arch Ophthalmol* 1968; 79:563–567.

116. McGavin DDM, Williamson J, Forrester JV, et al. Episcleritis and scleritis: a study of their clinical manifestations and association with rheumatoid arthritis. *BJO* 1976; 60:192–226.

117. Jayson MIV, Jones DEP. Scleritis and rheumatoid arthritis. *Ann Rheum Dis* 1971; 30:343–347.

118. Jayson MIV, Easty DL. Ulceration of the cornea in rheumatoid arthritis. *Ann Rheum Dis* 1977; 36:428–432.

119. Lyne AJ. "Contact lens" cornea in rheumatoid arthritis. *Br J Ophthalmol* 1970; 54:410–415.

120. Smith VA, Hoh HB, Easty DL. Role of ocular matrix metalloproteinases in peripheral ulcerative keratitis. *Br J Ophthalmol* 1999; 83:176–183.

121. Eiferman RA, Carothers DJ, Yankeelov JA. Peripheral rheumatoid ulceration and evidence for conjunctival collagenase production. *Am J Ophthalmol* 1979; 87:703–709.

122. Foster CS, Forstot SL, Wilson LA. Mortality rate in rheumatoid arthritis patients developing necrotizing scleritis or peripheral ulcerative keratitis. Effects of immunosuppression. *Ophthalmology* 1984; 91:1253–1263.

123. Donzis PB, Mondino BJ. Management of noninfectious corneal ulcers. *Survey Ophthalmol* 1987; 32:94–110.

124. Kenyon KR. Decision making in the therapy of external eye disease. Noninfected corneal ulcers. *Ophthalmology* 1982; 89:44–51.

125. Tauber J, Sainz de la Maza M, Hoang-Xuan T et al. An analysis of therapeutic decision making regarding immunosuppressive chemotherapy for peripheral ulcerative keratitis. *Cornea* 1990; 9:66–73.

126. Feder RS, Krachmer JH. Conjunctival resection for the treatment of the rheumatoid corneal ulceration. *Ophthalmology* 1984; 91:111–115.

127. Bernauer W, Ficker LA, Watson PG, Dart JKG. The management of corneal perforations associated with rheumatoid arthritis. *Ophthalmology* 1995; 102:1325–1337.

128. Easty DL, Madden P, Jayson MIV et al. Systemic immunosuppression in marginal keratolysis. *Trans Ophthalmol Soc UK* 1978; 98:410–417.

129. McCarthy JM, Dubord PJ, Chalmers A et al. Cyclosporine A for the treatment of necrotizing scleritis and corneal melting in patients with rheumatoid arthritis. *J Rheumatol* 1992; 19:1358–1361.

130. Weiss JL, Williams P, Lindstrom RL et al. The use of tissue adhesive in corneal perforations. *Ophthalmology* 1983; 90:610–615.

131. Wilson FM, Grayson M, Ellis FD. Treatment of peripheral corneal ulcers by limbal conjunctivectomy. *Br J Ophthalmol* 1976; 60:713–719.

132. Palay DA, Stulting RD, Waring GO et al. Penetrating keratoplasty in patients with rheumatoid arthritis. *Ophthalmology* 1992; 99:622–627.

133. Portnoy SL, Insler MS, Kaufman HE. Surgical management of corneal ulceration and perforation. *Survey Ophthalmol* 1989; 34:47–58.

10
Iatrogenic Limbal Stem Cell Deficiency

Gary S. Schwartz and Edward J. Holland

Introduction

A stable ocular surface depends upon the proper functioning of the limbal stem cells (SC). A limited number of disorders have been described that lead to ocular surface instability from abnormal stem cell function. Aniridia is a primary disorder in which improper development of the anterior segment results in a decreased number of SC. In all likelihood, the remaining cells, in addition to being decreased in number, are also dysfunctional. Aniridic patients are not born with abnormal ocular surfaces. As they become older, epitheliopathy develops in the peripheral cornea and slowly extends centrally. This advancement of surface disease indicates a progression of limbal SC dysfunction or loss.

Another cause of SC dysfunction is severe conjunctival deficiency. Examples of this category include patients with Stevens–Johnson syndrome (SJS) and ocular cicatricial pemphigoid (OCP), diseases resulting in inflammation of the conjunctiva and limbus. In these patients, the primary disease affects the conjunctiva, and the SC are involved secondarily. The corneal surface is almost always normal throughout the early stages of these disease processes. Only later, when the stem cell population is diminished from the constant conjunctival inflammation, does the corneal epithelium become abnormal. Eventually, if stem cell loss continues, conjunctivalization of the cornea will occur and the patient will show clinical signs of stem cell deficiency.

Other patients develop SC deficiency due to loss of stem cells from chemical or thermal injury. In this category are those patients with ocular surface disease secondary to alkali, acid, or thermal injury. These patients sustain loss of the majority of their SC populations at the time of the injury. In all likelihood, they sustain further, gradual SC loss in the period following injury, due to inflammation. The injury to the conjunctival tissue is another important factor that leads to the worsening of the stem cell function seen in these patients.

Yet another cause of ocular surface disease due to SC deficiency is contact-lens-induced keratopathy.[1] Contact-lens-induced keratopathy can lead to severe conjunctivalization of the cornea. Kenyon and co-workers evaluated one case of severe contact-lens-induced keratopathy and found migration of conjunctival epithelium and goblet cells into the corneal surface. The ocular surface disease here is most likely due to chronic injury to the limbal SC. The injury to the SC is probably due to chronic ischemia in these patients, since it is worst in the superior quadrants compared with all other quadrants.

Corneal intraepithelial neoplasia (CIN) is a less commonly described cause of ocular surface disease from limbal SC deficiency.[2] CIN thought to cause SC deficiency from replacement of normal SC with neoplastic ones. Typically, the ocular surface disease starts sectorally at the location of the limbal CIN. This abnormal corneal tissue then spreads circumferentially, and, if enough of the limbus is eventually involved, total ocular surface failure may result.

Etiology of Iatrogenic Limbal Stem Cell Deficiency

The above mentioned categories account for the vast majority of cases of limbal stem cell deficiency reported in the literature. However, another group of patients exists that have stem cell deficiency but yet do not fit into any of these categories. It is likely that many of these patients go undiagnosed with stem cell deficiency because they do not have a classically described cause for their stem cell dysfunction.

Tseng categorized stem cell deficiency etiologies according to whether they represented hypofunction or aplasia of stem cells.[3] Those etiologies resulting from stem cell hypofunction included aniridia, multiple endocrine deficiency, neurotrophic keratopathy, chronic lim-

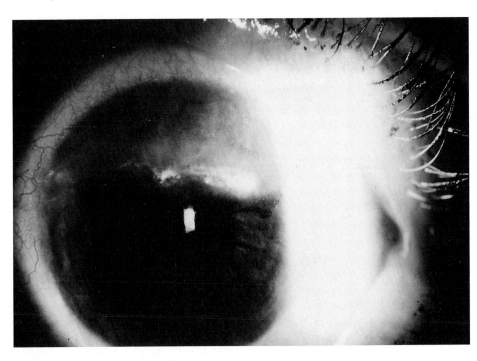

Figure 10.1. Patient 1. Slit-lamp photograph demonstrating a superior sectoral area of thickened, irregular epithelium with neovascularization and lipid keratopathy. Stem cell deficiency resulted from multiple surgeries for pterygium and the use of topical Mitomycin C.

bitis, pterygium, and pseudoterygium. Etiologies listed as stem cell aplasia included chemical/thermal injury, SJS, and multiple surgeries or cryotherapies to the limbal region. Although the latter category was named in Tseng's study, details of patients with this condition were not described.

In 1998, the authors described a group of patients with iatrogenic limbal stem cell deficiency.[4] These patients had stem cell disease not secondary to a known diagnosis. These patients were similar to the above patients in Tseng's "multiple surgeries or cryotherapies to the limbal region" group. Although these eyes do not have a known specific cause for stem cell deficiency, they do share similarities in past ocular history, clinical findings, and clinical course. All eyes demonstrated a chronic, progressive epitheliopathy that began in the peripheral cornea and progressed centrally (Figure 10.1). In some cases, the epitheliopathy was accompanied by fine neovascularization (Table 10.1). The clinical findings were not consistent with other causes of epitheliopathy such as keratoconjunctivitis sicca, blepharokeratoconjunctivitis, or toxic epitheliopathy. In addition, the epitheliopathy neither responded to standard therapies for dry eye management, nor resolved after reduction or cessation of topical medications.

Each of the eyes described had prior surgery involving the corneoscleral limbus, and the mean number of prior surgeries per eye was 2.6. We hypothesize that direct trauma to the limbus at the time of surgery results in loss of stem cells. Ocular surgery involving the corneoscleral limbus is, of course, quite common, yet limbal stem cell deficiency from prior surgery is quite rare. We believe that surgery to the limbus does not typically

cause loss of enough of the stem cell population to result in ocular surface disease. However, surgical manipulation of the limbus does initiate a localized loss of SC that predisposes patients to develop the clinical findings of limbal deficiency when exposed to further stem cell trauma.

In support of this argument, all of our patients were affected in the superior quadrant corresponding to the site of prior limbal surgery. It is well known that the superior limbus is richer in limbal stem cells than any other part of the ocular surface.[5] It is likely that both the length and location of the surgical incisions were influential in the development of stem cell deficiency. Two eyes of two patients had extracapsular cataract extraction (ECCE) utilizing an eleven millimeter limbal wound. Four eyes of three patients had previous intracapsular

Table 10.1. Sequelae of limbal stem cell deficiency.

Patient number	Quadrant of epitheliopathy	Central cornea affected	Stromal sequelae of epitheliopathy
1	superior	yes	stromal scarring, neovascularization, lipid keratopathy
2	R.E.: entire cornea	yes	stromal scarring
	L.E.: entire cornea	yes	stromal scarring
3	R.E.: superior	yes	none
	L.E.: superior	yes	none
4	superotemporal	yes	stromal scarring
5	superotemporal	no	none
6	superior	no	none

R.E., right eye; L.E., left eye

cataract extraction (ICCE) with wounds typically involving 180 degrees of the corneal perimeter (Figure 10.2). The anterior nature of ICCE and older ECCE wounds likely caused direct trauma to the limbal SC at the time of the surgery. It is interesting to note that none of the patients reported in this series had cataract surgery via phacoemulsification. It is very likely that phacoemulsification incisions, by nature of their being shorter than both the ECCE and ICCE incisions, result in significantly less trauma to the limbal SC population.

Another possible factor for the superior location of the stem cell damage is the contribution of the upper eyelids. Although difficult to evaluate, it is possible that mechanical forces elicited by the upper eyelids may cause localized ischemia and further stem cell damage.

The chronic use of topical medications including pilocarpine, beta blockers, antibiotics, and corticosteroids appeared to play a significant role in six eyes (Table 10.2). These topical medications are known to be toxic to the corneal epithelium. It is possible that chronic use

Figure 10.2. Patient 3, right eye. A. Slit-lamp photograph demonstrating abnormal limbal vascular pattern superiorly in patient with previous intracapsular cataract extraction, subsequent penetrating keratoplasty with trans-sclerally sutured posterior chamber lens. The patient also had a tube-shunt procedure. B. Fluorescein dye demonstrates abnormal epithelium of superior aspect of graft.

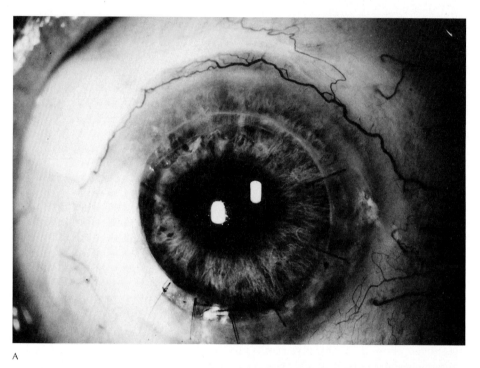

A

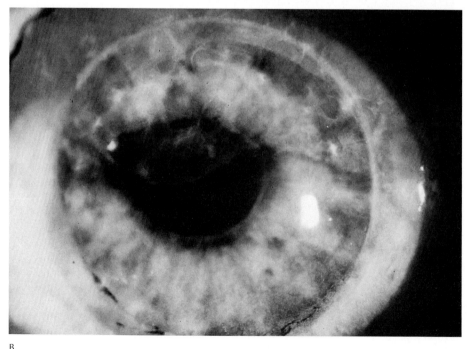

B

Table 10.2. Summary of clinical data.

Patient No., Age (years), Sex, Eye	Visual Acuity	Prior Surgeries	Contributing Ocular Conditions
1. 42, F, L.E.	20/70	pterygium excisions with conjunctival transplant × 3, superficial keratectomy	topical mitomycin QID × 30 days
2. 81, F, R.E.	20/400	ICCE	keratoconjunctivitis sicca, diabetes mellitus, chronic pilocarpine and beta blocker for many years
2. 81, F, L.E.	20/400	ICCE	keratoconjunctivitis sicca, diabetes mellitus, chronic pilocarpine and beta blocker for many years
3. 76, M, R.E.	20/200	ECCE PK with sulcus PCL tube-shunt procedure	rosacea, keratoconjunctivitis sicca, topical beta blocker × 5y, antibiotic/steroid × several years
3. 76, M, L.E.	HM	ICCE PK with TS-PCL	rosacea, keratoconjunctivitis sicca, antibiotic/steroid × several years
4. 82, F, R.E.	20/400	ICCE PK, repeat PK with TS-PCL	rubeola keratitis
5. 62, M, L.E.	20/30	PK × 3 ECCE with PCL	HSV keratitis, chronic viroptic, nasolacrimal duct obstruction
6. 66, F, L.E.	20/70	cataract needling, PK with TS-PCL repeat PK	aphakic corneal edema keratoconjunctivitis sicca

No., number; F, female; M, male; L.E., left eye; R.E., right eye; HM, hand motions; ICCE, Intracapsular cataract extraction; ECCE, extracapsular cataract extraction; PK, penetrating keratoplasty; PCL, posterior chamber lens; TS-PCL, trans-sclerally sutured posterior chamber lens; HSV, Herpes simplex virus.

is also toxic to the limbal SC. One eye was exposed to topical mitomycin C for 30 days. Mitomycin C is an antimetabolite that specifically targets dividing cells. The entire ocular surface was exposed to MMC, but the only site of stem cell decompensation was at the site of the previous conjunctival autograft. It is probable that the surgical trauma in combination with the antimetabolic toxicity led to irreversible stem cell damage and resulting ocular surface disease.

Other diagnoses that may have contributed to stem cell failure, and which were present in some of these patients, include keratoconjunctivitis sicca, rosacea, and HSV keratitis. It is possible that these disease entities led to stem cell dysfunction through chronic inflammation or increased epithelial turnover. It is interesting to note that, although penetrating keratoplasty (PK) does not cause specific surgical trauma to the limbal stem cells, 5 eyes in this study had a total of 8 prior PK's. The increased demand on the host epithelium to repopulate the donor graft was probably a factor for the development of limbal SC deficiency in these patients.

The patients with iatrogenic limbal stem cell deficiency are different from those with limbal stem deficiency from other causes, since there is not a single disease entity that leads to their limbal deficiency. Multiple factors, including surgery, topical medications, and external disease probably all contribute to limbal stem cell deficiency in these patients. It is likely that prior surgery, with its traumatic insult to the limbal stem cells,

the most important etiologic factor, since each patient within this study had undergone extensive surgery involving the corneoscleral limbus, and the area of stem cell deficiency always corresponded to the area of prior limbal surgery.

The clinical course of this disorder is a slowly progressive epitheliopathy beginning at the peripheral cornea and progressing centrally. It may be sectoral in an area corresponding to an area of previous limbal surgery. This sectoral nature can lead to the appearance of a wedge-shaped area of abnormal epithelium immediately adjacent to normal epithelium (Figure 10.3). By and large, the sectoral nature separates this form of limbal stem deficiency from those described previously, which tend to involve the entire limbus.

Medical Management

A certain percentage of iatrogenic limbal stem cell deficiency patients will require no therapy. These patients are either asymptomatic or mildly symptomatic, and the visual axis is not threatened. Therefore, the initial decision is whether to initiate treatment in a patient with iatrogenic limbal stem cell deficiency.

Because chronic use of topical medications is a probable etiologic agent, the first step in medical management is discontinuation of any unnecessary topical medications. These agents typically include antiglaucoma

Figure 10.3. Patient 4. A. Slit-lamp photograph demonstrating a wedge-shaped area of stromal scarring secondary to chronic epitheliopathy in a patient with prior intracapsular cataract extraction, penetrating keratoplasty, and repeat penetrating keratoplasty with trans-sclerally sutured posterior chamber lens. B. Fluorescein dye demonstrates that the abnormal epithelium originates from the superotemporal limbus and extends into the pupillary axis.

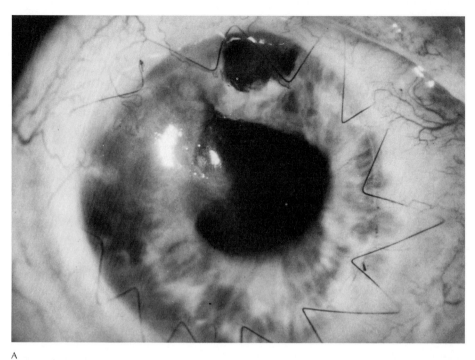

A

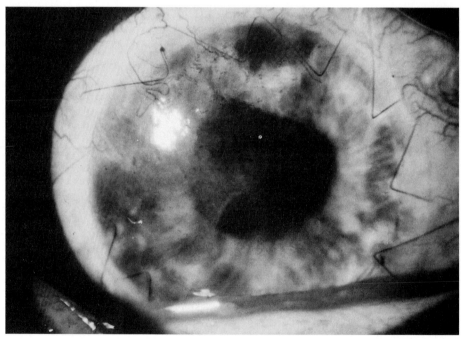

B

medications and antibiotics. Preserved artificial tear preparations should be either discontinued, or replaced by nonpreserved lubricants.

Topical corticosteroids appear to relieve discomfort and may cause some regression of clinical findings in select patients with mild disease. The mechanism for this is uncertain, but these patients do have chronic, low-grade inflammation, and the topical corticosteroids not only improve comfort, but also reduce inflammation and encourage regression of neovascularization.

Another possible beneficial medical therapy, although unproven, is topical retinoic acid. It has been our experience that this medication can prevent progression and, in some cases, even lead to regression of abnormal epithelial cells in patients with mild to moderate disease.

Surgical Management

If medical therapy fails, the first surgical technique to consider is sequential conjunctival epitheliectomy.[6] In this procedure, described by Dua, abnormal epithelium is scraped repeatedly, allowing normal epithelium to repopulate the corneal surface. This technique is described in detail in Chapter 14.

Amniotic membrane transplantation may also be used to manage iatrogenic limbal stem cell deficiency. Placement of this membrane at the time of superficial keratectomy provides scaffolding for the growth of new healthy epithelial cells.[7] It also may promote transdifferentiation of conjunctiva-like epithelium to corneal epithelium. Innate anti-inflammatory properties of the human amniotic membrane also likely work to improve the overall health of the ocular surface.

For severe disease resulting in visual loss, a stem cell transplant procedure may be required for visual rehabilitation.[8] If the fellow eye is unaffected, the procedure of choice is conjunctival limbal autograft (CLAU) and, in the future, possibly ex vivo expanded limbal autograft (EVELAU). Although the fellow eye may not manifest clinical findings of iatrogenic limbal stem cell deficiency, it often has had exposure to similar surgical trauma, chronic medications, and external disease factors, and may harbor a subclinical stem cell deficiency. These eyes should be approached cautiously, since using this otherwise asymptomatic eye as a donor for a CLAU may deplete it of necessary stem cells and cause symptomatic iatrogenic limbal stem cell deficiency in that eye as well. For these reasons, EVELAU may prove a superb option for these patients in the future.

For severe bilateral disease, one of the limbal allograft procedures is required for visual rehabilitation. These include living-related conjunctival limbal allograft, keratolimbal allograft, and living-related ex vivo expanded limbal allograft. Because iatrogenic limbal stem cell deficiency often manifests in a sectoral nature, it has been our experience that a partial keratolimbal allograft placed over the affected area of limbus will usually restore a healthy ocular surface.

Conclusions

Although little has been written about iatrogenic limbal stem cell deficiency, patients with this disorder are probably more common than the literature might suggest. It is important to recognize this disorder as a limbal deficiency, since standard medical therapies will not address its etiology. The sequelae of this condition include stromal scarring and significant loss of vision. Fortunately, phacoemulsification has replaced ECCE and ICCE as the procedure of choice for cataract extraction in many parts of the world. Because of its shorter, and often temporally placed, incision, phacoemulsification is probably less likely to lead to iatrogenic limbal stem cell deficiency. Hopefully we will be witnessing less iatrogenic limbal stem cell deficiency in the future.

References

1. Jenkins C, Tuft S, Liu C, et al. Limbal transplantation in the management of chronic contact-lens-associated epitheliopathy. *Eye* 1993; 7:629–33.
2. Erie JC, Campbell RJ, Liesegang TJ. Conjunctival and corneal intraepithelial and invasive neoplasia. *Ophthalmol* 1986; 93:176–83.
3. Tseng SCG, Chen JJY, Huang AJW, et al. Classification of conjunctival surgeries for corneal disease based on stem cell concept. *Ophthalmology Clinics of North America* 1990; 3:595–610.
4. Schwartz GS, Holland EJ. Iatrogenic limbal stem cell deficiency. *Cornea* 1998; 17(1):31–7.
5. Wiley L, SunderRaj N, Sun TT, et al. Regional heterogeneity in human corneal and limbal epithelia: An immunohistochemical evaluation. *Invest Ophthalmol Vis Sci* 1991; 32:594–602.
6. Dua HS, Azuara-Blanco A. Limbal stem cells of the corneal epithelium. *Surv Ophthalmol* 2000; 44(5):415–25.
7. Schwab IR. Cultured corneal epithelia for ocular surface disease. *Tr Am Ophth Soc* 1999; XCVII:891–986.
8. Holland EJ, Schwartz GS. The evolution of epithelial transplantation for severe ocular surface disease and a proposed classification system. *Cornea* 1996; 15(6):549–556.

Part IV

Management

11
Surface Stabilization Procedures

Marian S. Macsai, Mark J. Mannis, and Jason K. Darlington

Ocular surface dysfunction may result from a broad range of disease entities. Recurrent corneal erosion, non-healing epithelial defects, and corneal melts may ensue following injury, infection, or inflammatory disease. In this chapter, we will review those procedures that may be useful in stabilization and protection of the surface in a variety of disease states.

Indications

Specific surgical techniques for stabilization of the corneal surface should be included in the armamentarium of anterior segment surgeons. These techniques are almost always adjuncts to primary medical treatment including both topical and systemic regimens. For the most part, these are simple surgical maneuvers that are task-specific. Numerous different diagnostic indications for adjunct surgical intervention in the management of ocular surface disease exist. These include (1) keratoconjunctivitis sicca, (2) neurotrophic keratitis, (3) exposure keratitis, (4) corneal ulceration, (5) recurrent corneal erosion, (6) conjunctival ulceration, (7) scleromalacia, and (8) bullous keratopathy.

The techniques useful in management of these conditions are varied and include (1) punctal occlusion, (2) tarsorrhaphy, (3) conjunctival flaps, (4) anterior stromal puncture, (5) corneal cautery, (6) superficial keratectomy, and (7) phototherapeutic keratectomy (see Table 11.1).

Procedures

Punctal Occlusion (Temporary, Permanent, Excisional)

Temporary occlusion of the puncta can be achieved using a variety of techniques.[1,2,3] Insertion of dissolvable collagen plugs may be used either as a diagnostic maneuver prior to permanent occlusion, or as a temporary occlusive measure when augmentation of the tear film is desired for a short period of time. The same effect can be achieved using sections of cat gut suture material. In both instances, the plugs are inserted at the slit-lamp after instillation of a drop of topical anesthetic. Using smooth-tipped micro-tying forceps or jeweler's forceps, the plug is inserted into the punctal orifice and maneuvered into the upper and/or lower canaliculus. For longer-lasting effect, more than one plug can be placed sequentially in the same punctum. Depending on the degree of hydration desired, one or all of the puncta can be closed at the same time using this technique. The patient should be advised that the effect of collagen plugs is temporary, and that these will generally dissipate completely by 10 days after insertion.[4,5]

An alternative modality for temporary punctal occlusion is the placement of a small drop of cyanoacrylate glue at the punctal orifice.[6] A 30-gauge needle on a tuberculin syringe can be used to apply a microscopic amount of cyanoacrylate to the punctal orifice. Application of an excessive amount of glue may result in either conjunctival or corneal irritation.

Longer-lasting punctal occlusion can be achieved with the use of silicone plugs.[7] These devices provide a more long-term effect and remain in place until removed by the physician. The size of the plug needed is determined by visual inspection of the punctal orifice at the slit-lamp. After instillation of a drop of topical anesthetic, a punctal dilator may be used to stretch the punctal orifice. The silicone plug is then placed into position while the lid is fixated with the finger. An attempt should be made to place the largest plug that will fit into the punctum snugly, and the cap of the plug should be flush with the eyelid margin (Figure 11.1). Care should be taken to avoid insertion of the entire silicone plug, including the cap, into the canaliculus. The surgeon should check the placement of the plug at the slit-lamp to be sure of its stability, and to ensure that there is no conjunctival or corneal irritation.

After establishing a therapeutic benefit from temporary punctal occlusion with either dissolvable collagen plugs, cyanoacrylate occlusion, or silicone plugs, permanent punctal occlusion may then be indicated. Cauterization of the punctal orifice with the argon laser has

Table 11.1. Surgical techniques of surface stabilization.

Increased lubrication	Nonhealing epithelial defects	Recurrent erosions
Punctal occlusion	Punctal occlusion	Anterior stromal puncture
Collagen plugs	Tarsorrhaphy	Superficial keratectomy
Silicone plugs	Botulinum injection	PTK
Cyanoacrylate	Gold weight	
Punctal cautery	Conjunctival flap	
Canaliculectomy		

been suggested; however, often several applications are required to achieve consistent results. The potential advantage of argon laser cautery of the canaliculi is the potential reversibility of the procedure.[8,9]

Thermocauterization of the epithelial lining of the canaliculus can be achieved with either monopolar or bipolar cautery, and is a more permanent mode of punctal occlusion.[10] Anesthesia of the area can be achieved with a local injection of 1% lidocaine or prolonged application of a topical anesthetic. Injections of anesthetic agents may be subcutaneous, subconjunctival, or a regional nerve block (trochlear nerve) for the superior canaliculus. After anesthesia is achieved, the cautery tip is inserted into the canaliculus and cautery is applied to the point of blanching of the surrounding tissue (Figure 11.2). Avoidance of both the conjunctiva and the cornea is imperative to avoid an iatrogenic burn to the surrounding tissue. A successful procedure is usually signaled by the presence of a "cast" of canalicular epithelium on the cautery needle. Visible occlusion of the punctal orifice is not necessary to achieve a therapeutic benefit. After the canaliculus heals and fibrosis replaces

the epithelium removed by the cautery tip, occlusion of the punctal orifice will ensue.

If punctal occlusion has not been achieved with any of the above mentioned modalities, including punctal plugs, laser, thermocautery, canaliculectomy may be considered. Reversal of any of these permanent techniques for punctal occlusion is difficult and involves extensive surgical reconstruction of the lacrimal drainage system.

Tarsorrhaphy (Temporary, Partial, Total, Permanent)

Closure of the eyelids with a tarsorrhaphy, partial or total, will decrease the exposed area of the ocular surface, decrease the evaporation of the tear film and decrease trauma to the ocular surface resulting from friction during blinking of the eyelids. A partial tarsorrhaphy allows the patient to preserve central vision, at the same time allowing the surgeon to examine the ocular surface of the cornea and bulbar conjunctiva. A total tarsorrhaphy compromises both the patient's vision as well as the surgeon's ability to examine the eye.

Temporary ptosis of the upper eyelid can be induced with a botulinum injection to the upper eyelid. Although somewhat costly, this temporary occlusion of the eyelid may stabilize the ocular surface during the period of temporary paralysis of the upper-eyelid retractors. The paralytic effect may last 3 months in some patients, and if a therapeutic effect is achieved the injections may be repeated, or a more permanent form of tarsorrhaphy can be employed.

Temporary tarsorrhaphy can also be achieved through the application of cyanoacrylate to the eyelid

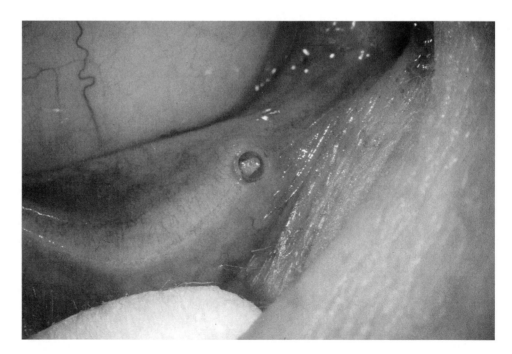

Figure 11.1. Silicone punctum plug in position in the inferior punctum.

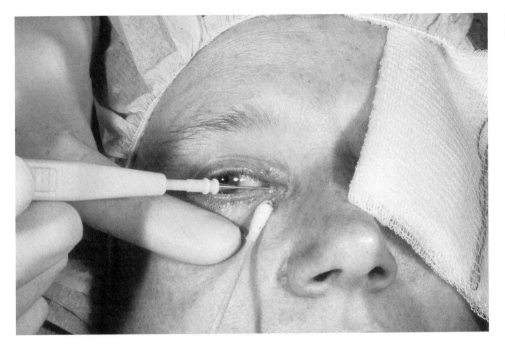

Figure 11.2. Electrocautery of the inferior punctum.

margin and intentional adhesion of the upper eyelid to the lower eyelid.[11] Using a 30-gauge needle on a tuberculin syringe, cyanoacrylate is applied sparingly to the eyelid margin and the lashes. Intentional adhesion of the upper and lower eyelids is achieved prior to drying the cyanoacrylate. Avoidance of irritation to the conjunctiva and cornea is imperative to prevent further damage to the ocular surface.

For short-term occlusion of the eyelids, a 6-0 silk mattress suture can be placed through the eyelids and tied over bolsters to prevent erosion of the suture through the eyelid. The surgeons must avoid full-thickness penetration of the eyelid to prevent rubbing of the suture on the cornea or conjunctiva and further irritation of the ocular surface.

A more permanent, but entirely reversible, tarsorrhaphy is achieved by suturing the eyelids closed after removal of the skin at the eyelid margin. Removal of the eyelid margin skin can be achieved with a carbon dioxide laser, or surgical excision. After peritarsal injection of local anesthesia, splitting of the eyelid down the gray line and surgical excision of the posterior eyelid margin with a Westcott scissors provides a raw surface for the formation of fibrosis and scar tissue after the surfaces are apposed with sutures. A 6-0 polyglactin or silk double-armed suture can be used to created a horizontal figure-eight suture through the upper and lower tarsus. The suture is tied tightly to appose the exposed surface of the eyelid margin, and the knot is placed at the lateral canthus. The ends of the suture are left long (Figure 11.3). Avoidance of inversion of the eyelashes is necessary to avoid further irritation of the ocular surface. If a larger tarsorrhaphy is indicated, then this technique of suture placement may be modified to include more than one suture to oppose the eyelid margins. The great advantage of this technique is that it can be performed easily at the bedside or in the office, is highly adjustable in terms of the amount of occlusion desired, and is more cosmetically acceptable, since it requires no bolsters or sutures visible on the skin.[12]

Decreased corneal exposure, decreased evaporation of the tear film and ptosis can also be achieved by application of a gold weight to the upper eyelid. An initial trial through adhesion of the gold weight to the external skin may demonstrate therapeutic results. Subcutaneous implantation of a gold weight into the upper eyelid is achieved with a minor surgical procedure. A regional nerve block of the upper eyelid is performed using 1% lidocaine. A small subcutaneous pocket is dissected anterior to the tarsus and the gold weight is implanted into the pocket. The subcutaneous tissues and the skin are closed over the weight and the skin sutures are removed in 7 days.[13] The gold weight is easily removed from those patients who recover adequate eyelid function and have resolution of their ocular surface disease.

Conjunctival Flap (Partial, Total)

The purpose of advancement of the conjunctiva over the cornea is to recruit conjunctival vasculature to a non-healing corneal defect, infection, or severe inflammatory focus. Advancement of the conjunctiva over the cornea may be partial (advancement or bucket-handle) or total (Gundersen) depending on the severity of the corneal lesion.

For a peripheral corneal lesion, a partial advancement or bucket-handle conjunctival flap may be indicated. A

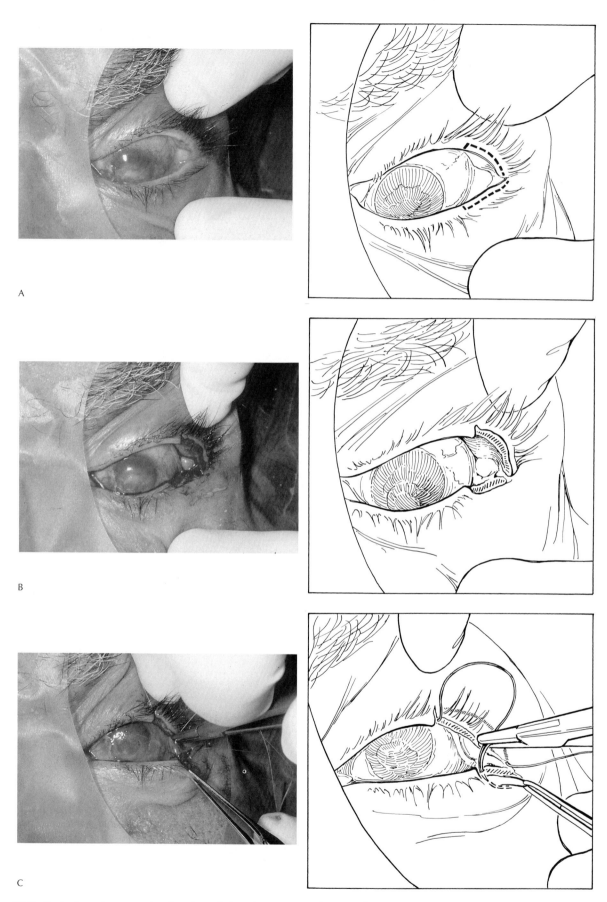

Figure 11.3. Technique for tarsorrhaphy: A. splitting the tarsus at the gray line, B. excision of a strip of posterior lid margin, C. placement of a vertical mattress or figure-eight suture in the tarsus.

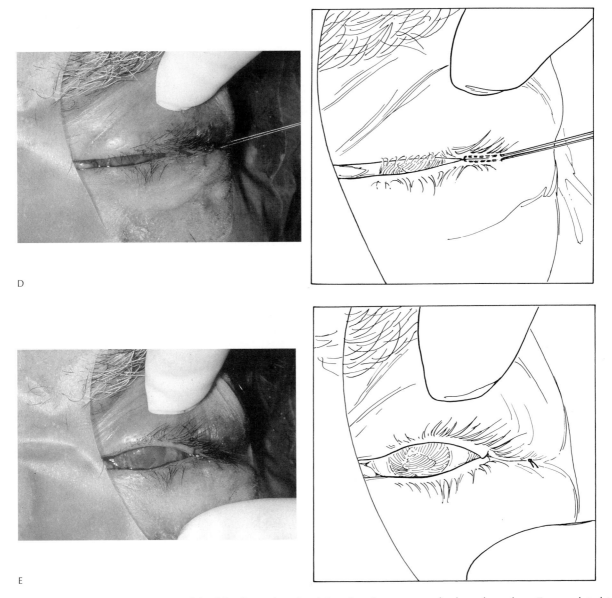

D

E

Figure 11.3. (*Continued*) D. apposition of the bleeding edges by tightening the suture at the lateral canthus, E. completed tarsorrhaphy.

subconjunctival injection of 1% lidocaine with a 30-gauge needle on a tuberculin syringe will provide anesthesia to the conjunctiva and assist in loosening the tissue for the underlying Tenon's capsule. The corneal epithelium must be removed completely from the area intended for conjunctival coverage. The area of conjunctiva is dissected loose from the underlying Tenon's capsule and an advancement of the flap is achieved. Alternatively, a bucket-handle pedicle can be formed and rotated into position to bring a local vascular supply to the peripheral cornea. The pedicle of conjunctiva is advanced over the area of cornea that is free from epithelium, and the conjunctiva is secured to the cornea using 10-0 nylon sutures (Figure 11.4).

In order to cover the cornea completely with a conjunctival flap, a bipedicle or Gundersen flap is necessary.[14,15] Fashioning such a flap requires regional anesthesia. A 360-degree conjunctival peritomy is performed with a Westcott scissors and the corneal epithelium is completely removed by debridement with a 64-Beaver blade. A suture is placed at the superior limbus in order to rotate the eye inferiorly and expose the superior bulbar conjunctiva. An area 15 mm superior to the superior limbus is marked with a gentian violet or methylene blue marker and a linear conjunctival incision is made parallel to the superior corneal limbus. The nasal and temporal bulbar conjunctiva are not incised. The conjunctiva is dissected off the underlying Tenon's

Figure 11.4. Conjunctival advancement flap: A. dissection of the conjunctiva to be advanced, B. advancement flap in position, bucket-handle flap: C. dissection of the conjunctiva to be rotated, D. rotated tissue sutured into position.

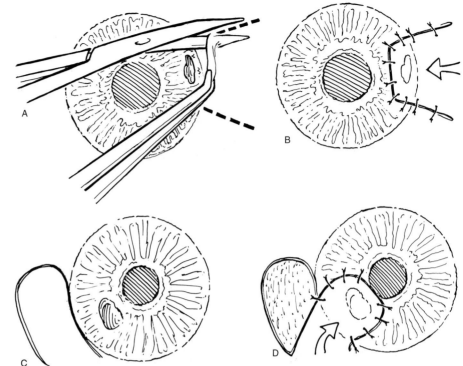

capsule taking extreme care to prevent perforation or creation of a "buttonhole" in the conjunctival flap. The conjunctival flap is then moved inferiorly to cover the cornea (denuded of epithelium) and secured to the corneal limbus with 8-0 polygalactin suture (Figure 11.5). The conjunctival vasculature at the nasal and temporal bulbar aspects of the conjunctival flap are preserved. An acceptable optical and cosmetic result is achieved if there is little Tenon's capsule adherent to the conjunctival flap and the flap is maintained thin. Unfortunately, failure to remove the corneal epithelium completely, or the creation of even a small buttonhole in the thin conjunctival flap, will spell failure, whether from nonadherence to the cornea, or the inevitable enlargement of the buttonhole.

Anterior Stromal Puncture

The technique of anterior stromal puncture was first described by McLean et al. in 1986.[16] Anterior stromal puncture or fixation is a simple technique used for the management of recurrent corneal erosion. It can be employed in post-traumatic, post-infectious, and dystrophic recurrent corneal erosion when medical therapy and/or therapeutic lenses have not been successful in stabilizing the ocular surface.[17] After placement of a topical anesthetic in the eye, the procedure is performed at the slit-lamp using a 25-, 27-, or 30-gauge needle. With direct slit-lamp visualization the ophthalmologist places a grid of anterior stromal punctures. The epithelium need not be intact over the area of the erosion, but care

should be taken to avoid deep penetration into the stroma or possible perforation of the cornea. A bend in the tip of the needle, either manually with a locking needle driver, or commercially pre-bent needles will help prevent deep penetration or perforation of the cornea (Figure 11.6).

Some have recommended the use of the YAG laser for the placement of anterior stromal punctures.[18–20] The mechanism of action of anterior stromal puncture is not simply implantation of nests of epithelium into the stroma to anchor the epithelium and prevent recurrent erosions. Rather, the traumatic rupture of Bowman's layer by the needle tip incites fibroblast transformation of the underlying keratocytes and fibrin deposition to enhance epithelial adhesion to Bowman's layer.[21–23]

Corneal Cautery (Salleras Procedure)

A similar concept of increased adhesion of epithelium through scar formation is the underlying principal of the Salleras procedure—thermal or electrocautery of Bowman's membrane. Originally described by Antonio Salleras, this is an older technique employed primarily in painful bullous keratopathy in cases in which penetrating keratoplasty is not an option.[24,25] Recurrent formation and rupture of the cornea epithelial bullae results in painful corneal erosions and increases the risk of corneal ulcer formation. The Salleras procedure facilitates epithelial adhesion through the formation of subepithelial cicatrix, but compromises corneal clarity. In patients with

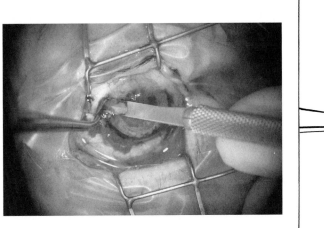
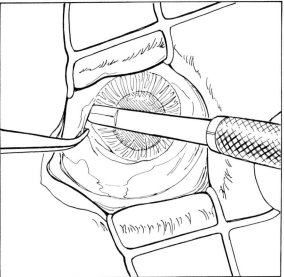

A

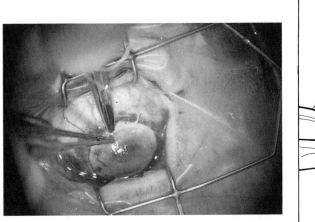
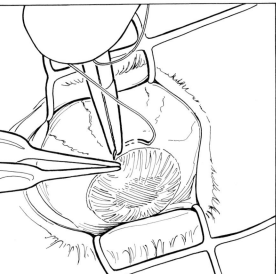

B

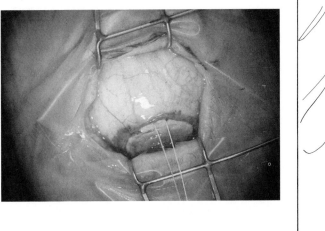
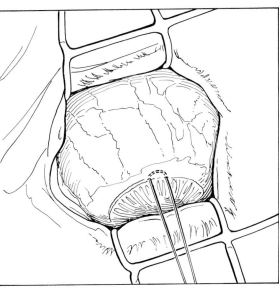

C

Figure 11.5. Gundersen flap technique: A. a 360-degree peritomy is performed at the limbus, B. a traction suture is placed at the superior limbus, C. the traction suture is used to rotate the eye inferiorly.

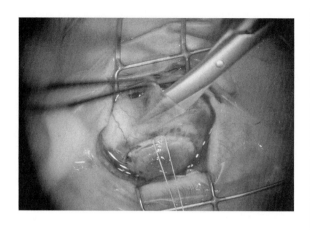

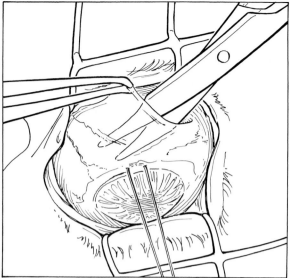

D

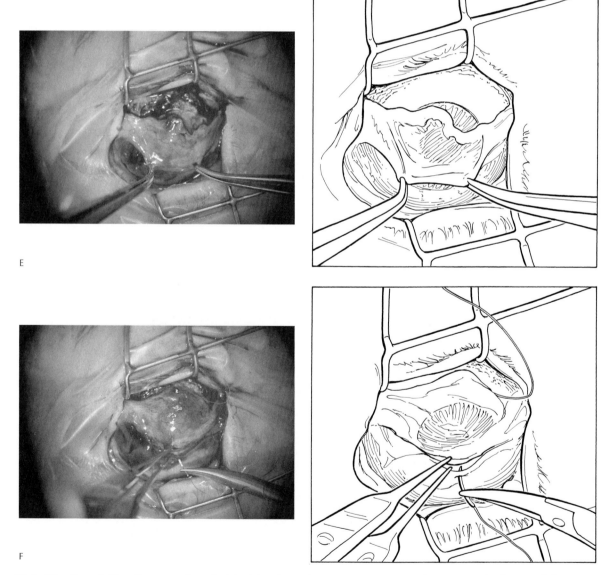

E

F

Figure 11.5. (*Continued*) D. a linear conjunctival incision is made 15 mm superior to the superior limbus, and the conjunctiva is dissected from the underlying Tenon's fascia down to the limbus, E. the bridge flap is positioned over the cornea, F. the flap is sutured into position.

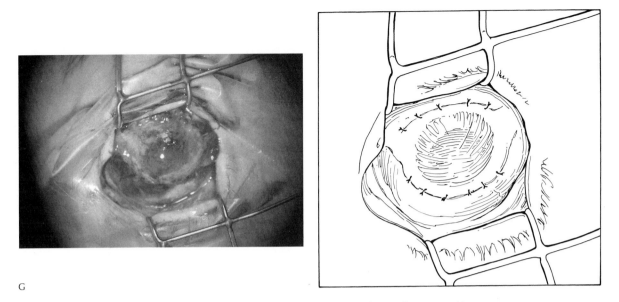

G

Figure 11.5. (*Continued*) G. completed Gundersen flap in position.

Figure 11.6. Anterior stromal puncture: A. the technique of anterior stromal puncture, B. a cornea with recurrent erosion syndrome treated with a grid of stromal punctures.

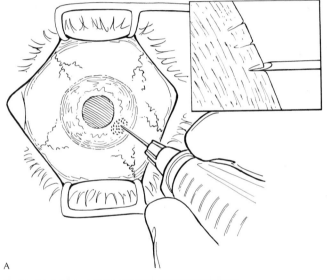

A

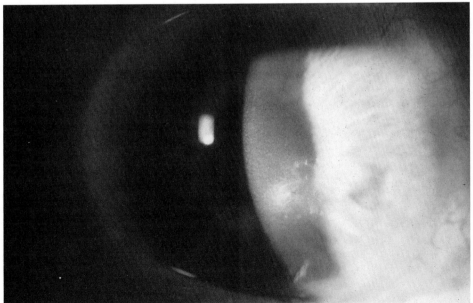

B

little visual potential, this technique may afford comfort and surface stabilization without major surgical intervention. As opposed to anterior stromal puncture, this technique is performed on the corneas after the epithelium has been removed. Under topical anesthesia, at the slit-lamp or under the operating microscope, the corneal epithelium is removed. Corneal cautery is performed using a disposable low-temperature battery-operated handheld cautery unit, or an electrocautery needle similar to that employed in punctal occlusion. The cautery is applied directly to the exposed Bowman's layer until a slight blanching of the surrounding tissue is seen. Frank

shrinkage of the underlying cornea is not necessary to achieve therapeutic results. The cautery marks should be adjacent to one another in the area of treatment, but need not be contiguous (Figure 11.7). Postoperatively, the eye should be treated with a long-acting cycloplegic drop and either patched with antibiotic ointment, or covered with a therapeutic lens until re-epithelialization is complete. The cautery will result in the formation of scar tissue in Bowman's layer with formation of a cicatrix between the epithelium and the underlying tissue. Although the cornea may be partially opacified from this procedure, the resultant stabilization of the corneal surface in an eye

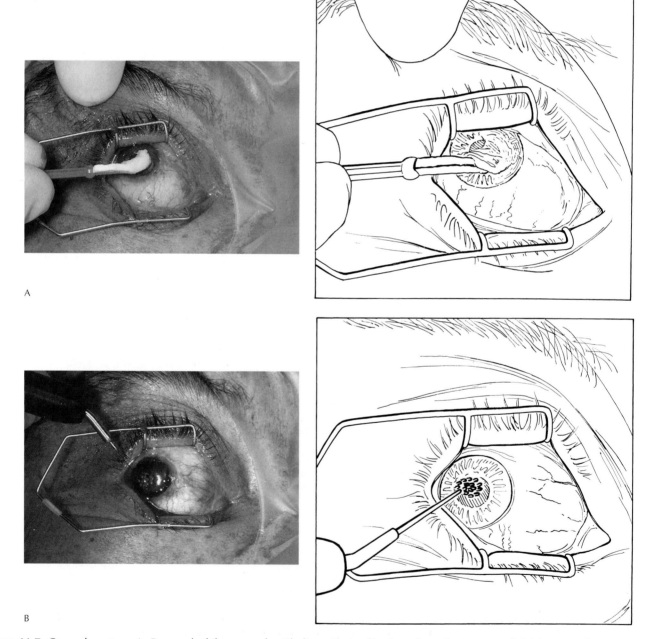

A

B

Figure 11.7. Corneal cautery: A. Removal of the corneal epithelium. B. Application of contiguous superficial burns to Bowman's layer.

with limited visual potential may obviate the need for more invasive surgical procedures.

Superficial Keratectomy

In certain cases of recurrent corneal erosions, the underlying problem is irregularity of the subepithelial tissue.[26,27] Smoothing of the subepithelial surface to enhance epithelial migration may be achieved in a variety of ways. Mechanical debridement of loose epithelium can be performed with a sharp instrument such as a 64 Beaver blade, and the underlying Bowman's layer may be mechanically smoothed. An alternative method involves the use of a rotating diamond burr. At the slit-lamp under topical anesthesia, the loose epithelium is removed. A rotating diamond burr is used to smooth the underlying surface of Bowman's layer. Re-epithelialization may be achieved through pressure patching of the eye or the use of a bandage contact lens. Adequate lubrication and attention to the external adnexa and possible lid disease are crucial to successful re-epithelialization (Figure 11.8).

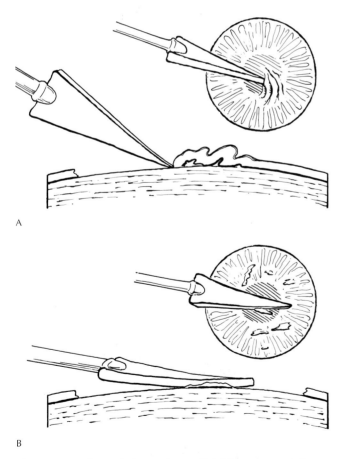

A

B

Figure 11.8. The technique of superficial keratectomy: A. removal of loose epithelium, B. removal of remaining adherent tissue.

Phototherapeutic Keratectomy

Phototherapeutic keratectomy (PTK) is an alternative treatment for recurrent corneal erosions.[28] Studies have demonstrated the efficacy of this technique in both traumatic and dystrophic corneal erosions.[29–34] As opposed to anterior stromal puncture, the epithelium must be removed before the procedure and allowed to repopulate the surface after application of the excimer laser. The mechanism of action of PTK in recurrent erosions is the smoothing of the subepithelial surface to enhance epithelial migration.

Mechanical debridement of the involved area of epithelium is performed under topical anesthesia with the patient in a supine position under the microscope of the excimer laser. Epithelial debridement is accomplished with a 64 Beaver blade, or a dry methylcellulose sponge. An ablation zone 6.5 mm in diameter is treated to an ablation depth of 5 microns in a random pattern to "paint" Bowman's layer, as it were. Care should be taken to avoid performing the ablation in a pattern that could result in a split of the visual axis. After the ablation, a bandage contact lens is applied to the denuded cornea and is left in place until re-epithelialization is complete. Temporary occlusion of the inferior punctum and the use of antibiotic solution that does not inhibit re-epithelialization aid in regeneration of the corneal epithelium. After removal of the contact lens, long-term (6 months) use of hyperosmotic 5% sodium chloride ointment at bedtime will decrease the likelihood of recurrence of the erosion. Comparative studies have demonstrated the efficacy of PTK for recurrent erosions, but due to the increased cost and decreased access to the excimer laser alternative therapies should be tried initially. Nonetheless, when the area of the recurrent erosion involves the visual axis, anterior stromal puncture may result in visually significant scarring and glare. Superficial PTK, as used in recurrent erosions, does not result in significant scar formation. Therefore, in patients with recurrent erosions involving the visual axis, PTK is probably preferable to anterior stromal puncture to decrease the risk of visually significant scarring.

Summary

Numerous surgical techniques exist that may aid in stabilization of the corneal surface. These techniques fall into three categories: (1) techniques that augment lubrication or decrease evaporation, (2) techniques to protect the ocular surface by occlusion, and (3) techniques to foster and stabilize epithelial adherence. These simple surgical techniques are task-specific and should be used as adjunct treatments in conjunction with standard medical therapy. Expansion of the anterior segment surgeon's repertoire to include these techniques will help avoid more invasive surgical intervention to stabilize the ocular surface.

References

1. Dohlman CH. Punctal occlusion in keratoconjunctivitis sicca. *Ophthalmol* 1978; 85:1277–1281.
2. Schwab IR. Keratoconjunctivitis Sicca. In: Abbott RL, ed. *Surgical Intervention in Corneal and External Diseases.* Orlando: Grune & Stratton, Inc., 1987: 51–58.
3. Lamberts DW. Punctal occlusion. *Int Ophthalmol Clin* 1994; 34:145–150.
4. Redmond JW. Punctal occlusion with collagen implants. *Ophthalmic Surg* 1992; 23:642.
5. Patel S, Grierson D. Effect of collagen punctal occlusion on tear stability and volume. *Advances in Experimental Medicine and Biology* 1994; 350:605–608.
6. Patten JT. Punctal occlusion with N-butyl cyanoacrylate tissue adhesive. *Ophthalmic Surg* 1976; 7:24–26.
7. Willis RM, Folberg R, Krachmer JH, Holland EJ. The treatment of aqueous deficiency dry eye with removal punctum plugs. A clinical and impression cytology study. *Opthalmol* 1987; 94:514–518.
8. Benson DR, Hemmady PB, Snyder RW. Efficacy of laser punctal occlusion. *Ophthalmol* 1992; 99:618–621.
9. Hutnik CM, Probst LE. Argon laser punctal therapy versus thermal cautery for the treatment of aqueous deficiency dry eye syndrome. *Can J Ophthalmol* 1998; 33:365–372.
10. Tuberville AW, Frederick WR, Wood TO. Punctal occlusion in tear deficiency syndromes. *Ophthalmol* 1982; 89: 1170–1172.
11. Donnenfeld ED, Perry HD, Nelson DB. Cyanoacrylate temporary tarsorrhaphy in the management of corneal epithelial defects. *Ophthalmic Surg* 1991; 22:591–593.
12. Stamler JF, Tse DT. A simple and reliable technique for permanent lateral tarsorrhaphy. *Arch Ophthalmol* 1990; 108:125–127.
13. Sobol SM, Alward PD. Early gold weight lid implant for rehabilitation of faulty eyelid closure with facial paralysis: an alternative to tarsorrhaphy. *Head and Neck* 1990; 12:149–153.
14. Gundersen T. Conjunctival flaps in the treatment of corneal disease with reference to a new technique of application. *Arch Ophthalmol* 1958; 60:880–888.
15. Sugar HS. The use of Gundersen flaps in the treatment of bullous keratopathy. *Am J Ophthalmol* 1964; 57:977–983.
16. McLean EN, MacRae SM, Rich LF. Recurrent Erosion. Treatment by anterior stromal puncture. *Ophthalmol* 1986; 93:784–787.
17. Rubinfeld R, Laibson PR, Cohen EJ, Arentsen JJ, Eagle RCJ. Anterior stromal puncture for recurrent erosion: further experience and new instrumentation. *Ophthalmic Surg* 1990; 21:318–326.
18. Geggel HS. Successful treatment of recurrent corneal erosion with Nd:YAG anterior stromal puncture. *Am J Ophthalmol* 1990; 110:404–407.
19. Geggel HS, Maza CE. Anterior stromal puncture with the Nd:YAG laser. *Invest Ophthalmol Vis Sci* 1990; 31:1555–1559.
20. Rubinfeld R, MacRae SM, Laibson PR. Successful treatment of recurrent corneal erosion with Nd:YAG anterior stromal puncture. *Am J Ophthalmol* 1991; 111:252–255.
21. Judge D, Payant J, Frase S, Wood TO. Anterior stromal micropuncture electron microscopic changes in the rabbit cornea. *Cornea* 1990; 9:152–160.
22. Hsu JK, Rubinfeld RS, Barry P, Jester JV. Anterior stromal puncture. Immunohistochemical studies in human corneas. *Arch Ophthalmol* 1993; 111:1057–1063.
23. Hashizume N, Saika S, Ooshima A, Yamanaka O, Okada Y, Ohnishi Y. Corneal epithelial basement membrane after experimental anterior stromal puncture in guinea pigs: immunohistochemical study. *Jpn J Ophthalmol* 1997; 41: 376–380.
24. Salleras A. Bullous keratopathy. In: King JHJ, ed. *The Cornea World Congress.* Washington: Butterworths; 1965: 292–295.
25. DeVoe AG. Electrocautery of Bowman's membrane. *Trans Am Ophthalmol Soc* 1966; 64:109–122.
26. Kenyon KR. Recurrent corneal erosion: Pathogenesis and therapy. *Int Ophthalmol Clin* 1979; 19:169–195.
27. Buxton JG, Constad WH. Superficial epithelial keratectomy in the treatment of epithelial membrane dystrophy. *Cornea.* 1987; 6:292–297.
28. Tuli SW, Azar DT, Stark WJ, Binder PS. Recurrent Erosion Syndrome. In: Azar DT, Steinert RF, Stark WJ, eds. *Phototherapeutic Keratectomy: Management of Scars, Dystrophies, and PRK Complications.* Baltimore: Williams & Wilkins; 1997: 133–142.
29. O'Brart DP, Muir MG, Marshall J. Phototherapeutic keratectomy for recurrent corneal erosions. *Eye.* 1994; 8:378–383.
30. Lohmann CP, Sachs H, Marshall J, Gabel VP. Excimer laser phototherapeutic keratectomy for recurrent erosions: a clinical study. *Ophthalmic Surg Lasers* 1996; 27:768–772.
31. Bernauer W, De Cock R, Dart JK. Phototherapeutic keratectomy in recurrent corneal erosions refractory to other forms of treatment. *Eye* 1996; 10:561–564.
32. Cavanaugh TB, Lind DM, Cutarelli PE, et al. Phototherapeutic keratectomy for recurrent erosion syndrome in anterior basement membrane dystrophy. *Ophthalmology* 1999; 106:971–976.
33. Morad Y, Haviv D, Zadok D, Krakowsky D, Hefetz L, Nemet P. Excimer laser phototherapeutic keratectomy for recurrent corneal erosion. *J Cat Refract Surg* 1998; 24: 451–455.
34. Jain S, Austin DJ. Phototherapeutic keratectomy for treatment of recurrent corneal erosion. *J Cataract Ref Surg* 1999; 25:1610–1614.

12
The Evolution and Classification of Ocular Surface Transplantation

Edward J. Holland and Gary S. Schwartz

The management of severe ocular surface disease (OSD) has benefited from major breakthroughs in recent years. Previously, patients with severe ocular surface disease had a poor prognosis. At one time, available techniques for visual rehabilitation consisted of lamellar and penetrating keratoplasty, tarsorrhaphy, and preserved artificial tears. Superficial keratectomy to remove abnormal epithelium typically resulted in reinvasion of the corneal surface with conjunctiva-like cells (conjunctivalization). A penetrating or lamellar keratoplasty resulted in a stable surface only for as long as the donor epithelium was present. However, after the eventual donor epithelial sloughing, the ocular surface failed due to conjunctivalization.

Modern treatment of severe ocular surface disease is quite different. Advances in microsurgical techniques and understanding of the role of the limbal stem cells have led to great improvements in both visual acuity and quality of life for these patients. Progress in this area has occurred in a stepwise fashion. What follows is a chronological review of the major advancements in the treatment of severe OSD.

Evolution of Ocular Surface Transplantation

Conjunctival Transplantation

The first transplantation procedure for severe OSD was described by Thoft in 1977 when he proposed "conjunctival transplantation" for monocular chemical burns.[1] In his procedure, he used several pieces of bulbar conjunctiva from the normal fellow eye (Figure 12.1). This conjunctival autograft procedure was based on the theory of conjunctival transdifferentiation. In two publications, Thoft reported 22 eyes in which 19 obtained an improved ocular surface; however, two subsequent penetrating keratoplasties went on to fail.

Although a conjunctival autograft is useful in re-establishing an intact ocular surface in patients with conjunctival scarring, concerns exist as to whether this procedure truly results in normal corneal epithelium.[2] Tsai et al.[3] compared the results of limbal transplantation and conjunctival transplantation in a rabbit model of OSD. They reported a significant decrease in corneal neovascularization with limbal transplantation and the resultant corneal epithelium displayed the corneal phenotype. Conjunctival transplantation resulted in a corneal epithelium with the phenotype of conjunctiva.

The technique of conjunctival autograft remains a valuable procedure for the management of fornix reconstruction as well as primary and recurrent pterygium. The success of conjunctival transplantation for the establishment of the corneal surface when a source of limbal stem cells is not available remains to be determined.

Keratoepithelioplasty

In 1984, Thoft described the first allograft procedure for the management of severe OSD (Figure 12.2). He called this procedure keratoepithelioplasty (KEP).[4] His procedure involved the use of lenticules of peripheral cornea from a cadaveric donor globe as a source of epithelium. A whole globe was used to obtain four pieces of partial-thickness cornea. Lenticules were carved from the midperipheral cornea and consisted of epithelium and a thin layer (0.2 mm) of stroma that served as a carrier for the delicate epithelium. The four lenticules were placed evenly around the corneoscleral limbus and sutured to the sclera. Limbal cells were not used in this technique. The epithelium from the lenticules spread and covered the recipient cornea.

Because cadaveric eyes, rather than the fellow eye, were used for the donor tissue, this technique was useful in treating patients with bilateral OSD. Four patients were reported in Thoft's study. Three patients had bi-

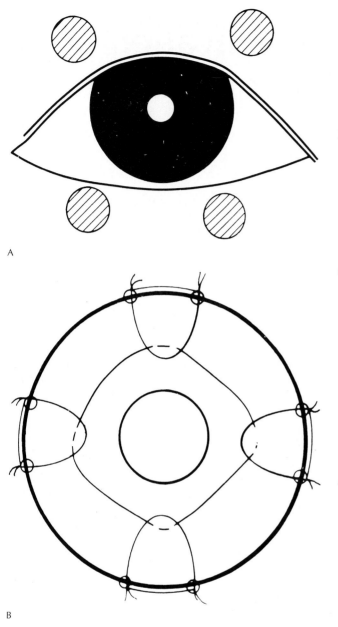

Although Thoft did not describe obtaining limbus with his KEP procedure, since there was not a good understanding of the stem cell theory at that time, it is possible that some stem cells were harvested with the peripheral corneal lenticules. In 1990, Turgeon and co-workers, including Thoft, reported on 13 additional patients managed with KEP.[5] The technique described was modified from Thoft's original procedure to include limbal tissue with the peripheral corneal tissue in an at-

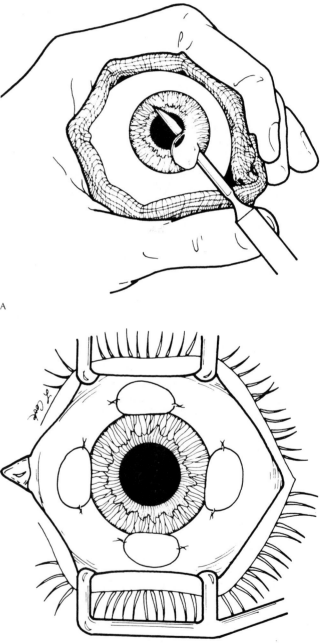

Figure 12.1. Thoft's conjunctival autograft. A. Grafts are taken from uninjured fellow eye in four quadrants from areas normally covered by eyelid. B. Placement of conjunctival grafts. (Reproduced with permission from the *Archives of Ophthalmology.*)

lateral chemical burns, and the fourth had severe atopic keratoconjunctivitis with symblepharon formation and persistent epithelial defects of both corneas. Following keratoepithelioplasty, the three chemical-burn patients developed a stable ocular surface and improved vision. The atopic keratoconjunctivitis patient, however, underwent a penetrating keratoplaty two months after keratoepithelioplasty, and the graft failed secondary to a bacterial infection. The range of follow-up was 9 to 30 months, and the median could not be determined from the data reported.

Figure 12.2. Thoft's keratoepithelioplasty. A. Preparation of lenticules from donor globe. B. Placement of lenticules around the corneoscleral limbus. (Reproduced with permission from the *American Journal of Ophthalmology.*)

tempt to transplant limbal stem cells. Of the 11 patients with at least 6 months' follow-up, 7 had a stable ocular surface, and 7 had improved visual acuity.

Limbal Stem Cell Theory

The single most important breakthrough in managing severe OSD was the understanding of the location and function of the limbal stem cells. In 1971, Davenger and Evenson[6] speculated that the source for replacing the corneal epithelium lay at the limbus when they observed that pigmented limbal cells moved centrally. Schermer and co-workers[7] studied patterns of cornea-specific 64K keratin expression and discovered that the corneal limbus basal cells are less differentiated than those found in other areas of the corneal epithelium.

Cell kinetic studies of the hematopoietic system, intestine, and epidermis indicate that stem cells and transient amplifying cells (TAC) make up the proliferating cells of epithelium.[8,9] Stem cells are present in all self-renewing tissues.[10] They compose a small subpopulation of the total tissue and make up 0.5% to 10% of the total cell population.[11,12] Stem cells are long-lived, have a long cell cycle time, have an increased potential for error-free proliferation with poor differentiation, and demonstrate a capability to divide in an asymmetric manner.[8,13,14] This asymmetric cell division allows one of the daughter cells to remain a stem cell while the other differentiates to become a TAC. The TAC then differentiates into postmitotic cells (PMC), and finally to terminally differentiated cells (TDC). Both the PMC and TDC are incapable of cell division.[13] Schermer and co-workers[7] proposed the cell proliferation scheme for the cornea as follows: limbal basal cells (stem cells) → basal corneal epithelium (TAC) → suprabasal corneal epithelium (TDC).

Cotsarelis and co-workers[15] provided additional evidence that stem cells were located at the limbus when they found that tritiated thymidine was incorporated for long time intervals into limbal basal cells. This labeling indicated that these cells exhibited a long cell cycle. Ebato and associates[16] reported that human ocular limbal epithelial cells grew better in culture and had higher rates of mitotic activity than peripheral corneal epithelial cells.

Many factors must be in balance in order for the limbal stem cells to thrive. The palisades of Vogt pass close to the corneal limbus and likely provide the limbal stem cells with both increased nutrition and greater interaction with blood-borne cytokines.[17] The basement membrane of the limbus is also different from that of the central cornea. There are more anchoring fibrils, a rough undulating surface,[17] and an abundance of type IV collagen.[18]

Understanding the role of the conjunctiva is also important in successfully managing OSD. The bulbar conjunctiva consists of 6 to 9 layers of stratified squamous cells organized in an irregular fashion. The forniceal conjunctival epithelium is 2 to 3 cell layers thick over the superior, and 4 to 5 layers thick over the inferior, tarsus. The normal conjunctival epithelium contains unicellular mucin-secreting goblet cells that account for 5% to 10% of the total number of basal cells. The function of the hydrophilic mucin secreted by the goblet cells is to coat the surface of the otherwise hydrophobic epithelium, thus making it wettable. The exact location of stem cells for conjunctival goblet and nongoblet epithelial cells is not currently known, although studies have shown that they are most likely located in the conjunctival fornices.[19–21]

Limbal Autograft

In 1989, Kenyon and Tseng[22] were the first to take the limbal stem cell theory and apply it clinically. They built on the work of Thoft by modifying his conjunctival autograft surgery to include limbal stem cells. In this way, their procedure was the first to specifically transplant limbal epithelial stem cells for severe OSD. In this procedure, conjunctival and limbal tissue from a normal fellow eye was used to manage diffuse limbal deficiency in unilateral ocular surface disease, or focal limbal deficiency in unilateral or bilateral disease (Figure. 12.3). Their technique used grafts of bulbar conjunctiva that extended approximately 0.5 mm onto the clear cornea centrally, thus containing limbal cells. The authors reported data on 21 cases with 6 months or more of follow-up. Preoperative diagnoses included acute and chronic chemical injuries, thermal injury, contact-lens-induced keratopathy, and iatrogenic limbal stem cell deficiency. The results were impressive with rapid surface healing in 19 cases, stable ocular surface in 20 cases, improved visual acuity in 17 cases, and arrest of regression of corneal neovascularization in 15 cases. No complications developed in the donor eyes. Seven of seven patients underwent simultaneous or subsequent successful penetrating or lamellar keratoplasty.

One major concern is the risk for the fellow eye, which acts as the donor. A recent study has shown that partial removal of full-thickness limbal zone will compromise the donor surface.[23] When a large corneal epithelial defect was subsequently introduced in these eyes, a clinical picture consistent with limbal deficiency occurred. In addition, it has been shown that even the removal of partial-thickness limbal epithelium could cause a milder form of limbal deficiency and abnormal corneal epithelial wound healing.[24]

Keratolimbal Allograft

Tsai and Tseng reported a modification of Thoft's keratoepithelioplasty procedure in 1994.[25] They described an "allograft limbal transplantation" procedure that utilized a whole globe to provide a keratolimbal graft. A

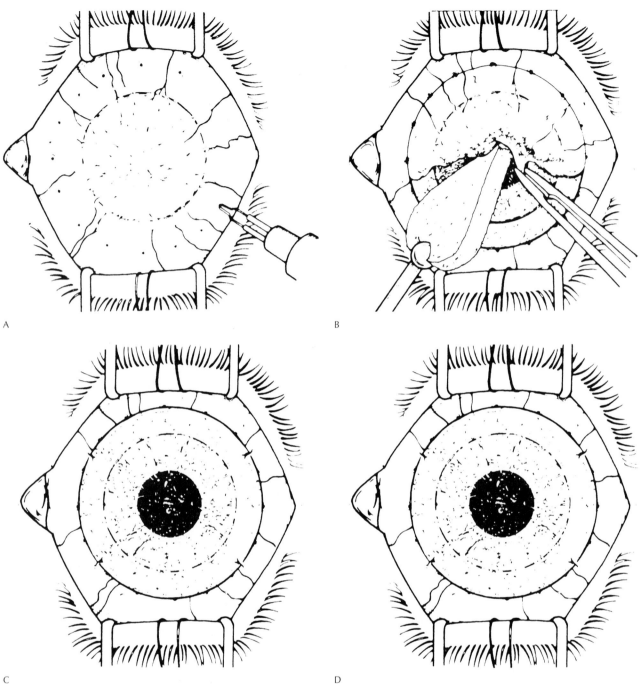

A

B

C

D

Figure 12.3. Kenyon and Tseng's conjunctival autograft. A. Area of bulbar conjunctival to be resected is marked approximately 2 mm posterior to the limbus. B. Abnormal corneal epithelium and fibrovascular pannus are stripped by blunt dissection. C. Additional surface polishing smoothes the stromal surface and improves clarity. D. Superior and inferior limbal autografts are delineated.

suction trephine was used to make mid-peripheral and scleral incisions, resulting in a continuous ring of keratolimbal tissue. The resultant keratolimbal ring was divided into three equal pieces and transferred to the recipient eye. Postoperatively, all patients were treated with oral cyclosporin A (CsA) in addition to topical corticosteroids.

In 1995, Tsubota and colleagues reported a technique they termed "limbal allograft transplantation," another variation of a keratolimbal allograft.[26] Their technique was the first report of using stored corneoscleral rims for stem cell transplantation. By using stored tissue, they afforded patients several days with which to coordinate surgery after acquisition of suitable donor tissue.

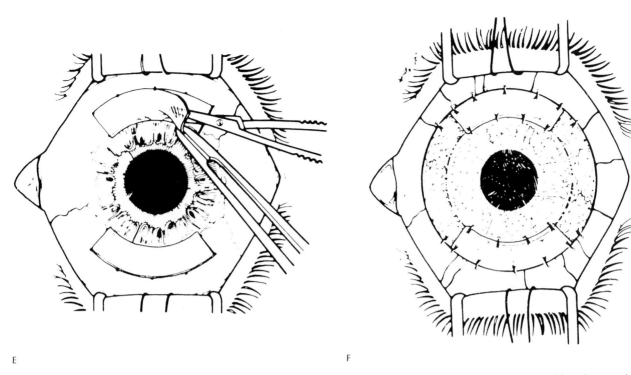

E   F

Figure 12.3. (*Continued*) E. Bulbar conjunctival portion of the autograft is undermined and thinly dissected free from its limbal attachments. F. The limbal autografts are transferred to their corresponding sites in the recipient eye. (Reproduced with permission from *Ophthalmology*.)

To increase the total number of transplanted limbal stem cells, the authors modified Tsubota's technique to utilize two stored corneoscleral rims (Figure 12.4). We transplant three of the four harvested 180-degree crescents to each host eye to accomplish two things. First, we completely surround the host limbus with transplanted tissue, allowing this tissue to act as a barrier to

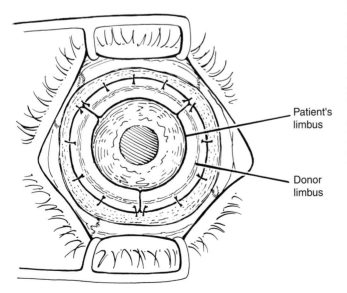

Patient's
limbus

Donor
limbus

Figure 12.4. Schematic diagram of recipient eye with KLAL crescents sutured in place.

block any gap areas through which conjunctival tissue can otherwise migrate. Second, we supply each host eye with 1½ times the transplanted limbal stem cells as it could receive from a single donor eye.[27,28]

Living-Related Conjunctival Allograft

In 1995, Kwitko and co-workers described a technique called allograft conjunctival transplantation.[29] In this report, they were the first to utilize a living relative as a source of donated ocular surface tissue. They harvested conjunctival tissue, and made a specific point of stating that they did not transplant limbal tissue. Donor conjunctiva was obtained from siblings, and if tissue could not be obtained from a sibling, a parent was used.

Kenyon and Rapoza described a technique they called limbal allograft transplantation in which they transplanted limbal tissue with a conjunctival carrier from a living related donor.[30] This technique was similar to Kenyon and Tseng's technique of limbal autograft, except that the donor tissue was obtained from a living relative as opposed to the fellow eye. This technique differs from Kwitko's living related conjunctival allograft technique in that Kenyon and Rapoza transplanted limbal tissue along with conjunctival. Postoperative management included topical corticosteroids in all cases, with topical and/or systemic CsA predominantly for HLA haplo-identical or -incompatible cases. The use of oral CsA ranged from 3 to 34 months with a mean of 11.25 months for those treated.

Human Amniotic Membrane Transplantation

Further strategies to reconstruct the ocular surface have included the use of human amniotic-membrane transplantation (AMT). AMT had been previously used for dermal burns and as a means to prevent tissue adhesion in abdominal, pelvic, vaginal, and oral surgery. De Rotth, in 1940, described the use of amniotic membrane for the repair of conjunctival defects and symblepharon.[31] In 1995, Kim and Tseng used amniotic membrane for ocular surface reconstruction in a rabbit model of OSD.[32] In their studies, they demonstrated that AMT facilitated epithelialization without allowing host fibrovascular ingrowth onto the membrane, and suggested that this procedure might be clinically useful for ocular surface reconstruction.

Following on this work, in 1996 Tsubota and co-workers were the first to reconstruct human eyes with severely diseased ocular surfaces and limbal deficiency utilizing AMT.[33] They combined AMT with a limbal stem cell allograft in 14 eyes of 11 patients with Stevens–Johnson syndrome and ocular cicatricial pemphigoid.

Human amniotic-membrane transplantation is useful in conjunction with epithelial transplantation because it promotes epithelial growth without fibrovascular growth and reduces ocular surface inflammation.[34] It supports differentiation of epithelial cells, is nonantigenic, and is resorbed in vivo.[35] However, one must bear in mind that, when a true limbal stem cell deficiency exists, AMT should not be performed alone as an alternative to limbal stem cell transplantation.

Ex Vivo Expansion of Limbal Stem Cells

In 1997, Pellegrini and co-workers described a procedure using autologous cultivated corneal epithelium to restore the ocular surfaces of two patients with unilateral alkali injury.[36] They based their procedure on tissue culture work that had been done by Lindberg and co-workers in 1993.[37] Pellegrini's group used a 1–2 mm^2 full-thickness limbal specimen from the healthy fellow eye to create sheets of corneal epithelial cells in tissue culture. These epithelial sheets were then transplanted to the injured eye. Both patients were followed for more than two years, and both retained a stable ocular surface, implying that stem cells had been transplanted. One patient went on to have PK and obtained visual acuity of 20/30. Because this procedure represents an autograft technique, these patients were not treated with systemic immunosuppression.

In 2000, Tsai and co-workers[38] and Schwab and co-workers[39] separately published their results using ex vivo expanded limbal stem cells grown on human amniotic membrane. Tsai's group expanded limbal epithelium on human amniotic membrane prepared as described by Lee and Tseng,[40] and six eyes of six patients showed epithelialization within four days. Patients were followed for a minimum of one year; 5 patients obtained 20/50 vision or better, and the sixth, an alkali-injury patient with stromal scarring, achieved 20/200 vision.

Schwab's group grew harvested limbal stem cells on human amniotic membrane that had been denuded of native epithelium in a technique described by Schwab the previous year.[41] Seven patients had OSD from limbal stem cell deficiency, and 7 patients had "other corneal surface disease" such as CIN and recurrent pterygium. Four of the limbal stem cell deficiency patients received ex vivo expanded tissue derived from a living relative, while the other 3 received tissue derived from their fellow eye. Minimum follow-up for these patients was 6 months. All allograft patients received oral and topical cyclosporin A during the postoperative period. The ocular surface reconstruction was considered successful in all allograft patients, and in one of the three autograft patients. One allograft patient with alkali injury subsequently underwent successful penetrating keratoplasty.

Systemic Immunosuppression

Another important advancement in the evolution of ocular surface transplantation is the use of systemic immunosuppression. Ocular surface failure following limbal stem cell transplantation tends to fall within one of three clinical presentations.[27,42] First, patients who have a severely inflamed ocular surface, such as a recent chemical injury, or Stephens–Johnson syndrome with persistent inflammation, can demonstrate a marked increase in inflammation during the immediate postoperative period that causes destruction of the transplanted cells. This reaction is not truly "rejection" in the classic sense; rather, it represents direct damage of the transplanted cells from the high level of inflammation present in the host eye. Second, there is the patient who has minimal preoperative inflammation, but who develops an acute allograft rejection reaction seen as intense injection at the graft-host junction and subsequent conjunctivalization of the ocular surface in the area of the rejection. An epithelial rejection line can sometimes be seen in these cases. The third type of failure is seen in patients who appear to have a successful KLAL with the appearance of healthy epithelium. They then go on to develop a gradual, progressive conjunctivalization, either sectorally or completely, without evidence of increase in inflammation. This reaction represents either chronic, low-grade rejection, or stem cell exhaustion. The reason for failure cannot be determined by clinical examination; rather, it will probably require histologic study.[42]

The first two presentations are secondary to inflammation, and the third occurs for unknown reasons, possibly immunologic. Therefore, it is imperative that all patients be treated aggressively with immunosuppression following limbal stem cell transplantation for severe OSD. The ophthalmologist must remember that transplanting limbal stem cells differs greatly from transplanting a corneal button for a penetrating keratoplasty. The fundamental difference lies in the fact that during PK, avascular corneal tissue, with a relatively low presence of antigen, is transplanted into an avascular recipient bed. Limbal tissue, however, with its preponderance of Langerhans cells, has a much higher presence of antigen than central corneal tissue.

We believe the use of systemic immunosuppression significantly improves the outcomes of ocular surface allograft procedures. Evaluation of our data of 62 patients who had undergone limbal stem cell allograft found that patients who received systemic immunosuppression demonstrated statistically significant improvement when compared to those not receiving systemic immunosuppression.[43] Rao and co-workers reported 9 eyes of 8 patients who underwent living-related conjunctival limbal allograft. All received the best HL-A match available. Systemic immunosuppression was not used, and all ocular surfaces went on to fail. The authors felt that the cause of ocular surface failure was secondary to immune-mediated rejection.[44] Daya recently presented a series of patients with living-related conjunctival limbal allograft. He described 10 eyes of 8 patients. All received the best HL-A match available, and all received systemic immunosuppression. Eight eyes survived.[45]

Our current immunosuppression protocol consists of a combination of topical and systemic agents. The specific regimen will be discussed in detail in Chapter 22 of this text.

Classification of Ocular Surface Transplantation

As described above, a variety of techniques have been reported for surgical repair for the management of severe OSD. Multiple terms have been used in previous studies, including conjunctival transplantation,[1] autologous conjunctival transplantation,[46] allograft conjunctival transplantation,[29] limbal conjunctival autograft,[47] limbal transplantation,[48] limbal allograft transplantation,[26,30] homotransplantation of limbal stem cells,[12] keratoepithelioplasty,[4,49] and allograft limbal transplantation.[25]

All of the procedures share the common goal of stabilization of the ocular surface. Although the different techniques have similar goals, they vary based on the source of the donor tissue, and whether the procedure is primarily a conjunctival or a limbal transplantation. Limbal transplantation procedures also vary depending on the carrier tissue used for the transfer of the limbal stem cells. Carrier tissue is needed in limbal transplantation because it is not technically possible to transfer limbal stem cells alone.

The source of donor tissue for epithelial transplantation can be the fellow eye (autograft), a cadaveric whole globe (allograft), a cadaveric corneoscleral rim (allograft), or a living relative (allograft). Conjunctival transplants transfer conjunctiva only. Limbal transplants, on the other hand, utilize either conjunctiva or cornea as a carrier tissue for fragile limbal stem cells. What follows is a classification of surgical procedures for the treatment of OSD based on the source of donor tissue, the carrier tissue employed, and whether the procedure is a conjunctival transplant or a limbal transplant (Table 12.1).[50]

Conjunctival transplantation procedures can be either autografts or allografts, depending on the source of donor tissue. A conjunctival autograft (CAU) utilizes tissue from the fellow eye. A conjunctival allograft can utilize donor tissue from a cadaver or living relative and be designated as a cadaveric conjunctival allograft (c-CAL) or living related conjunctival allograft (lr-CAL).

Limbal transplantation procedures can be subdivided based on the donor and the carrier tissue. A conjunctival limbal autograft (CLAU) utilizes tissue from the fellow eye, and conjunctiva is the carrier. A cadav-

Table 12.1. Classification for surgical procedures for the management of severe OSD.

Procedure	Abbrev.	Donor	Transplanted tissue
Conjunctival transplantation			
Conjunctival autograft	CAU	fellow eye	Conjunctiva
Living-related conjunctival allograft	lr-CAL	living relative	Conjunctiva
Limbal transplantation			
Conjunctival limbal autograft	CLAU	fellow eye	Limbus/conjunctiva
Cadaveric conjunctival limbal allograft	c-CLAL	cadaveric whole globe	Limbus/conjunctiva
Living-related conjunctival limbal allograft	lr-CLAL	living relative	Limbus/conjunctiva
Keratolimbal allograft	KLAL	cadaveric stored tissue	Limbus/cornea
Ex vivo expanded limbal autograft	EVELAU	fellow eye	Ex vivo expanded limbal cells
Living-related ex vivo expanded limbal allograft	lr-EVELAL	living relative	Ex vivo expanded limbal cells
Amniotic membrane transplantation	AMT	Stored human amniotic membrane	Human amniotic membrane

eric conjunctival limbal allograft (c-CLAL) utilizes a cadaveric donor for conjunctiva and limbus. A living related conjunctival limbal allograft (lr-CLAL) is a procedure in which a living relative donates conjunctiva and limbal tissue. A keratolimbal allograft (KLAL) utilizes a cadaveric donor, and peripheral cornea is used to transfer the limbal stem cells.

Ex vivo expanded limbal transplantation is the newest technique to provide a source of donor limbal tissue. Using this technology, limbal tissue from a donor is expanded in culture prior to transplantation. In ex vivo expanded limbal autograft (EVELAU), the source of tissue is the patient's own limbal stem cells. In living-related ex vivo expanded limbal allograft (lr-EVELAL), the source of tissue is the limbus of a living relative.

Amniotic membrane is harvested from human placenta. This tissue can be stored frozen for extended periods of time. Amniotic membrane provides basement membrane and can be used for conjunctival replacement, or as an adjunct to limbal stem cell transplantation. This tissue provides substrate for epithelial growth without providing epithelial stem cells.

The choice of which procedure is best for an OSD patient is dependent on preoperative diagnosis, laterality and severity of disease, and availability of a living related donor. The role of these factors in selection of the appropriate surgical technique is discussed fully elsewhere in this text.

References

1. Thoft RA. Conjunctival transplantation. *Arch Ophthalmol* 1977; 95:1425–1427.
2. Kruse FE, Chen JJ, Tsai RJ, et al. Conjunctival transdifferentiation is due to incomplete removal of limbal basal epithelium. *Invest Ophthalmol Vis Sci* 1990; 31:1903–1913.
3. Tsai RJ-F, Sun T-T, Tseng SCG. Comparison of limbal and conjunctival autograft transplantation in corneal surface reconstruction in rabbits. *Ophthalmology* 1990; 97:446–455.
4. Thoft RA. Keratoepithelioplasty. *Am J Ophthalmol* 1984; 97:1–6.
5. Turgeon PW, Nauheim RC, Roat MI, et al. Indications for keratoepithelioplasty. *Arch Ophthalmol* 1990; 108:33–36.
6. Davanger M, Evensen A. Role of the pericorneal papillary structure in renewal of corneal epithelium. *Nature* 1971; 229:560–561.
7. Schermer S, Galvin S, Sun T-T. Differentiation-related expression of a major 64K corneal keratin in vivo and in culture suggests limbal location of corneal epithelial stem cells. *J Cell Biol* 1986; 103:49–62.
8. Lathja LG. Stem cell concepts. *Differentiation* 1979; 14:23–34.
9. Kinoshita S, Friend J, Thoft RA. Biphasic cell proliferation in transdifferentiation of conjunctival to corneal epithelium in rabbits. *Invest Ophthalmol Vis Sci* 1983; 24:1008–1014.
10. Potten CS, Loeffler M. Epidermal cell proliferation. I. Changes with time in the proportion of isolated, paired, and clustered labeled cells in sheets of murine epidermis. *Virchows Arch* [B] 1987; 53:286–300.
11. Potten CS, Morris RJ. Epithelial stem cells in vivo. *J Cell Sci* 1988; 10(suppl):45–62.
12. Pfister RR. Corneal stem cell disease; concepts, categorization, and treatment by auto- and homotransplantation of limbal stem cells. *CLAO J* 1994; 20:64–72.
13. Leblond CP. The life history of cells in renewing systems. *Am J Anat* 1981; 160:114–158.
14. Potten CS. Epithelial proliferative subpopulations. *Stem Cells and Tissue Homeostasis*. Cambridge University Press, 1978, p. 317.
15. Cotsarelis G, Dong G, Sun T-T, et al. Differential response of limbal and corneal epithelial to phorbol myristate acetate (TPA). *Invest Ophthalmol Vis Sci* 1987; 28(suppl):1.
16. Ebato B, Friend J, Thoft RA. Comparison of limbal and peripheral human corneal epithelium in tissue culture. *Invest Ophthalmol Vis Sci* 1988; 29:1533–1537.
17. Zieske JD. Perpetuation of stem cells in the eye. *Eye* 1994; 8:163–169.
18. Kolega J, Manabe M, Sun T-T. Basement membrane heterogeneity and variation in corneal epithelial differentiation. *Differentiation* 1989; 42:54–63.
19. Wei ZG, Sun T-T, Lavker RM. Rabbit conjunctival and corneal epithelial cells belong to two separate lineages. *Invest Ophthalmol Vis Sci* 1996; 37:523–533.
20. Wei ZG, Wu RL, Lavker RM, Sun T-T. In vitro growth and differentiation of rabbit bulbar, fornix, and palpebral conjunctival epithelia. Implications on conjunctival epithelial transdifferentiation and stem cells. *Invest Ophthalmol Vis Sci* 1993; 34:1814–1828.
21. Lavker RM, Wei ZG, Sun T-T. Phorbol ester preferentially stimulates mouse forniceal conjunctival and limbal epithelial cells to proliferate in vivo. *Invest Ophthalmol Vis Sci* 1998; 39:301–307.
22. Kenyon KR, Tseng SCG. Limbal autograft transplantation for ocular surface disorders. *Ophthalmology* 1989; 96:709–723.
23. Chen JJ, Tseng SC. Corneal epithelial wound healing in partial limbal epithelium. *Invest Ophthalmol Vis Sci* 1990; 31:1301–1314.
24. Chen JJ, Tseng SC. Abnormal corneal epithelial wound healing in partial thickness removal of limbal epithelium. *Invest Ophthalmol Vis Sci* 1991; 32:2219–2233.
25. Tsai RJF, Tseng SCG. Human allograft limbal transplantation for corneal surface reconstruction. *Cornea* 1994; 13:389–400.
26. Tsubota K, Toda I, Saito H, et al. Reconstruction of the corneal epithelium by limbal allograft transplantation for severe ocular surface disorders. *Ophthalmology* 1995; 102:1486–1495.
27. Holland EJ. Epithelial transplantation for the management of severe ocular surface disease. *Trans Am Ophthalmol Soc* 1996; 19:677–743.
28. Croasdale CR, Schwartz GS, Malling JV, Holland EJ. Keratolimbal allograft: recommendations for tissue procurement and preparation by eye banks, and standard surgical technique. *Cornea* 1999; 18:52–58.
29. Kwitko S, Raminho D, Barcaro S, et al. Allograft conjunc-

tival transplantation for bilateral ocular surface disorders. *Ophthalmology* 1995; 102:1020–1025.

30. Kenyon KR, Rapoza PA. Limbal allograft transplantation for ocular surface disorders. *Ophthalmology* 1995; 102 (suppl):101–102.

31. De Rotth A. Plastic repair of conjunctival defects with fetal membrane. *Arch Ophthalmol* 1940; 23:522–525.

32. Kim JC, Tseng SCG. Transplantation of preserved human amniotic membrane for surface reconstruction in severely damaged rabbit corneas. *Cornea* 1995; 14:473–484.

33. Tsubota K, Satake Y, Ohyama M, et al. Surgical reconstruction of the ocular surface in advanced ocular cicatricial pemphigoid and Stevens–Johnson syndrome. *Am J Ophthalmology* 1996; 122(1):38–52.

34. Tseng SC, Prabhasawat P, Barton K, Gray T, Meller D. Amniotic membrane transplantation with or without limbal allografts for corneal surface reconstruction in patients with limbal stem cell deficiency. *Arch Ophthalmol* 1998; 116:431–441.

35. Schwab IR, Isseroff RR. Bioengineered corneas—the promise and the challenge (ed). *N Engl J Med* 2000; 343:136–138.

36. Pellegrini G, Traverso CE, Franzi AT, et al. Long-term restoration of damaged corneal surfaces with autologous cultivated corneal epithelium. *Lancet* 1997; 349:990–993.

37. Lindberg KL, Brown ME, Chaves HV, et al. In vitro propagation of human ocular surface epithelial cells for transplantation. *Invest Ophthalmol Vis Sci* 1993; 34:2672–2679.

38. Tsai RJ-F, Li L-M, Chen J-K. Reconstruction of damaged corneas by transplantation of autologous limbal epithelial cells. *N Engl J Med* 2000; 343:86–93.

39. Schwab IR, Reyes M, Isseroff RR. Successful transplantation of bioengineered tissue replacements in patients with ocular surface disease. *Cornea* 2000; 19(4):421–426.

40. Lee SH, Tseng SCG. Amniotic membrane transplantation for persistent epithelial defects with ulceration. *Am J Ophthalmol* 1991; 123:303–312.

41. Schwab IR. Cultured corneal epithelia for ocular surface disease. *Tr Am Ophth Soc* 1999 SCVII:891–986.

42. Holland EJ, Schwartz GS. Epithelial stem-cell transplantation for severe ocular surface disease, editorial. *N Engl J Med* 1999; 340(22):1752–1753.

43. Djalilian AR, Bagheri MM, Schwartz GS, et al. Keratolimbal allograft for the treatment of limbal stem cell deficiency. Presented at Scientific Program at Castroviejo Cornea Society, Orlando, FL, October 23, 1999.

44. Rao SK, Rajagopal R, Sitalakshmi G, Padmanabhan P. Limbal allografting from related live donors for corneal surface reconstruction. *Ophthalmology* 1999; 106(4):822–828.

45. Daya SM, Living-related conjunctivo-limbal allograft (lr-CLAL) for the treatment of stem cell deficiency: an analysis of long-term outcome. *Ophthalmology* 1999; 106(10) suppl, p. 243.

46. Vastine DW, Stewart WB, Schwab IR. Reconstruction of the periocular mucous membrane by autologous conjunctival transplantation. *Ophthalmology* 1982; 89:1072–1081.

47. Ronk JF, Ruiz-Esmenjaud S, Osorio M, et al. Limbal conjunctival autograft in a subacute alkaline corneal burn. *Cornea* 1994; 13:465–468.

48. Jenkins C, Tuft S, Liu C, et al. Limbal transplantation in the management of chronic contact-lens-associated epitheliopathy. *Eye* 1993; 7:629–633.

49. Turgeon PW, Nauheim RC, Roat MI, et al. Indications for keratoepithelioplasty. *Arch Ophthalmol* 1990; 108:233–236.

50. Holland EJ, Schwartz GS. The evolution of epithelial transplantation for severe ocular surface disease and a proposed classification system. *Cornea* 1996; 15(6):549–556.

13
Preoperative Staging of Disease Severity

Gary S. Schwartz, José A.P. Gomes, and Edward J. Holland

Introduction

Diseases that affect the ocular surface are multifactorial and present different stages of severity. Choice of treatment and visual prognosis are dependent upon a wide variety of factors. The most important features to consider in evaluating these patients include the degree of limbal stem cell (SC) loss, the extent of conjunctival disease, and presence and etiology of conjunctival inflammation. Other contributing factors include tear film abnormalities, the presence or absence of keratinization, eyelid abnormalities, laterality of disease, and the general health and age of the patient. The additional need for subsequent penetrating or lamellar keratoplasty will also affect the likelihood of successful ocular surface and visual rehabilitation.

Because so many factors will determine not only a patient's symptomatology, but also the choice of treatment and prognosis for success, it is important to establish a preoperative staging system that defines disease severity based on these critical factors. If we are going to recommend appropriate treatment and suitably evaluate outcomes, it is imperative that patients from one staging group be compared to patients within the same group. For example, it is well understood that patients with active conjunctival inflammation and total limbal stem cell deficiency, as is seen in severe Stevens–Johnson syndrome (SJS), will have a much worse prognosis than patients with total stem cell deficiency without conjunctival involvement, such as in aniridia.[1,2] Not only will the SJS patient have more significant symptoms on presentation, but he or she will have less likelihood of successful ocular surface and visual rehabilitation. In addition, both of these patients will have more significant disease than the patient with only partial limbal stem cell deficiency and no conjunctival involvement, as in iatrogenic limbal stem cell deficiency.

When reviewing the literature, it is imperative to consider these preoperative factors in order to compare the efficacy of one surgical management with another appropriately. For example, let us compare two studies that appeared in the *New England Journal of Medicine* thirteen months apart. In June of 1999, Tsubota and colleagues described their results for 43 eyes of 39 patients with severe ocular surface disease using a technique of keratolimbal allograft (KLAL).[3] The source of tissue in all cases was a single cadaver globe. They noted that 22 of 43 eyes (51%) achieved corneal epithelialization and mean visual acuity improved to 0.02 (20/1000). Thirteen months later, in July of 2000, Tsai and co-workers described their results on 6 eyes of 6 patients using transplantation of autologous ex vivo expanded limbal stem cells (EVELAU) that had been grown on human amniotic membrane.[4] Their results showed complete epithelization of all six eyes within four days of transplantation. Five of 6 patients' final visual acuity averaged 20/45, and the remaining patient with an opaque cornea improved from counting fingers to 20/200.

A quick read of these two studies would seem to demonstrate that Tsai's EVELAU procedure is far superior to Tsubota's KLAL. However, a more careful evaluation of the patients enrolled in these two reports shows that this conclusion cannot be drawn based upon these two studies alone. Tsubota's study evaluated 39 patients. Twenty-five patients had SJS or ocular cicatricial pemphigoid (OCP) and 14 patients had chemical or thermal injury. All patients in Tsubota's study had abnormal conjunctiva, and 25 of the 39 patients (64%) had a diagnosis consistent with chronic, active conjunctival inflammation. It is well known that these disease entities carry the worst prognosis for ocular surface rehabilitation, and 50% success in these classes of patients can be considered exceptional.[5]

In contrast, Tsai's study included only 6 cases, and none had either SJS or OCP. One patient had "congenital pterygium," one had "pseudo-pterygium," one had phlyctenular disease, two had partial limbal deficiency from chem-

158

ical burns, and one had total limbal deficiency from a chemical burn. Tsai's patients had significantly milder forms of ocular surface disease than Tsubota's and demonstrated a greater likelihood of re-epithelization and ocular surface stabilization regardless of the chosen treatment. It is also difficult to compare these two studies because of the vast difference in patients enrolled in them. For these reasons, it is impossible to compare these two techniques based solely on these two articles. It is imperative that clinicians consider disease severity when comparing studies involving different surgical procedures; otherwise, they may inadvertently arrive at conclusions not truly supported by the results.

What follows is a discussion of the preoperative factors one must consider when evaluating severe ocular surface disease (OSD) patients. This chapter concludes with a system for staging ocular surface disease patients.

Preoperative Factors for Staging Disease Severity

Laterality of Disease

The most significant preoperative factor of visual function and quality of life is laterality of disease. Patients with unilateral disease, no matter how severe in the affected eye, have the opportunity for normal vision in the fellow eye. These patients, therefore, suffer less morbidity from their disease than do patients with bilateral disease and often do not need to undergo surgery to restore driving or reading vision.

Many patients with monocular disease will opt to undergo surgery to restore binocular vision for treatment of a chronically painful or cosmetically unacceptable diseased eye (Figure 13.1). For these patients, the normal fellow eye serves as a potential source of stem cells for transplantation to the diseased one, thereby potentially eliminating the need for an allograft. One autograft is preferred over an allograft for two important reasons. First, patients undergoing autograft do not need to be placed on systemic immunosuppression and thus avoid the potential serious complications associated with these medications. Second, autograft patients do not carry the risk of graft rejection, which is the principal cause of limbal stem cell graft failure.

Extent of Limbal Stem Cell Deficiency

Severity of disease is dependent upon the extent of limbal stem cell deficiency. Patients with partial loss of the limbal stem cells typically have a better prognosis than those with total loss. If there are residual normal stem cells, there is an opportunity for ocular surface rehabilitation without the need for transplantation. Patients with partial stem cell deficiency may be treated successfully with medical management or sequential conjunctival epitheliectomy with or without amniotic membrane transplantation (Chapters 14 and 20). Patients with more extensive stem cell deficiency cannot populate their corneal surfaces with remaining stem cells and most often require limbal stem cell transplantation to restore a healthy ocular surface. In this way, patients with sectoral epitheliopathy from iatrogenic limbal stem cell deficiency or partial chemical injury have treatment options unavailable to the aniridic patient with total limbal stem cell deficiency, and thus have a better chance for ocular surface stabilization with less invasive treatment.

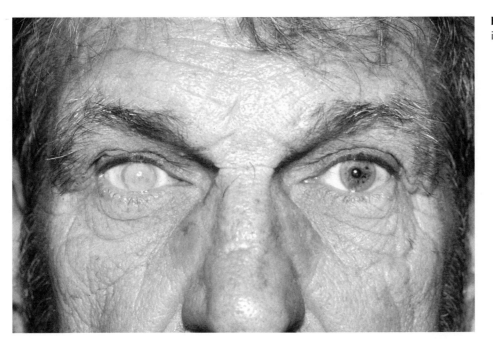

Figure 13.1. Unilateral chemical injury.

Extent of Conjunctival Disease

The most severe forms of OSD occur when limbal stem cell disease occurs in combination with conjunctival disease. A normally functioning conjunctiva is essential for a properly functioning limbus and corneal surface. Therefore, in patients with combined limbal and conjunctival disease, all of the problems encountered in limbal deficiency will be present and compounded by the conjunctival epithelial and goblet cell deficiency. Mucin tear deficiency, subepithelial fibrosis, symblepharon, ankyloblepharon, foreshortening of the conjunctival fornix, and, in the most severe cases, keratinization of the entire surface are all manifestations of conjunctival disease. Each will worsen the symptomatology, prognosis, and likelihood for surgical success in severe OSD patients.

For example, a patient with aniridia has a total limbal stem cell deficiency with a normal conjunctiva, while a patient with a severe alkali injury has a total limbal stem cell deficiency with extensively diseased conjunctiva (Figure 13.2). Not only will the alkali-injury patient be more symptomatic on presentation, but the chance for successful ocular surface rehabilitation will be greatly reduced regardless of which surgical procedure is chosen. The presence of conjunctival disease not only limits the treatment options, but also increases the chance for stem cell failure from immunologic as well as nonimmunologic reasons.

Etiology of Conjunctival Inflammation

The next important contributing factor is the nature of the patient's conjunctival disease. A strong distinction exists between patients with abnormal conjunctiva from prior inflammation and patients who currently have active inflammation. Patients with active conjunctival inflammation have more immune mediators and cells in their ocular surfaces. These agents can exacerbate postoperative inflammation after stem cell transplantation, thus increasing the risk for transplant failure. If possible, preoperative management of these patients includes postponement of surgery until inflammation can be controlled through topical and systemic medications. Postponing surgery is especially important for alkali- and acid-injured patients whose conjunctival inflammation will decrease with time, especially if treated with a regimen of anti-inflammatory medications (Figure 13.3).

Patients with active autoimmune disease, such as OCP and SJS may have persistent inflammation despite systemic immunosuppression. Although alkali- and acid-injured patients will eventually quiet over time, SJS and OCP patients typically have chronic active inflammation that may last for years (Figure 13.4).[6,7] This inflammation likely leads to progression of the limbal stem cell deficiency with further loss of stem cells from direct injury from inflammatory agents. In addition, it is this inflammation that places these patients in the worst prognostic group, because the inflamed eye does not provide a stable environment for the transplanted limbal stem cells.

Reflex Tearing

Treating severe dry eye is critical to the success of ocular surface reconstruction, especially for OCP and SJS patients. In addition to lubrication, tears supply important components for corneal and conjunctival epithelial

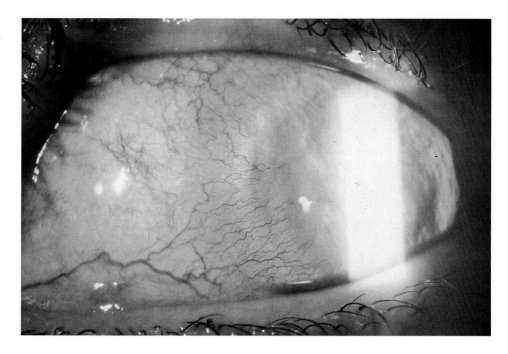

Figure 13.2. Aniridic keratopathy patient has conjunctivalization of cornea, but a relatively healthy conjunctiva.

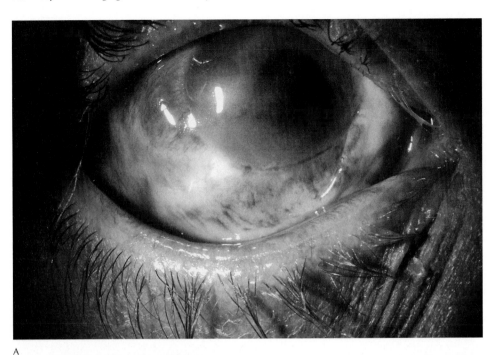

A

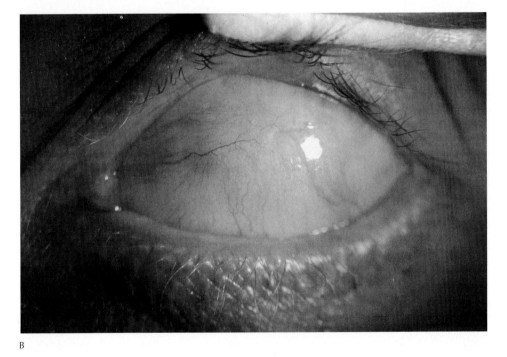

B

Figure 13.3. Acute acid injury. A. Notice active conjunctival inflammation. B. Ten-year-old alkali injury. Although there is total conjunctivalization and opacification of cornea, the eye is relatively uninflamed.

cells, such as epidermal growth factor, electrolytes, and vitamin A. Most non-Sjögren's type dry-eye patients can produce reflex tears in response to nasal stimulation, even though they may have nonstimulated Schirmer test results of 0 mm.[8] Tsubota and co-workers considered patients to have severe dry eye when the results of their Schirmer tests with nasal stimulation were less than 10 mm.[9] Because these patients are lacking the important factors normally found in tears, they are incapable of proper wound healing and have a worse prognosis for ocular surface reconstruction.

Keratinization

In 1996, Holland described keratinization of the conjunctiva as a risk factor for failure of keratolimbal allograft (KLAL).[1] Patients with preoperative conjunctival keratinization had significantly poorer outcomes when compared to those without keratinization (Figure 13.5). Aqueous tear production was another useful parameter to predict outcome. Patients with a Schirmer test of 2 mm, or less at 5 minutes without anesthesia, had a significantly poorer prognosis. However, using logistic re-

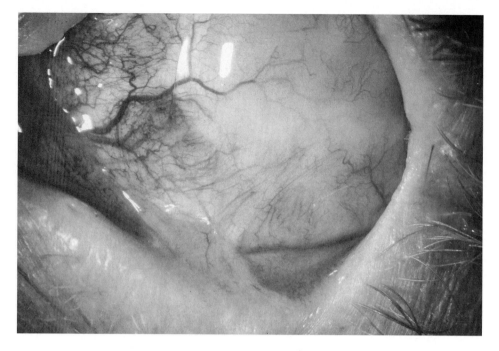

Figure 13.4. Chronic conjunctival inflammation and symblepharon formation due to Stevens–Johnson syndrome.

gression, the combination of both keratinization and low Schirmer testing demonstrated that only keratinization was a significant risk factor. It is possible that an abnormally low Schirmer test is also an independent risk factor, but this study did not have any patients with a low Schirmer test without keratinization to support this theory.

Need for Penetrating Keratoplasty

It is our experience that roughly half of patients undergoing limbal stem cell transplantation for severe OSD will need no further surgical procedure. However, half of patients will need to undergo penetrating or lamellar keratoplasty for visual rehabilitation. The presence of a corneal graft potentially increases the demand for the limbal stem cells to repopulate the corneal surface. This extra demand may very well stress a marginally functional transplanted stem cell population, further placing the patient at risk for chronic epitheliopathy.

If a corneal graft is needed and the endothelium is normal, lamellar keratoplasty is preferable to penetrating keratoplasty for patients who have had limbal stem cell transplantation previously. Performing penetrating

Figure 13.5. Stevens–Johnson syndrome patient with severe surface failure and keratinization.

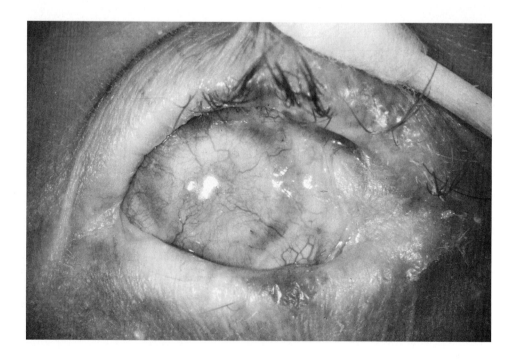

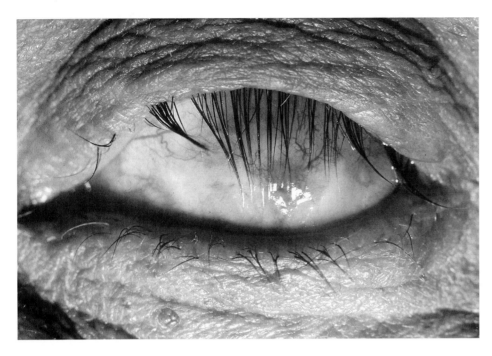

Figure 13.6. Severe trichiasis secondary to entropion as a result of an alkali injury.

keratoplasty adds the additional risk of endothelial rejection which, in some cases, can be more difficult to control than limbal stem cell rejection and can ultimately lead to loss of the patient's vision.

Mechanical Eyelid Problems

The status of the eyelids and ocular adnexa can also play an important role in the health of the ocular surface. Diseases that affect the function of the conjunctiva and limbal stem cell will often result in eyelid abnormalities. The eyelid abnormalities that can be seen include trichiasis, distichiasis, entropion, ectropion, and lagophthalmos (Figure 13.6). These abnormal lid conditions can lead to exposure keratitis, epithelial defects, and scarring of the cornea. It is important to address any eyelid abnormalities surgically before or during ocular surface transplantation. We find it useful to perform a tarsorrhaphy at the time of limbal stem cell transplantation in the majority of patients to promote healing of the ocular surface.

Systemic Health of the Patient

The use of systemic immunosuppression significantly increases the success rate of ocular surface allografts.[10] Patients with complicating medical conditions such as renal disease, advanced age, diabetes mellitus, and hypertension may not tolerate chronic systemic immunosuppression and therefore have a higher likelihood for graft rejection.

Age of the Patient

The very young patient with stem cell disease presents unique challenges to the clinician. A younger patient will typically have more inflammation than an older patient with the same disease process. As previously stated, increased inflammation will worsen not only the symptoms and prognosis, but also the likelihood of any surgical success.

Pediatric patients are difficult to examine in the eye clinic. It may take a team of assistants to comfort or restrain a child so that the clinician can conduct a proper examination. A portable slit-lamp is a necessity in examining small children, and a strong set of eyelids or a good Bell's phenomenon will foil even the best-equipped and well-intentioned ophthalmologist. Repeat examinations under anesthesia to monitor progress are often required in small children with severe OSD.

In addition, medication administration is difficult in small children. They will often exhibit significant blepharospasm when approached with eyedrops, and once the drops are administered, they commonly cry and in so doing, dilute the necessary medications.

Staging of Ocular Surface Disease

A practical approach at staging severe OSD is outlined in Table 13.1. In this system, staging is determined by status of both the limbal stem cells and conjunctiva. First the patient is categorized based upon the extent of limbal stem cell depletion. If there is partial limbal stem cell deficiency with depletion of less than half of the stem cell population, the patient is classified as stage I. If greater than half of the limbus is deficient, the patient is classified as stage II.

Next, the patient is categorized based on the condition of the conjunctiva. If the conjunctiva is normal, the

Table 13.1. Classification of ocular surface disease based on number of lost stem cells and presence or absence of conjunctival inflammation.

	Normal conjunctiva (stage a)	Previously inflamed conjunctiva (stage b)	Inflamed conjunctiva (stage c)
Partial stem cell deficiency (Stage I)	Iatrogenic, CIN, contact lens (Stage Ia)	History of chemical or thermal injury (Stage Ib)	Mild SJS, OCP, recent chemical injury (Stage Ic)
Total/subtotal cell deficiency (Stage II)	Aniridia, severe contact lens and iatrogenic (Stage IIa)	History of severe chemical or thermal injury (Stage IIb)	Severe SJS, OCP, recent chemical or thermal injury (Stage IIc)

patient is staged as "a." If the conjunctiva is abnormal from previous inflammation, but is currently quiet, the patient is staged as "b." If the conjunctiva is currently inflamed, the patient is staged as "c." For example, a patient with total limbal stem cell deficiency with normal conjunctiva, is staged as IIa. A patient with total limbal stem cell deficiency with actively inflamed conjunctiva will be staged as IIc.

Examples of conditions that fit the classification of stage Ia include iatrogenic limbal stem cell deficiency (Figure 13.7),[11] contact lens-induced keratopathy, and conjunctival intraepithelial neoplasia. Stage IIa signifies total limbal stem cell deficiency with normal conjunctiva. Patients exhibiting stage Ia disease can progress to IIa with further loss of limbal stem cells. Therefore, iatrogenic limbal stem cell deficiency, contact lens keratopathy, and CIN can also progress to stage IIa. Aniridia, a primary SC disorder that appears to result from a deficiency in the development or maintenance of limbal SCs, is another entity that belongs in the IIa group (Figure 13.8).[12–14] Aniridic patients are not born with abnormal ocular surfaces; rather, a chronic epitheliopathy

develops peripherally with age and slowly extends centrally leading to potentially profound visual loss.

Stage Ib represents patients with partial limbal stem cell deficiency with conjunctiva that was previously inflamed, but currently quiet (Figure 13.9). Patients with a history of chemical or thermal injury with less than 50% limbal deficiency fall into this group. The severity of the injury depends on the nature of the chemical and the duration and surface area of exposure to the offending chemical. These patients have significant inflammation around the time of their injury, but the inflammation will quiet over time with judicious use of immunosuppressive agents. When planning surgery for these patients, it is best to wait for the inflammation to quiet down if possible, performing surgery when they are a stage Ib rather than a Ic.

Patients with greater than 50% limbal stem cell depletion with previously inflamed conjunctiva that is now quiet are grouped in stage IIb. This group is composed of patients with a history of chemical or thermal injury affecting greater than half of the limbus (Figure 13.10). Similar to the pathophysiology seen in those in

Figure 13.7. OSD Stage Ia. Sectoral stem cell deficiency due to previous limbal surgery and topical glaucoma medications.

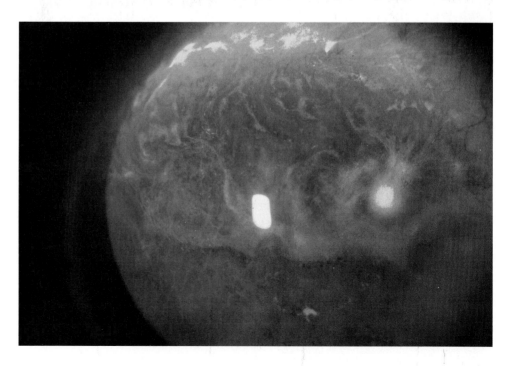

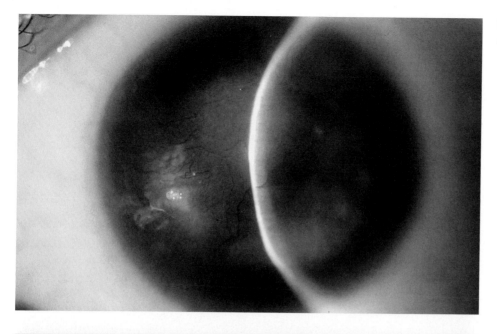

Figure 13.8. OSD Stage IIa. Aniridic keratopathy.

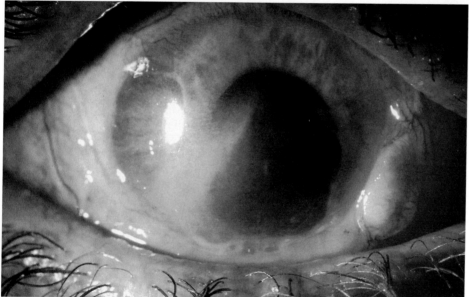

Figure 13.9. OSD Stage Ib. Partial limbal deficiency from previous acid injury.

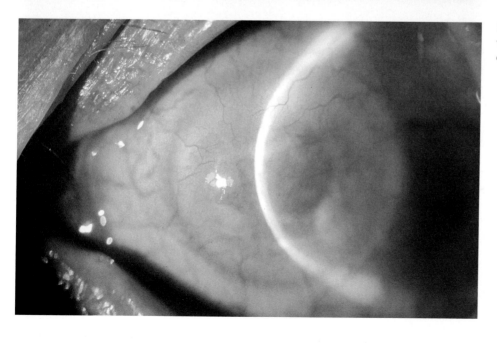

Figure 13.10. OSD Stage IIb. Previous alkali injury chronic stem cell failure.

Figure 13.11. OSD Stage Ic. Superior limbal deficiency secondary to topical mitomycin C.

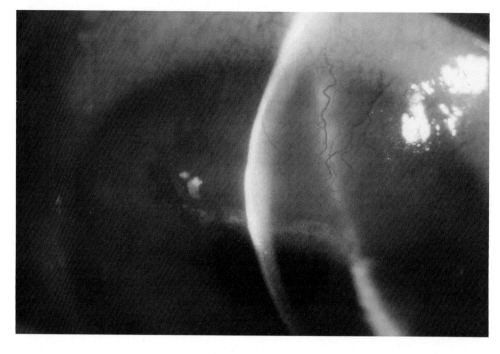

group Ib above, these patients are staged as IIc around the time of their exposure, and move to the IIb category when the conjunctiva becomes uninflamed.

Patients with active conjunctival inflammation can develop subsequent partial limbal stem cell deficiency, and this represents stage Ic. One group within this stage is the conjunctival inflammatory disorders that have not reached the severe stage, such as mild SJS and OCP. Conjunctival inflammation leads to conjunctival scarring, aqueous tear deficiency, and the eventual loss of partial limbal function.[15] The other patients in this group are those with alkali, acid, or thermal burns with only partial limbal stem cell depletion who have not had the opportunity for the conjunctiva to quite down (Figure 13.11). As stated earlier, with time and proper treatment, the inflammation in these patients will usually diminish and these patients will move from stage Ic to Ib.

The most severe forms of OSD involve total limbal stem cell deficiency with active conjunctival inflammation. These cases make up stage IIc and includes severe SJS, OCP, and recent chemical injuries (Figure 13.12). In these cases, total limbal stem cell deficiency is compli-

Figure 13.12. OSD Stage IIc. Total ocular surface failure due to Stevens–Johnson syndrome.

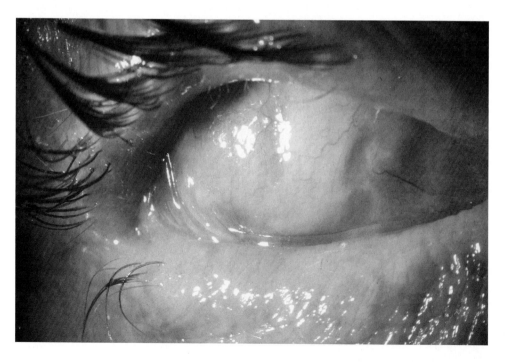

cated by conjunctival inflammation and scarring, decreased mucin and aqueous tear production, and potential for keratinization of the ocular surface. These patients have the poorest prognosis for surgical rehabilitation.[1]

Summary

It is important for the clinician to understand the contributions of both the limbal stem cells and conjunctival disease in selecting the surgical options for a patient's rehabilitation. As stated before, it is imperative that this concept be understood when evaluating clinical studies comparing treatment modalities, since patients with one stage of disease should be compared only with patients at the same stage. Recommendations for treatment based on staging will be covered in Chapter 26.

References

1. Holland EJ. Epithelial transplantation for the management of severe ocular surface disease. *Trans Am Ophthalmol Soc* 1996; 94:677–743.
2. Tseng SCG, Prabhasawatt P, Barton K, et al. Amniotic membrane transplantation with or without limbal allografts for corneal surface reconstruction in patients with limbal stem cell deficiency. *Arch Ophthalmol* 1998; 116:431–441.
3. Tsubota K, Satake Y, Kaido M, et al. Treatment of severe ocular-surface disorders with corneal epithelial stem-cell transplantation. *N Engl J Med* 1999; 340:1697–1703.
4. Tsai RJ-F, Li L-M, Chen J-K. Reconstruction of damaged corneas by transplantation of autologous limbal epithelial cells. *N Engl J Med* 2000; 343:86–93.
5. Holland EJ, Schwartz GS. The evolution of epithelial transplantation for severe ocular surface disease and a proposed classification system. *Cornea* 1996; 15:549–556.
6. Foster CS, Fong LP, Azar D, et al. Episodic conjunctival inflammation after Stevens–Johnson syndrome. *Ophthalmol* 1998; 95:453–462.
7. Heiligenhaus A, Schaller J, Mauss S, et al. Eosinophil granule proteins expressed in ocular cicatricial pemphigoid. *Br J Ophthalmol* 1998; 82:312–317.
8. Tsubota K. The importance of the Schirmer test with nasal stimulation. *Am J Ophthalmol* 1991; 111:106–108.
9. Tsubota K, Satake Y, Ohyama M, et al. Surgical reconstruction of the ocular surface in advanced ocular cicatricial pemphigoid and Stevens–Johnson syndrome. *Am J Ophthalmol* 1996; 122:38–52.
10. Djalilian AR, Bagheri MM, Schwartz GS, et al. Keratolimbal allograft for the management of limbal stem cell deficiency. Paper presented at scientific program at Castroviejo Cornea Society, Orlando, FL, October 23, 1999.
11. Schwartz GS, Holland EJ: Iatrogenic limbal stem cell deficiency. *Cornea* 1998; 17:31–57.
12. Mackman G, Brightbill FS, Optiz JM. Corneal changes in aniridia. *Am J Ophthalmol* 1979; 87:497–502.
13. Margo CE. Congenital aniridia; a histopathologic study of the anterior segment in children. *J Ped Ophthalmol Strabismus* 1983; 20:192–198.
14. Nelson LB, Spaeth GL, Nowinski T, et al. Aniridia, a review. *Surv Ophthalmol.* 1984; 28:621–642.
15. Tugal-Tutkun I, Akova YA, Foster CS. Penetrating keratoplasty in cicatrizing conjunctival diseases. *Ophthalmology* 1995; 102:576–585.

14

Sequential Sectoral Conjunctival Epitheliectomy (SSCE)

Harminder S. Dua

Introduction

The limbal epithelium, with its repository of stem cells, acts as a barrier that exerts an inhibitory growth pressure, preventing the migration of conjunctival epithelial cells onto the cornea.[1] When an ocular surface epithelial defect involves the cornea and limbus, this barrier is lifted and conjunctival epithelium often migrates across the denuded limbus to cover the corneal surface. The participation of conjunctival epithelium in the healing of corneal epithelial wounds has been known for a long time.[2] It was believed that conjunctival epithelium covering the cornea undergoes a slow transformation to assume characteristics resembling corneal epithelium, a process referred to as conjunctival transdifferentiation.[3–8] However, several investigators are of the opinion that complete conjunctival transdifferentiation probably does not occur. The consensus from most animal studies is that, although morphological transdifferentiation is possible, biochemically and functionally it is far from satisfactory.[1,9–11] Moreover, it has also been suggested that, in animal studies supporting conjunctival transdifferentiation, transdifferentiation could have occurred due to incomplete removal of limbal basal epithelium.[12] This incomplete removal would explain how regenerated epithelium could demonstrate both corneal and conjunctival features without one actually changing into the other. Long-term follow-up of conjunctivalized corneas in humans has revealed that clinical transdifferentiation of the conjunctival epithelial phenotype into corneal epithelial phenotype does not occur.[13] Impression cytology studies have revealed persistence of goblet cells in areas of conjunctivalization.

The corneal surface covered by conjunctival epithelium is characterized by the presence of goblet cells and is usually vascularized.[14] It appears thin, irregular, and is prone to recurrent erosions.[15] When it covers the pupillary area, vision can be significantly impaired.

It therefore follows that, in ocular surface defects, conjunctival epithelium should be prevented from covering the corneal surface, or if unavoidable or already established at the time of presentation, it should be removed at a later date to facilitate corneal epithelial cover for the cornea. Removal of conjunctival epithelium may have to be staged or repeated until the desired end point is attained. *Sequential sector conjunctival epitheliectomy (SSCE)* describes the above procedure, wherein conjunctival epithelium, covering a sector of the cornea and limbus, or adjacent bulbar conjunctiva, is removed and prevented from crossing the limbus until the denuded surface is covered by corneal epithelium derived cells.[13]

Indications for SSCE

Following are the indications for SSCE:

1. During the healing of acute ocular surface defects involving the cornea and limbus to prevent conjunctivalization of the cornea.
2. In patients with partial limbal stem cell deficiency with established conjunctivalization of the cornea.
3. In patients undergoing limbal allografts (including living-related tissue) and limbal autografts for total stem cell deficiency.
4. Following excision of limbal lesions.

It is well established that large ocular surface epithelial defects, involving the cornea, limbus, and adjoining conjunctiva heal by centripetal migration of epithelial cells from the remaining intact corneal and conjunctival epithelium, and by circumferential migration of limbal epithelial cells along the limbus, arising from the two ends of the remaining intact limbal epithelium.[16] The circumferentially migrating limbal epithelial sheets meet to reestablish the limbal epithelial

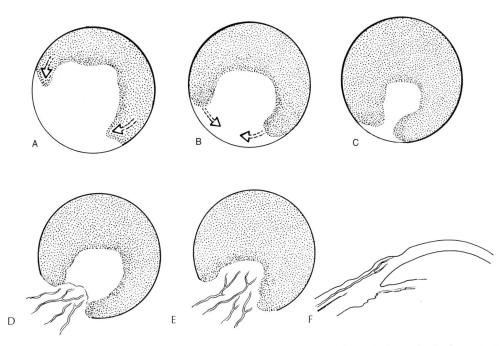

Figure 14.1. Diagrammatic representation of the healing of an ocular surface defect involving the limbus. (A) Arrowheads indicate the formation of tongue-shaped epithelial sheets, from the remaining intact epithelium, at either end of the limbal defect (hatched area represents fluorescein staining). (B) Arrows indicate the circumferential migration of tongue-shaped sheets along the limbus. (C) Limbal cover is always re-established before the central defect heals. (D) Conjunctival epithelium (solid black) may extend across the limbus to cover the cornea and inhibit further migration of the limbal epithelial sheets. (E and F) Area covered by limbal epithelium is sharply demarcated from normal corneal epithelium, is thin, irregular, and attracts new blood vessels. (Dua HS et al. *Brit J Ophthalmol* 1994; 78:402. Reproduced with permission from the BMJ Publishing Group.)

barrier (Figure 14.1). It has been postulated that this preferential circumferential migration along the limbus may represent a repopulation of the limbus with stem cells.[15,16] Centripetal migration also occurs from this newly established limbal epithelium to eventually close the central corneal epithelial defect, following a pattern similar to that occurring in patients with a central corneal epithelial defect and an intact limbus.[17] Often, however, the centripetally migrating healing conjunctival epithelium reaches the limbus and crosses it to cover the cornea to a variable extent. This conjunctival epithelial sheet contact inhibits the circumferentially migrating limbal epithelium, and the area of limbus covered by it remains "conjunctivalized" and devoid of limbal stem cells.[16]

The same migration patterns are seen following limbal allo- and autografts used in the management of total stem cell deficiency. Cells derived from the limbal explants following autologous and living-related donor transplants migrate centripetally and circumferentially along the limbus. Here too, despite peritomy and conjunctival recession, conjunctival epithelium often reaches the limbus and encroaches on the corneal surface.[18,19] The conjunctival encroachment results in an admixture of limbal explant-derived corneal cells and conjunctival cells. When cadaveric donor limbal tissue is used, the transplanted limbal tissue is more complete through 360 degrees of the recipient eye, and centripetal migration is predominantly observed. However, depending on the technique used, gaps may exist and provide an avenue for conjunctival cells to reach the limbus and encroach on the cornea.

In the circumstances described above, SSCE is performed to prevent conjunctival epithelium from reaching the limbus. It is effectively held back until repopulation of the limbus from surviving limbal cells or donor limbus is achieved. Similarly, if conjunctivalization has already occurred, the epithelium over the affected area of the cornea and limbus is removed to allow healing from healthy limbus-derived cells.

The same principles will apply following resection of limbal lesions and other surgical procedures performed during ocular surface reconstruction.

Contraindications for SSCE

Following are the contraindications for SSCE:

1. Total limbal involvement.
2. Dense fibrovascular pannus.
3. Thin underlying stroma.
4. Very dry eye.
5. Anaesthetic cornea.

Total limbal involvement with conjunctivalization of the cornea is a definite contraindication for SSCE. Removal of conjunctival epithelium from the cornea will only result in more conjunctival cells coming in, since there is no surviving limbus to provide corneal epithelial cells. In such situations, a limbal transplant procedure is the primary intervention.

The presence of a dense fibrovascular pannus with partial stem cell deficiency is a relative contraindication. A fibrovascular pannus requires excision. The underlying stromal bed, if healthy, may support epithelialization from limbus-derived corneal epithelial cells. If not it may result in a persistent epithelial defect with exposed stromal collagen. In such instances, an amniotic membrane transplant may need to be combined with SSCE.[20] In patients in whom the ocular surface is very dry, the corneal stroma under the fibrovascular pannus is very thin. If corneal sensation is markedly reduced, removal of an established cover, albeit abnormal, can lead to a persistent defect, exposure, and stromal melt risking perforation.

Preoperative Considerations

The preoperative workup of a patient for SSCE involves asking the following questions:

1. What is the extent of conjunctivalization of the cornea?
2. How many clock hours of the limbus are involved?
3. Is the visual axis covered with abnormal epithelium?
4. Is the patient symptomatic?

Examination to determine the tear function, corneal sensation, and thickness of the underlying stroma should also be carried out.

The extent of conjunctivalization of the cornea is determined by clinical examination. Instillation of a drop of 2% fluorescein will highlight the abnormal epithelium with a green fluorescence in blue light. The abnormal epithelium shows a stippled staining pattern and may also show filaments and small erosions. Another key clinical sign is late fluorescein staining of abnormal epithelium. This dull green appearance occurs a few minutes after instillation and is to be differentiated from the immediate bright green positive stain of an epithelial defect. The demarcation between abnormal and normal (limbus derived) epithelium is readily identified by the presence of tiny "protrusions" or "buds" of corneal epithelium all along the line of contact of the two epithelial phenotypes. Pooling of dye is also seen along this line of contact, since the abnormal epithelial sheet is thinner than the adjacent healthy normal corneal epithelium (Figures 14.2 and 14.3). Impression cytology helps to identify goblet cells, and confirm the conjunctival nature of the abnormal epithelium.

It is important to determine the clock hours of surviving limbus. If less than 3 clock hours of limbus survive, the strategy of SSCE may need to be modified such that it aims to achieve only visual axis cover with normal epithelium, rather than trying to establish normal cover for the entire cornea. There is a theoretical risk of "stretching the surviving limbus too far." Extensive SSCE may provide a good result in the short term, but eventually could lead to stem cell exhaustion.

Involvement of the visual axis invariably affects vision, and SSCE is certainly an option to be considered. If, however, the visual axis is not involved and vision is reasonable, one may consider no intervention, only observation over the long term. Studies have shown that corneal and conjunctival epithelial phenotypes can co-exist on the corneal surface over prolonged periods of time.[13] At times, however, the patient's symptoms may dictate intervention. Recurrent erosions and filamentary keratitis are the common associations when SSCE may be considered, even if the visual axis is not involved.

Surgical Technique

The surgical technique is a superficial mechanical debridement of the abnormal epithelium maintaining, as far as possible, the integrity of the underlying stroma.[13] When describing the procedure to the patient, the word "scraping" should be avoided. The alternative of "brushing off" the abnormal cells is more acceptable. Patients should be forewarned about the pain that may be experienced in the first 24 to 48 hours postoperatively.

The eye is first anaesthetized with a topical anaesthetic agent. A drop of 2% fluorescein is instilled immediately before the procedure. At the slit-lamp, the abnormal epithelium is gently brushed or peeled off using a surgical blade or crescent knife. An assistant may be required to hold the lids apart, or a wire speculum may be inserted. Usually, however, the surgeon can manage alone. In established cases of conjunctivalization of the cornea, it is important to include the edge of the existing corneal epithelial sheet, i.e., the removal should extend a millimeter beyond the contact line into normal corneal epithelium (Figure 14.4). After initial removal of the bulk of the epithelium with a surgical instrument, the denuded surface is wiped firmly with a dry absorbent surgical sponge. When more than 3 clock hours of normal limbus are preserved, the entire corneal area with abnormal epithelium, the corresponding limbus, and the adjacent conjunctiva for approximately 3 to 5 mm, are denuded. When less than 3 clock hours of limbus is present, only an area corresponding to the pupillary aperture, to include the visual axis, is denuded.

When SSCE is used as a preventive measure, as after limbal transplantation, denudation of conjunctival epithelium is carried out when it approaches to within a

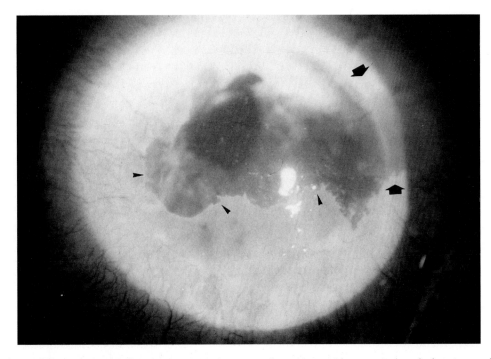

Figure 14.2. Slit-lamp diffuse view of a fluorescein-stained cornea of a patient with a corneal graft showing a clear demarcation between corneal and conjunctival epithelial phenotypes. The conjunctival epithelium shows light staining with fluorescein and blood vessels can be seen extending on the conjunctivalized epithelium. Tiny "buds" of corneal epithelium can be seen along the line of contact between corneal and conjunctival epithelium (arrowheads). The pupillary area is covered by corneal epithelium with is "sustained" by 2 clock hours of intact limbus (between large arrows). The best corrected visual acuity was 6/12. SSCE is not usually necessary in such cases (where visual axis is not involved) (×10). (Dua HS *Brit J Ophthalmol* 1998; 82:1408. Reproduced with permission from the BMJ Publishing Group.)

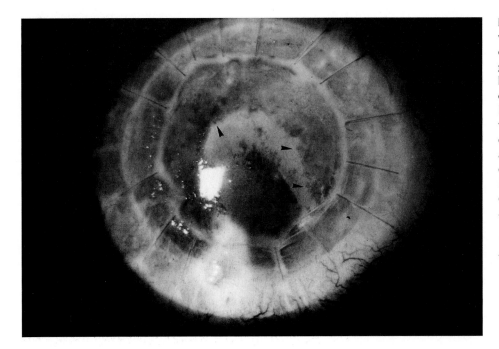

Figure 14.3. Slit-lamp diffuse view of a fluorescein-stained cornea of a patient with a corneal graft showing a clear demarcation between corneal and conjunctival epithelial phenotypes. The pupillary area is covered by conjunctival epithelium. Tiny "buds" of corneal epithelium can be seen along the line of contact between corneal and conjunctival epithelium (arrowheads) (×10). In such cases, visual acuity is impaired and SSCE is beneficial. (Dua HS *Brit J Ophthalmol* 1998; 82:1407. Reproduced with permission from the BMJ Publishing Group.)

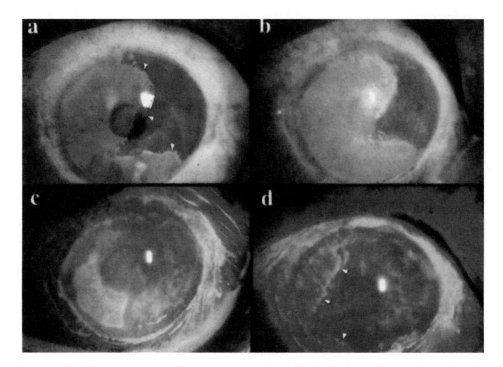

Figure 14.4. (A). Photograph of fluorescein-stained cornea of a patient who had presented several months after a chemical injury, showing a clear demarcation between corneal and conjunctival epithelial phenotypes (arrowheads). The pupillary area is almost entirely covered by conjunctival epithelium. Tiny "buds" of corneal epithelium can be seen along the line of contact between corneal and conjunctival epithelium. The patient's vision was 3/18 (×10). (B) The eye after SSCE. All conjunctival epithelium from the corneal surface and limbus was removed (×10). (C) The eye on day 3 following SSCE. The corneal sheet has covered the pupillary area, but the conjunctival epithelium has encroached on the cornea along the temporal limbus (×10). (D) The eye after complete healing. A new line of contact is established between corneal and conjunctival epithelial phenotypes (arrowheads), but the pupillary area is covered by healthy corneal epithelium. The patient's vision improved to 6/9 (×10). (Dua HS *Brit J Ophthalmol* 1998; 82:1410. Reproduced with permission from the BMJ Publishing Group.)

couple of millimeters of the healing corneal epithelium (Figures 14.5 and 14.6). In all cases, a bandage contact lens is inserted after the procedure. In individuals who are apprehensive about the procedure at the slit-lamp, it can be performed under the operating microscope with the patient lying down.

Postoperative Management

Immediately following the procedure, the eye is treated with preservative-free drops of antibiotics, a corticosteroid such as prednisolone acetate 0.5%, and nonsteroidal anti-inflammatory drugs (ketorolac tromethamine 0.5%) as prophylaxis against infection, inflammation, and pain. When more than 50% of the corneal surface is denuded, autologous serum drops may provide added benefit. Nonsteroidal anti-inflammatory drops are discontinued after 2 to 3 days, and the remaining medications are continued until epithelial healing is complete.

Close monitoring of the healing epithelium with regular follow-up every 24 to 48 hours is the key to the success of SSCE. Migration of conjunctival epithelium to-

ward or onto the limbus can be anticipated by close observation of the healing ocular surface and can be prevented by repeating the procedure when required, until corneal epithelial cover for the cornea is reestablished. As mentioned previously, it is not always necessary to aim for coverage of the entire cornea with phenotypic corneal cells. SSCE can be terminated as soon as a reasonable proportion of the cornea, including the visual axis, is covered by corneal epithelial cells.[21]

SSCE and the principle of preventing conjunctival epithelium from encroaching on the corneal surface is essential in establishing appropriate epithelial cover for the corneal surface during epithelial wound healing, and particularly following limbal transplantation. It must be remembered, however, that conjunctival epithelial cover is better than no epithelial cover. Hence, in severe ocular surface injury, when the entire limbus is affected or involved, it is prudent to allow the conjunctival epithelium to cover the cornea. This situation can be maintained until the acute phase settles and appropriate surgical intervention can be undertaken with an enhanced chance of success.

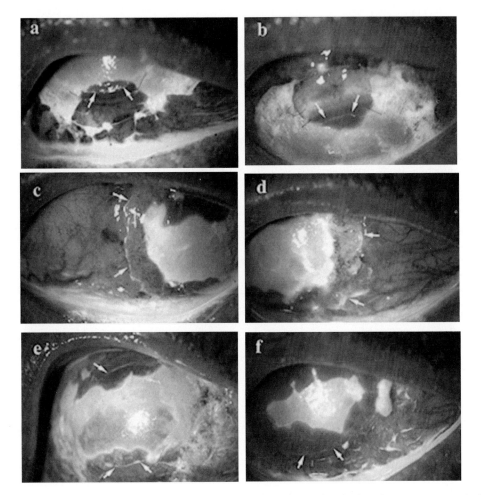

Figure 14.5. Photographs of fluorescein-stained ocular surface of recipient eye that had undergone conjunctival limbal autograft. On day 2 following surgery, donor epithelial cells can be seen migrating onto the recipient surface from the explants placed at the 6 o'clock (A) and 12 o'clock (B) positions. Arrows indicate the anterior edge of the explants. On day 4 following surgery, host conjunctival epithelial cells can be seen migrating from the edge (arrows) of the recessed conjunctiva on both the temporal (C) and nasal (D) sides. SSCE of the advancing conjunctival epithelial sheets was carried out with a surgical blade (E), leaving behind the limbal-explant derived expanding corneal epithelial cells (arrows). (F). The circumferentially migrating limbal-explant derived corneal epithelial cells have met temporally and nasally. The large corneal epithelial defect healed with corneal cells and the small nasal conjunctival defect healed with conjunctival cells. Healing was complete by day 8. (Dua HS and Azuara-Blanco A *Brit J Ophthalmol* 2000; 84:275. Reproduced with permission from the BMJ Publishing Group.)

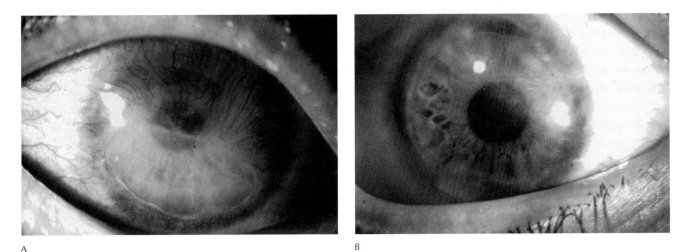

A   B

Figure 14.6. (A) Clinical slit-lamp diffuse photograph of eye of patient described in Figure 14.5. The photograph illustrates the large persistent epithelial defect following alkali burn. (B) The same eye following autolimbal transplant and SSCE. The corneal surface is completely derived from (auto)limbal explant corneal epithelial cells. (Dua HS and Azuara-Blanco A *Brit J Ophthalmol* 2000; 84:276. Reproduced with permission from the BMJ Publishing Group.)

References

1. Tseng SCG. Concept and application of limbal stem cells. *Eye* 1989; 3:141–157.
2. Friedenwald JS. Growth pressure and metaplasia of conjunctival and corneal epithelium. *Doc Ophthalmol* 1951; 6:184–192.
3. Shapiro MS, Friend J, Thoft RA. Corneal re-epithelialization from the conjunctiva. *Invest Ophthalmol Vis Sci* 1981; 21:135–142.
4. Tseng SCG, Hirst LW, Farazdaghi M, Green WR. Goblet cell density and vascularization during conjunctival transdifferentiation. *Invest Ophthalmol Vis Sci* 1984; 25:1168–1176.
5. Tseng SCG, Hirst LW, Farazdaghi M, Green WR. Inhibition of conjunctival transdifferentiation by topical retinoids. *Invest Ophthalmol Vis Sci* 1987; 28:538–542.
6. Tseng SCG, Farazdaghi M, Rider AA. Conjunctival transdifferentiation induced by systemic vitamin A deficiency in vascularized rabbit corneas. *Invest Ophthalmol Vis Sci* 1987; 28:1497–1504.
7. Aitken D, Friend J, Thoft RA. Corneal re-epithelialization from the conjunctiva. *Invest Ophthalmol Vis Sci* 1988; 29:224–231.
8. Huang AJW, Watson BD, Hernandez E, Tseng SCG. Induction of conjunctival transdifferentiation on vascularized corneas by photothrombotic occlusion of corneal vascularization. *Ophthalmology* 1988; 95:228–235.
9. Thoft RA, Friend J. Biochemical transformation of regenerating ocular surface epithelium. *Invest Ophthalmol* 1977; 16:14–20.
10. Kinoshita S, Friend J and Thoft RA. Biphasic cell proliferation in transdifferentiation of conjunctival to corneal epithelium in rabbits. *Invest Ophthalmol Vis Sci* 1983; 24:1008–1014.
11. Harris TM, Berry ER, Pakurar AS, Sheppard LB. Biochemical transformation of bulbar conjunctiva into corneal epithelium: An electrophoretic analysis. *Exp Eye Res* 1985; 41:597–605.
12. Kruse FE, Chen JJY, Tsai RJF, Tseng SCG. Conjunctival transdifferentiation is due to incomplete removal of limbal basal epithelium. *Invest Ophthalmol Vis Sci* 1990; 31:1903–1913.
13. Dua HS. The conjunctiva in corneal epithelial wound healing. *Br J Ophthalmol* 1998; 82:1407–1411.
14. Thoft RA, Friend J, Murphy HS. Ocular surface epithelium and corneal vascularization in rabbits. I. The role of wounding. *Invest Ophthalmol Vis Sci* 1979; 18:85–92.
15. Dua HS, Gomes JAP, Singh A. Corneal epithelial wound healing. *Br J Ophthalmol* 1994; 78:401–408.
16. Dua HS, Forrester JV. The corneoscleral limbus in human corneal epithelial wound healing. *Am J Ophthalmol* 1990; 110:646–656.
17. Dua HS, Forrester JV. Clinical patterns of corneal epithelial wound healing. *Am J Ophthalmol* 1987; 104:481–489.
18. Dua HS, Azuara-Blanco A. Allo-limbal transplantation in patients with limbal stem-cell deficiency. *Br J Ophthalmol* 1999; 83:414–419.
19. Dua HS, Azuara-Blanco A. Autologous limbal transplantation in unilateral stem cell deficiency. *Br J Ophthalmol* 2000; 84:273–278.
20. Tseng SCG, Prabhasawat P, Barton K, Gray T, Meller D. Amniotic membrane transplantation with or without limbal allografts for corneal surface reconstruction in patients with limbal stem cell deficiency. *Arch Ophthalmol* 1998; 116:431–441.
21. Dua HS, Azuara-Blanco A. Limbal stem cells of the corneal epithelium. *Surv Ophthalmol* 2000; 44:415–425.

15
Conjunctival Autograft

Donald T.H. Tan

Introduction

Conjunctival autograft transplantation is a form of ocular surface transplantation in which an autologous free conjunctival graft is obtained from the superior bulbar conjunctiva and sutured to the scleral bed (Figure 15.1). Conjunctival autografting is now extensively employed in pterygium surgery, in which the conjunctival graft is most often obtained from the same eye, but may be obtained from the opposite eye if previous surgery or scarring is present in the affected eye. This procedure is considered by many to set the standard in the surgical treatment of pterygium today, since the procedure can provide excellent cosmesis, is safe, and has been reported to have a low rate of recurrence. However, poor surgical technique resulting from a lack of understanding of basic surgical principles may result in a poor outcome and higher rates of recurrence. This chapter outlines the history and development of conjunctival autograft transplantation and the important surgical principles that allow for consistently successful surgery.

History and Development of Conjunctival Autograft Transplantation

In 1977, Thoft described the procedure of conjunctival transplantation which is now recognized as the forerunner of modern ocular surface transplantation surgery.[1] Although the importance of the limbus as the source of limbal stem cells for repopulation of corneal surface epithelium has now resulted in various forms of limbal transplantation, conjunctival transplantation is still commonly performed in pterygium surgery, in which the procedure is termed conjunctival autografting. The use of a free conjunctival autograft to cover a bare scleral defect after pterygium excision was first described in 1931 by Gómez-Márquez, who utilized superior bulbar conjunctiva from the contralateral eye. However, it was Kenyon who in 1985 proposed the current conjunctival autograft transplantation technique for ad-

vanced and recurrent pterygium which is now considered to be the gold standard procedure.[2,3] Today, the basic surgical techniques of conjunctival autografting may also be applicable to a range of other conjunctival disorders including traumatic or chemically induced symblepharon with conjunctival cicatrization and forniceal shortening and for wide excision of potentially premalignant conjunctival lesions.

In 1985, Kenyon originally suggested that conjunctival autografting could be reserved for advanced or recurrent pterygium, since it is more time-consuming and technically difficult compared to simple excision or the use of excision combined with adjunctive therapy such as mitomycin C or beta-irradiation.[3] However, conjunctival autograft has been widely accepted as the procedure of choice for primary pterygium due to (1) the excellent cosmesis and low recurrence rate that can be achieved if correct surgical principles are adhered to (Figure 15.2), (2) the realization that simple excision results in unacceptably high rates of recurrence, and (3) the recognition of infrequent, but potentially sight-threatening, long-term complications reported with mitomycin C and beta-irradiation therapies.

Efficacy of Conjunctival Autografting

We previously performed a randomized controlled trial in Singapore comparing conjunctival autografting with bare sclera excision for primary and recurrent pterygium. Our results demonstrated that conjunctival autografting could achieve a low recurrence rate (2%) in a tropical population in which the bare-sclera recurrence rate was 61% for primary pterygium, and 82% for recurrent pterygium (Figure 15.3).[4] However, this was a single surgeon efficacy trial, and analysis of conjunctival autografting among 23 surgeons in the same institution revealed a wide variation in recurrence rates ranging from 5% to 83%.[5] In addition, there was a clear trend correlating prior surgical experience and recurrence rate, with surgeons who had performed fewer au-

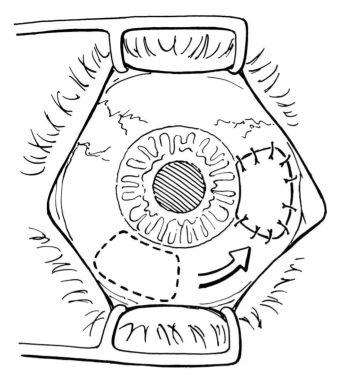

Figure 15.1. Diagram illustrating the principle underlying conjunctival autografting: suturing of a free conjunctival graft from the superior bulbar conjunctiva over the scleral bed of an excised pterygium.

tografts prior to study entry producing higher recurrence rates (Table 15.1). This suggests that conjunctival autografting is a relatively demanding procedure that has a significant learning curve and may explain the wide range of recurrences reported.

Other published studies on conjunctival autografting report varying recurrence rates from 2% to 39%.[6–16] This range of recurrence rates compares favorably with bare sclera excision and mitomycin C application (0% to 38%),[15,17–19] while recurrence rates reported for simple bare-sclera excision are considerably higher (24% to 89%).[4,6,8,15–22] It is likely that differing surgical technique may account for the wide range of recurrences reported in pterygium surgery, while inconsistency in defining recurrence and varying periods of follow-up remain additional factors to consider when comparing these studies. Sánchez-Thorin and co-workers performed meta-analysis comparing baresclera resection with and without mitomycin C, and conjunctival autograft for primary pterygium. They demonstrated that the odds for recurrence are 6 and 25 times higher if no autograft is performed or if mitomycin C is not used, but acknowledged study limitations imposed by the relative paucity of randomized controlled trials in the pterygium literature and the possibility of publication bias.[23] The potential of conjunctival autografting as the superior procedure of choice is demonstrated in Figure 15.4, in which recurrence of a pterygium occurred after lamellar keraplasty had been performed. Prior to lamellar keratoplasty, 2 previous surgeries had been attempted: bare-sclera excision and conjunctival autografting with an inadequate surgical technique (a thick, small graft that retracted after surgery). Initial success was achieved with lamellar keratoplasty (Figure 15.4A), but aggressive recurrence over the graft area occurred within 4 months of surgery (Figure 15.4B). A repeat conjunctival autograft utilizing the appropriate surgi-

Figure 15.2. Conjunctival autograft transplantation. Front view showing excellent cosmetic result with no evidence of recurrence.

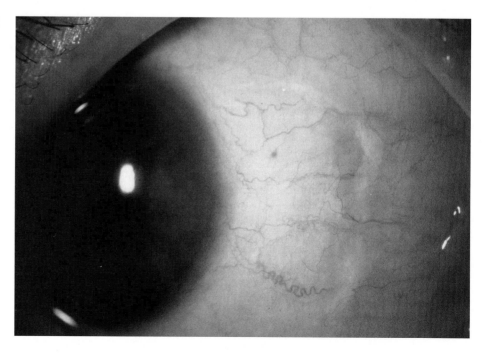

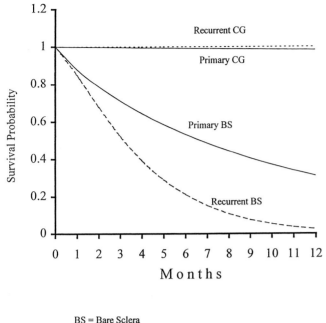

BS = Bare Sclera
CG = Conjunctival Autograft

Figure 15.3. Weibull survival-curve analysis comparing success of conjunctival autografting with bare scleral excision in reducing pterygium recurrence. (Reproduced with permission from *Archives of Ophthalmology* 1997; 15:1235–1240.)

cal technique outlined below resulted in an excellent cosmetic result, with no evidence of recurrence at 2 years (Figure 15.4C).

Surgical Technique

Conjunctival autografting for pterygium involves 2 main steps: (1) removal of the pterygium from the corneal and scleral surfaces, and (2) harvesting and suturing in place a free conjunctival graft from the superior bulbar conjunctiva. Correct surgical technique for the former will result in minimal damage to adjacent ocular structures, while careful attention to basic principles in conjunctival surgery for the latter ensures a successful autograft.

Table 15.1. Individual surgeons' recurrence rates compared with previous experience with conjunctival autografting, from a single ophthalmic institution.

Surgeon	No. of conjunctival autografts prior to study entry	Recurrence rate in study
A	10	5%
B	5	10%
C	4	14%
D	1	17%
E	1	30%
F–I	0	20–83%

Pterygium Excision Technique

The aim is to ensure complete pterygium tissue removal without excessive adjacent tissue damage or scarring. Incomplete removal of remnant pterygium tissue may result in residual scarring obscuring the visual axis, or optical degradation of the precorneal tear film with a proud scar, while incomplete removal at the limbus and conjunctival aspects may increase the risk of pterygium recurrence. In addition, excessive tissue removal at the time of surgery may result in irregular corneal astigmatism or scleral thinning and dellen formation. Excision of recurrent pterygium is inherently more difficult, since scarring obliterates tissue planes and there is, therefore, a higher risk of extraocular muscle damage and scleral or corneal tissue loss.

The principles of pterygium excision are:

1. complete removal of all pterygium tissue at Bowman's plane and the sclera
2. minimizing scarring and astigmatism at the cornea
3. minimizing scleral damage

For recurrent pterygium, one further principle should be prior identification or isolation of the medial or lateral rectus muscle to prevent inadvertent muscle damage and disinsertion.

Anesthesia
Subconjunctival or regional anesthesia can be utilized. For autografting, retrobulbar or peribulbar anesthesia is preferable to allow for careful and controlled harvesting of the graft. General anesthesia may be indicated in cases of recurrent pterygium with marked muscle restriction and scarring.

Exposure/Stabilization of the Globe
A corneal traction suture at the 12 o'clock limbus provides good control of the globe both horizontally during pterygium excision and vertically during subsequent harvesting of a superior autograft. A superior rectus bridle suture should be avoided, since this will limit the extent and site of the graft harvesting.

Excision of Pterygium Tissue
Pterygium fibers run radially toward the central cornea and are most adherent at the limbus and at the pterygium head, but are often minimally adherent to the sclera, unless previous surgery has been performed. As such, a clean plane between pterygium tissue and underlying sclera is easily achieved if dissection is initiated at the scleral aspect, or body of the pterygium (Figure 15.5). Care should be taken not to initiate pterygium body dissection too far from the limbus, since horizontal tissue retraction occurs in all cases. An excision 3 to 4 mm away from the limbus, for example, will result in an adequate bare scleral defect measuring 6 to 8 mm horizontally.

Figure 15.4. Conjunctival autografting after failure of lamellar keratoplasty for pterygium. A. initial surgical result after lamellar keratoplasty for recurrent pterygium; B. aggressive recurrence within 4 months; C. conjunctival autografting successfully performed for recurrence after lamellar keratoplasty—no recurrence 2 years following autografting.

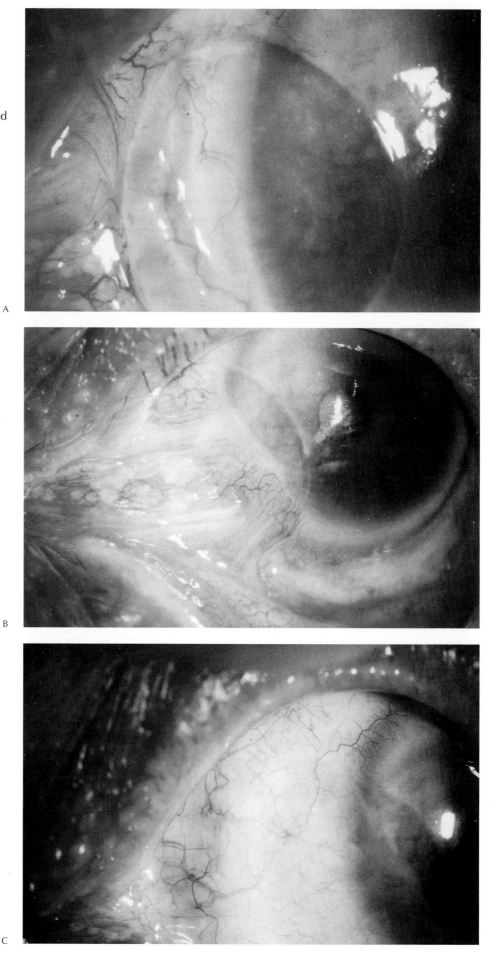

A

B

C

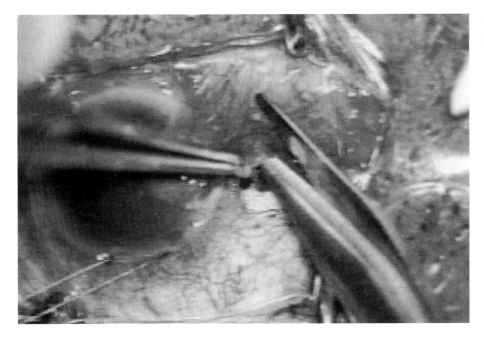

Figure 15.5. Pterygium excision technique: initial incision site at body of pterygium.

Reflection of the pterygium tissue toward the corneal aspect next exposes limbal attachments, which may then be firmly detached or scraped away using a #64 Beaver microblade to peel pterygium tissue from the sclera and limbus. Using the microblade oriented perpendicularly to the cornea, but scraping horizontally, will allow peeling or scraping of pterygium tissue off Bowman's layer in a lamellar fashion (Figure 15.6), while reducing the risk of cutting deeper into healthy stroma. One should attempt to detach all pterygium tissue in one piece, which will reduce the risk of leaving remnant tissue tags on the cornea. In some cases, pterygium tissue may be more deeply rooted beyond Bowman's layer and into the corneal stroma. Care

should be taken to avoid deep dissection in these cases, which will result in excessive tissue loss nearer the head of the pterygium, which lies closer to the visual axis.

All fibrovascular pterygium tissue should be removed at the scleral bed and limbus to reduce the risk of recurrence. A wide excision technique is therefore employed, necessitating removal of a thin strip of normal conjunctiva above and below the pterygium body. Additional fibrovascular tissue may be removed at the conjunctival edges by exerting traction on subepithelial fibers and undermining the overlying conjunctival epithelium. However, this also results in further tissue retraction and a larger scleral bed defect.

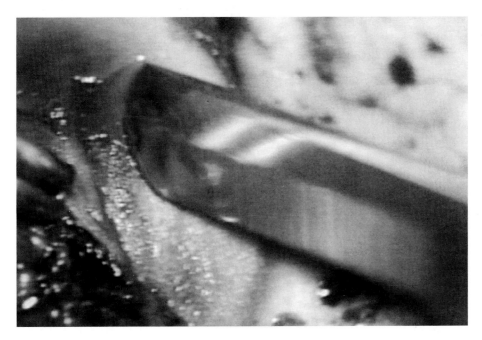

Figure 15.6. Pterygium excision technique: peeling/scraping pterygium tissue from Bowman's layer.

Figure 15.7. Pterygium morphology grading system: A. grade T1: atrophic pterygium (episcleral vessels unobscured); B. grade T2: intermediate pterygium (episcleral vessels partially obscured); C. grade T3: fleshy pterygium (episcleral vessels totally obscured). (*Archives of Ophthalmology* 1997; 15:1235–1240, with permission.)

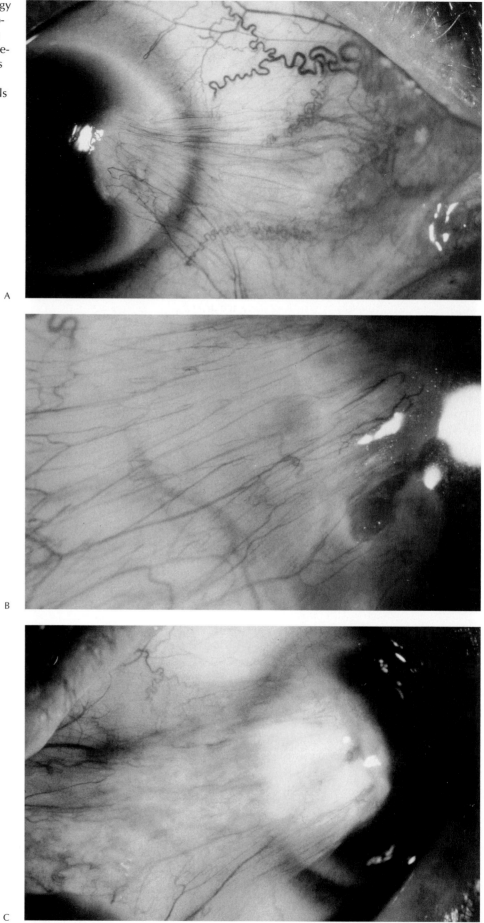

Importance in Removing All
Fibrovascular Pterygium Tissue

Evidence exists that pterygium fibroblasts are transformed and exhibit high cellular proliferative characteristics. They may, therefore, be involved in pterygium recurrence, and it is important to attempt to remove as much fibrovascular pterygium tissue as possible. Chen and co-workers cultured conjunctival fibroblasts from normal conjunctiva and pterygium specimens and showed that pterygium-derived fibroblasts acquired a transformed phenotype with more aggressive growth characteristics.[24] Flow-cytometry measurements of DNA content and cellular proliferation rates in primary and recurrent pterygia in our laboratory have also confirmed this finding (see Chapter 6, Pterygium).[25] Finally, the clinical role of the fibrovascular component of pterygium in relation to surgical recurrence is demonstrated in our randomized clinical trial, in which recurrence after bare scleral excision was clearly found to be related to the degree of fibrovascular tissue in the pterygium.[4] A clinical slit-lamp grading scale was developed, based on relative translucency of the body of the pterygium. Grade T1 (atrophic) denoted a pterygium in which episcleral vessels underlying the body of the pterygium were unobscured and clearly distinguished (Figure 15.7). Grade T3 (fleshy) denoted a thick pterygium in which episcleral vessels underlying the body of the pterygium were totally obscured by fibrovascular tissue. All other pterygia that did not fall into these two categories (i.e., episcleral vessel details were indistinctly seen or partially obscured) fell into Grade T2 (intermediate). The study clearly showed that recurrence correlated well with translucency, with fleshy pterygium having the highest capacity for recurrence, while atrophic pterygium had the lowest. The difference in recurrence rates was highly significant for both primary and recurrent pterygia (Figure 15.8).

Recurrent Pterygium Excision

Recurrent pterygium surgery should be performed by an experienced surgeon, since surgery may be difficult or hazardous. Previous surgery usually results in significant fibrous scarring and adherence to the underlying sclera throughout the body of the pterygium, with obliteration or distortion of planes and landmarks. In the most severe instances, scarring may obliterate the fornix and cause symblepharon with adherence of the lid margin to the cornea (Figure 15.9). Adherence to the corneal stroma will also be encountered if previous excision occurred deep into Bowman's layer. Loss of tissue planes makes division of pterygium scar tissue from normal sclera and corneal stroma more difficult, and care should be taken to avoid an excessively deep dissection.

In many instances, the rectus muscle sheath may also be encased in dense fibrous scar tissue. Occasionally, tractional forward migration of the insertion of the af-

fected rectus muscle may occur, leading to the possibility of inadvertent damage or detachment of the muscle. Isolation of the involved rectus muscle posterior to the pterygium scar is, therefore, important prior to dissection of scar tissue. Dissection of all scar tissue around the muscle is required to prevent ocular motility restriction. Lid symblepharon, if present, should also be released, to allow the globe to fall back away from the

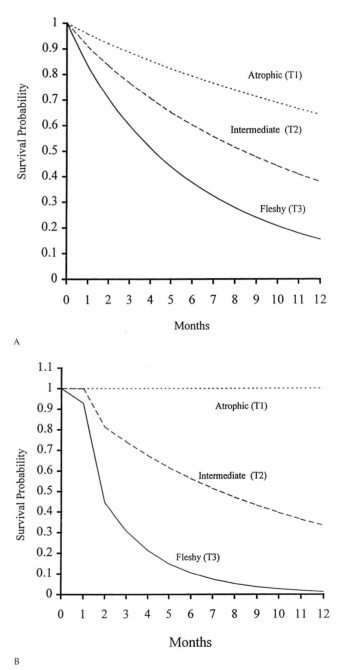

Figure 15.8. Weibull survival-curve analysis according to pterygium morphology grade: A. primary pterygium; B. recurrent pterygium. (*Archives of Ophthalmology* 1997; 15:1235–1240, with permission.)

Figure 15.9. Aggressive pterygium recurrence with symblepharon and lower eyelid adhesion to the cornea following bare sclera excision of a primary pterygium.

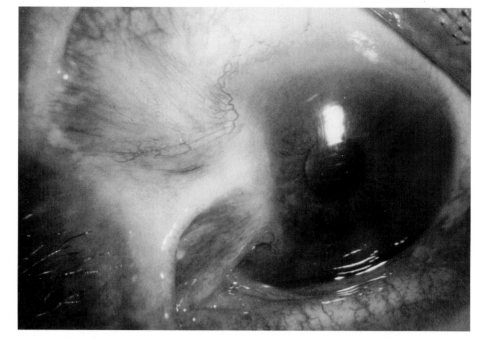

eyelid. It is generally unnecessary to close a forniceal or tarsal conjunctival defect after symblepharon release, since symblepharon or forniceal obliteration will not recur in the presence of an adequate conjunctival graft covering the bulbar conjunctival defect.

Harvesting of the Conjunctival Autograft

The most important step to successful autograft surgery is the careful harvesting of a thin, Tenon-free conjunctival graft which is of adequate size. Since this graft is integral to prevent pterygium recurrence, meticulous surgical technique to harvest the autograft is needed to ensure a consistently low rate of recurrence.

Harvesting Site

After completion of pterygium excision, the globe is rotated inferiorly to expose the superior bulbar conjunctiva which is the usual site for harvesting of the conjunctival graft (inferior bulbar conjunctiva may occasionally be utilized, but there may be inadequate tissue for a large graft, and inferior symblepharon with forniceal shortening may occur). A site far from the pterygium excision site is usually chosen in order to leave a significant quadrant of untouched conjunctiva in the event of the need for future filtration surgery. For instance, if a nasal pterygium is excised, the graft should be obtained from the superotemporal bulbar conjunctiva (Figure 15.10).

Superficial Dissection Technique

An essential factor for success is to obtain a thin, Tenon-free conjunctival graft. A natural tissue plane exists between Tenon's layer and the episclera, and this is the usual deep plane for conjunctival dissection in glaucoma filtration or strabismus surgery. Unfortunately, no such distinct tissue plane exists between Tenon's layer and the conjunctival epithelium, and superficial dissection to separate these layers requires practice. A fine nick of the epithelial layer initially allows epithelium to be lifted up without inclusion of Tenon's layer, and conjunctival scissors achieves separation of the two layers. Careful lifting of the epithelium allows Tenon's layer to be lifted and put on stretch, and Tenon's fibers are cut close to the epithelium, allowing the subepithelial tissues to retract away. Blunt-tipped conjunctival forceps and scissors prevent inadvertent buttonholing of the graft, but once adequate surgical skills are acquired it is possible to obtain a thinner graft with fine-tipped Vannas scissors (but at a higher risk of buttonholing). Dissection is carried forward to the superior limbus.

This superficial dissection technique has the advantage of reducing conjunctival hemorrhage, and cautery is rarely needed. In addition, if Tenon's layer is minimally disturbed and cautery is not employed, wound healing occurs without significant conjunctival scarring, and it is possible to reharvest conjunctiva from the same site.

Size of Conjunctival Autograft

Despite superficial dissection, some graft retraction will still occur as it is not possible to exclude subepithelial fibrous tissue completely. One should therefore aim to oversize the graft in relation to the donor site by approximately 1 mm in each diameter. Initially, careful measurement and marking of recipient bed and donor is useful to assist in accurate graft and scleral bed proportions. Cautery should not be utilized to mark the bed, since tearing of the graft originating from a cautery site may occur with minimal graft traction.

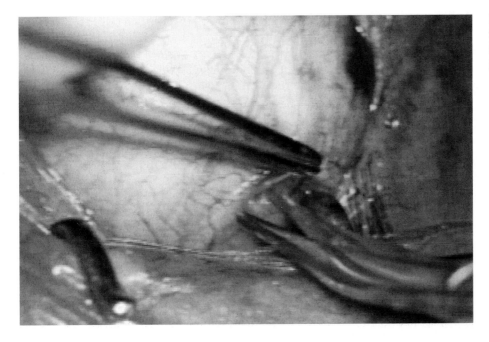

Figure 15.10. Initial incision site for harvesting: superotemporal bulbar conjunctiva for a nasal pterygium.

Orientation of Conjunctival Autograft

Although the theory of transplanting limbal stem cells by maximizing inclusion of limbal epithelium is attractive, no evidence exists that superficial conjunctival dissection is capable of including deep-lying limbal stem cells within the graft and, clinically, anatomical limbus-to-limbus orientation of the graft also does not appear to be essential for graft success. However, it is essential that the conjunctival graft be correctly positioned with the epithelium uppermost, and we recommend that, after completion of the harvesting, the graft be carefully slid into place from the superior harvest site to the bare sclera bed without any upward lifting away from the cornea. Inadvertent inversion of the graft will result in sloughing several days after surgery. Graft inversion may be recognized on the first postoperative day by the presence of a white opaque graft, which stains heavily with fluorescein. This graft may still be viable if surgical inversion is immediately carried out within 24 to 48 hours of the original surgery. Graft inversion detected at later periods after surgery is unlikely to be viable, and sloughing will ensue (Figure 15.11). At this stage, removal of graft remnants should be done and the bed left to re-epithelize naturally. Alternatively, amniotic membrane transplantation, if available, would be a useful procedure.

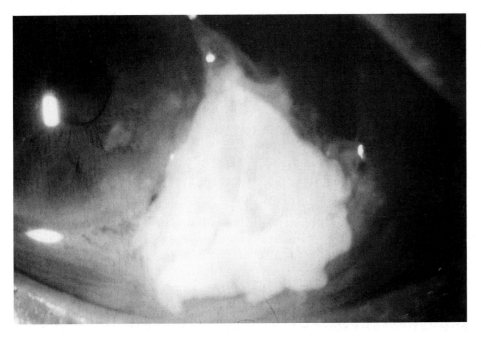

Figure 15.11. Graft inversion. A pale, opaque graft is noted 4 days after surgery.

Securing the Conjunctival Autograft

The conjunctival autograft is secured in place with interrupted sutures. 10-0 Vicryl or 8-0 virgin-silk sutures are preferred. Initial suture placement should involve the limbal limits of the graft, followed by the superior and inferior edges of the graft. It is important that the graft be sutured to underlying episclera over these sites, to prevent graft displacement during ocular movements. Suturing of the graft overlying the rectus muscle should not include underlying muscle tissue. Finally, a central limbal suture is also necessary to prevent forward migration, or bowstringing, of the graft onto the cornea. A subconjunctival antibiotic/steroid injection (away from the graft bed) completes the procedure. A final check should be made to ensure that the graft remains well secured to the globe despite rotation of the eye.

Other Techniques

Deliberate cuts within the graft at the end of the procedure are aimed at reduction of postoperative graft edema by providing drainage sites for edema fluid to escape. However, these cuts rapidly re-epithelize within days of surgery, and edema reaccumulates.

The combined use of conjunctival autografting with intraoperative application to the bed of the sclera has been reported. Wong and Law compared conventional conjunctival autografting with conjunctival autografting after a 1 minute application of 0.25 mg/ml of mitomycin C to the scleral bed in a series of 159 eyes, and reported recurrences rates of 26% and 76%, respectively.[13] No autograft complications, scleral necrosis or thinning were noted within the one year follow-up period. However, since the latter complications relating to mitomycin C therapy may occur many years after surgery, the absolute safety of combining mitomycin C with conjunctival autograft remains in question.

Postoperative Regime

Topical steroid/antibiotic eyedrops are usually required for a month after surgery because significant ocular surface inflammation occurs with conjunctival autografting. Care should be taken to identify steroid responders during this period, especially since conjunctival autografting compromises the success of future glaucoma filtration surgery. Topical nonsteroidal anti-inflammatory agents may be used as an alternative to steroids, but they are generally less effective in reducing inflammatory symptoms. Graft edema occurs to some degree in all cases, and should only be a cause for concern if severe enough to cause adjacent corneal dellen formation. Graft hemorrhage may also occur, and drainage or clot removal may be indicated in rare instances of severe hemorrhage. Premature suture breakage with localized graft retraction requires early resuturing, as a localized pterygium recurrence will occur. The superior bulbar conjunctival harvest site, which rapidly re-epithelizes, should also be inspected, since occasionally

granuloma formation may occur, requiring more aggressive steroid therapy, and occasionally, granuloma excision. Significant scarring with granuloma formation usually occurs only when a thick graft is harvested, involving removal of Tenon's tissue.

Causes of Recurrence After Conjunctival Autografting

The morphological appearance of pterygium recurrence after conjunctival autografting suggests several factors, which may lead to graft failure. Recurrence of the pterygium may occur at the superior or inferior margins of the conjunctival graft, suggesting that either inadequate peripheral excision of pterygium tissue occurred, or insufficient graft size are contributing factors. A thick graft with inclusion of underlying Tenon's tissue may lead to graft retraction and scalloping of the graft edge in the early postoperative period, causing exposure of bare sclera at the margins of the graft, which subsequently becomes the site of recurrence. Early breakage of sutures will also lead to localized graft retraction and localized recurrence at that site. However, it should be noted that in certain cases, a well-aligned and -sutured, thin conjunctival graft may itself subsequently transform into a recurrent pterygium at the region of the limbus, suggesting that a corneal or limbal factor may be responsible for recurrence in this instance (Figure 15.12).

Essential Factors for Successful Conjunctival Autografting

Based on the mechanisms of recurrence associated with conjunctival autograft failure, the important surgical principles of conjunctival autografting may be inferred and reemphasized:

1. obtaining a generous graft (measuring 6 to 8 mm horizontally and vertically)
2. adequate removal of all surrounding fibrovascular tissue
3. obtaining a thin, Tenon's-free graft (by superficial dissection techniques) to ensure minimal graft retraction
4. adequate stabilization of graft with anchoring sutures at the limbus, superior and inferior edges of the graft

Complications of Conjunctival Autografting

Conjunctival autografting is generally considered a safe procedure, since no serious sight-threatening complications are associated. However, complications relating to surgery may occur, both intraoperatively or in the early or late postoperative period, and awareness of these problems will enable appropriate preventive or therapeutic measures to be performed.

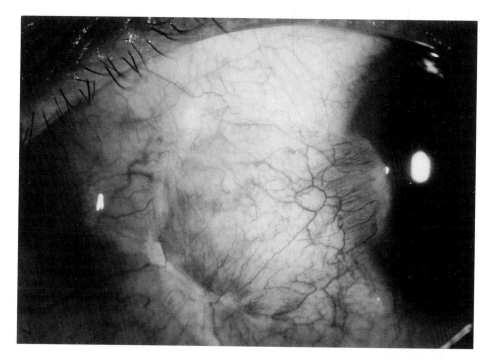

Figure 15.12. Recurrence after conjunctival autografting—one of the rare situations when the autograft itself transforms into a pterygium, leading to recurrence stemming from the graft itself. Note persistence of ocular surface inflammation as a possible causative factor.

1. Intraoperative Complications

a. Corneoscleral Perforation

This is an extremely rare complication that can occur only from inadvertent and excessive removal of corneal, limbal or scleral tissue. This may occur during excision of severe recurrent cases, in which excessive tissue was previously resected. Alternatively, perforation may occur in cases of misdiagnosed pseudopterygium, in which the primary pathology was an inadequately resected congenital limbal or epibulbar dermoid. In suspicious cases, a careful history to exclude the pre-existence of a dermoid-like limbal mass should be excluded, and if in doubt, the surgeon should have corneal or scleral donor tissue at hand with which to perform a lamellar corneoscleral patch graft.

b. Rectus Muscle Disinsertion

This is also a rare complication that would generally occur in severe recurrent pterygia, where previous scarring has resulted in obliteration and distortion of landmarks and tissue planes. In these cases, it may be difficult to identify muscle tissue that may be encased in thick scar tissue, and therefore prior isolation and tagging of the muscle should be tried before surgery on pterygium scar tissue is attempted. Identification of the muscle may be made by entering the sub-Tenon's space in the inferomedial or superomedial quadrant (where no scar tissue exists), and hooking the muscle with a squint hook. Traction with a muscle suture by an assistant then helps to maintain orientation of where the muscle is likely to lie, at the same time increasing exposure for dissection. During pterygium scar dissection, one should attempt to carefully dissect the scar tissue in superficial layers, and the first hint of muscle dam-

age is often a sudden profuse hemorrhage. Once a portion of the rectus muscle is identified, it is relatively simple to divide away the fibrous scar tissue encasing the muscle sheath. In the event of muscle damage, this should be carefully repaired and hemostasis secured before proceeding with further dissection. If the ultimate disaster occurs and the muscle is totally detached, locating the retracted muscle will be necessary. The various techniques utilized to perform this are outside the scope of this chapter but are fully described in strabismus surgery texts.

2. Early Postoperative Complications

a. Graft Edema (Figure 15.13)

Edema will occur to a certain extent in all cases after surgery and may persist for up to 3 weeks after surgery. Excessive edema will cause concern to patients and may result in adjacent corneoscleral dellen formation, requiring topical lubricants. Factors contributing to excessive edema are likely to be excessive surgical manipulation and prolonged surface drying of the graft. As outlined above, vertical cuts may be made intraoperatively, or in the early postoperative period, to allow egress of edema fluid, but reaccumulation of fluid usually occurs. Since excessive edema does not appear to influence graft survival, no treatment is necessary for this self-limiting condition.

b. Graft Hemorrhage (Figure 15.14)

Graft hemorrhage may be noted on the first postoperative day and is usually due to poor hemostasis of the scleral bed. Mild cases do not need surgical intervention, but a severe hematoma may lead to excessive graft elevation and dellen formation and is amenable to sim-

Figure 15.13. Graft edema with dellen formation.

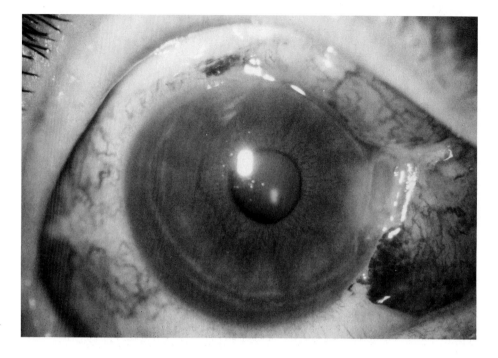

ple drainage through a fine needle puncture, performed at the slit-lamp.

c. Graft Retraction/Suture Breakage

Suture breakage during the first few days after surgery will result in graft retraction and may ultimately result in a conjunctival recurrence in that area. Within the first few days, it is advisable to resuture and attach the graft in place. Rarely, trauma or excessive eye rubbing may result in physical sloughing of the graph.

d. Graft Inversion and Necrosis

As discussed earlier, a graft that has been inadvertently inverted with the epithelial surface facing the scleral bed will appear white, opaque, and stains with fluorescein. Graft necrosis and sloughing will eventually occur. Correct replacement of the graft may be successfully performed within 24 to 48 hours of surgery. Beyond that, an amniotic membrane graft, a sliding conjunctival flap, or a graft from the opposite eye may be required. Alternatively, the necrotic graft may be simply removed

Figure 15.14. Graft hemorrhage.

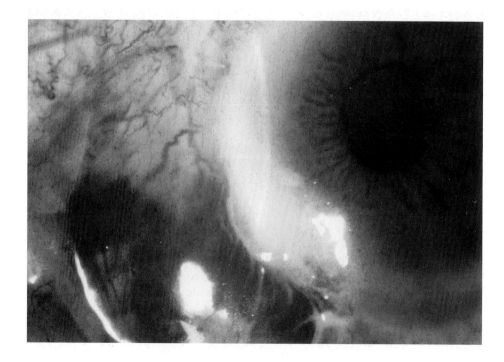

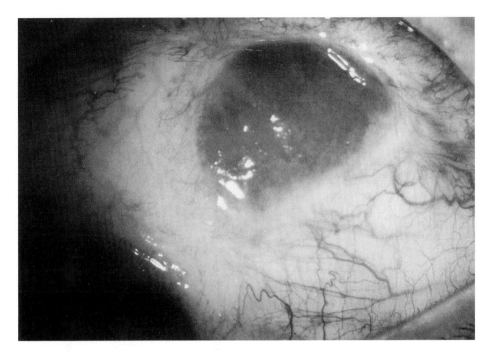

Figure 15.15. Granuloma formation at the graft harvest site, leading to subconjunctival fibrosis and scarring.

and the scleral bed left to re-epithelize as in a bare excision procedure, although this will be likely to lead to pterygium recurrence.

e. Corneoscleral Dellen

Dellen formation may occur after conjunctival autografting, either in the cornea adjacent to the graft, or in the scleral bed next to a retracted, edematous or hemorrhagic graft. Dellen may be treated conservatively with lubricants, ointments or eye patching. Dellen should be distinguished from scleral or corneal melting, which will not resolve with lubrication.

f. Conjunctival Granulomas (Figure 15.15)

Tenon's granuloma formation may occur within a week after pterygium surgery as a proliferative, inflammatory lesion; it is a form of pyogenic granuloma. Due to excessive inflammation and localized irritation occurring at the site of exposed Tenon's tissue, granulomas may occur at the graft harvest site, in the recipient bed adjacent to the autograft, or as a stitch granuloma. In our clinical trial comparing bare sclera excision with conjunctival autografting, the incidence of granuloma formation at the pterygium excision site was 19%.[4] In contrast, no granulomas occurred at the donor site with our superficial dissection technique. Minimal disturbance of Tenon's layer during superficial dissection will, therefore, greatly reduce the incidence of granuloma formation at the donor site. Small granulomas may spontaneously resolve with frequent application of steroid eyedrops, but larger granulomas are amenable to simple excision by virtue of their pedunculated structure.

3. Late Postoperative Complications

a. Epithelial Inclusion Cysts (Figure 15.16)

Cysts may occur in the graft and usually appear several weeks after surgery. Cysts are the result of inadvertent implantation of epithelium beneath the graft and are generally innocuous and self-limiting. Cyst puncture and drainage is a simple procedure, but the fluid often reaccumulates. Rarely, if recurrent and symptomatic, marsupialization, in which the cyst is laid open and the walls resected, may be required.

b. Conjunctival Scarring (Subconjunctival Fibrosis) at the Donor Site

Dense fibrotic scarring may occur at the donor site and often follows a prolonged healing process, excessive inflammation or granuloma formation at the donor site.[26] Scarring is more likely to be present if Tenon's tissue is excised at the time of graft harvesting, and is rare if superficial dissection is successful. Donor site scarring is asymptomatic, however, and is only of consequence if repeat grafting is required (scarring precludes harvesting of conjunctiva from the same site), or in the event of the patient developing glaucoma requiring filtration surgery. The presence of superior conjunctival scarring reduces the success of filtration surgery, and a superior temporal site for harvesting should be selected to reserve the superomedial quadrant as a site for future filtration surgery.

c. Steroid-induced Ocular Hypertension

The significant degree of ocular surface inflammation occurring after conjunctival autografting exceeds that which occurs after cataract surgery, necessitating the use of topical steroids for several weeks after surgery. In our clinical trial of conjunctival autografting, the ste-

Figure 15.16. Epithelial cyst occurring within the autograft.

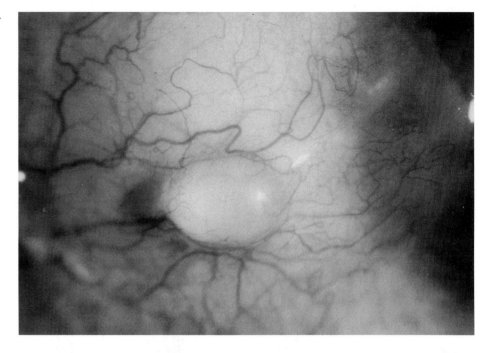

roid responder rate was 7%, and, therefore, monitoring of intraocular pressure after pterygium surgery is mandatory, especially as donor-site harvesting affects the success of future filtration surgery.

d. Corneal Astigmatism and Scarring
Careful excision of the pterygium, as discussed above, reduces iatrogenic scarring and induced astigmatism from either corneal tissue loss or from surface remnants of pterygium scar tissue. However, stromal scarring from lipid deposition often occurs in deeply invasive pterygia. Advanced pterygia are more likely to induce larger degrees of astigmatism and scarring within the visual axis. Localized changes in the precorneal tear film may in part be responsible for the localized flattening in the affected quadrant noted on corneal topography,[27] and partial regression of astigmatism may occur after successful conjunctival autografting.[28–31] In cases of severe scarring, lamellar keratoplasty is indicated.

Variants of Conjunctival Autografting

Certain situations may not permit conventional conjunctival autografting. Since an integral part of the procedure is to obtain healthy tissue from the superior bulbar conjunctiva, in eyes with prior damage or scarring, harvesting of donor tissue may not be possible. In addition, in cases in which several quadrants of limbus are involved, for example, broad pterygia, or combined medial and temporal pterygia, conventional autografting may not be feasible. In these situations, the modified techniques of conjunctival rotational autografting and annular conjunctival autografting are suggested. Note that these procedures are more advanced forms of

conjunctival autografting that should be attempted only after mastering conventional conjunctival autografting. An alternative to these procedures would be to obtain a free autograft from an unaffected opposite eye or a transposition flap from the inferior bulbar conjunctiva.[32]

1. Conjunctival Rotational Autografting

The major disadvantage of conjunctival autografting lies in the fact that harvesting a graft from the superior bulbar conjunctiva inevitably results in further ocular surface surgery in an eye with an already existing focal ocular surface disorder. In certain situations, surgery involving superior bulbar conjunctiva is contraindicated, or not possible. These situations include glaucoma patients with pre-existing drainage surgery blebs or seton surgery, glaucoma patients in which filtration surgery may possibly be indicated in future, or preexisting scarring in which harvesting a thin conjunctival graft would be very difficult. Alternatively, in cases in which excessively large, or several, grafts are required, for example in combined nasal and temporal pterygium surgery, or in combined cataract and pterygium surgery, conventional autografting may not be ideal.

We have described a modified procedure of conventional autografting, in which superior bulbar conjunctiva need not be utilized, which is termed conjunctival rotational autografting.[33] In this technique, conjunctival epithelium overlying the pterygium itself is carefully dissected and laid aside. After removal of the underlying fibrovascular pterygium tissue, this epithelium is replaced over the bare sclera after a 180-degree rotation so that normal nasal canthal epithelium can be applied to the limbal area (Figure 15.17).

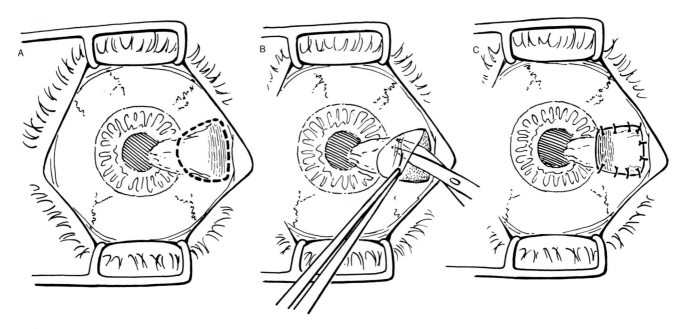

Figure 15.17. Stages of conjunctival rotational autografting: A. the area of conjunctival epithelium to be harvested is outlined by the black dotted line; B. The epithelial layer (with minimal subepithelial tissue) is dissected free taking care not to include the underlying fibrovascular pterygium tissue; C. The epithelial layer is replaced with a 180-degree reorientation onto the bared scleral bed (epithelial surface up). (*Ophthalmology* 1999; 106.1:67–71, with permission from Elsevier Science.)

A "rotated island graft" was first described by Spaeth in the 1920s.[34] Blatt in 1931 suggested that a 180-degree rotation of the graft displaces abnormal epithelium at the head of the pterygium away from the limbus, which in turn receives relatively normal epithelium from the nasal canthus.[35] Our prospective single-surgeon case series of 51 consecutive rotational autografts for 46 primary and 5 recurrent pterygia revealed a recurrence rate of 4% at a mean follow-up period of 12 months (range 2–22 months), suggesting that the efficacy of this procedure in reducing recurrence may be similar to that of conventional conjunctival autografting.[33] Indications for rotational autografting in this series included glaucoma patients, superior conjunctival scarring, simultaneous nasal and temporal pterygium surgery, and combined cataract and pterygium surgery.

It should be noted, however, that rotational autografting is significantly more difficult to do, since thin dissection of pterygium epithelium with separation of underlying pterygium fibrovascular tissue is difficult. In addition, oversizing of the graft is not possible. As such, conjunctival rotational autografting should only be attempted by surgeons who are already skilled in conventional conjunctival autografting. Other disadvantages of this procedure are prolonged graft hyperemia in some cases and increased epithelial pigmentation in highly pigmented conjunctiva. However, in the majority of cases, rotational autografting may achieve excellent cosmesis, if properly performed (Figure 15.18).

2. Annular Conjunctival Autografting

In extreme cases of pterygium, two or more quadrants of limbus may be destroyed by fibrovascular pterygium invasion. In cases of severe combined nasal and temporal pterygium, close proximity of lesions, either superiorly or inferiorly, results in virtual merging of pterygia, which again involves a large area of limbus. In these instances, the conventional technique of graft harvesting in conjunctival autografting may be inadequate to cover the subtotal limbal defect. We have, therefore, described a modification of conjunctival autografting whereby an elongated segment of conjunctiva is applied to the limbus to ensure full coverage of the annular limbal defect.[33] To obtain an elongated strip of conjunctiva, a large conventionally shaped rectangular graft is first harvested from the superior bulbar conjunctiva. This graft is then partially divided in its long axis to form an elongated strip (Figure 15.19A). This strip may now be carefully wrapped around the limbus to cover the scleral defect and sutured in place (Figure 15.19B). Figure 15.20 illustrates the successful implementation of annular conjunctival autografting in an advanced pterygium involving most of the cornea and limbus. The elongated strip of conjunctiva is clearly seen 1 week after surgery (Figure 15.20B). Six months after pterygium surgery, no recurrence was noted, and the patient subsequently underwent successful penetrating keratoplasty (Figure 15.20C,D).

Figure 15.18. Conjunctival rotational autograft in a patient with pterygium and preexisting glaucoma. A. preoperative state; B. 9 days after pterygium excision with rotational autografting; C. 17 months after surgery—no recurrence with good cosmetic result. (*Ophthalmology* 1999; 106.1:67–71, with permission from Elsevier Science.)

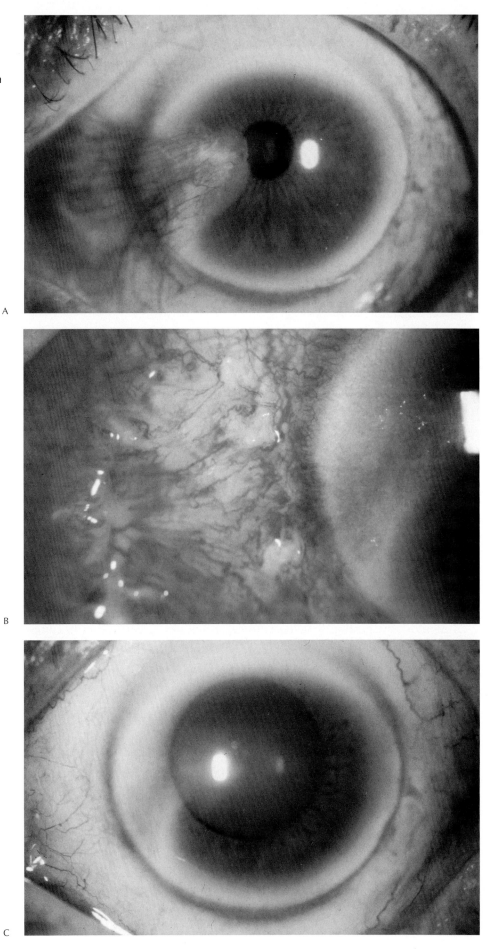

A

B

C

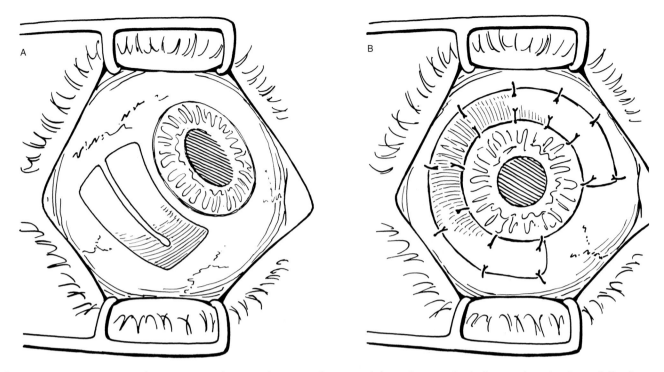

Figure 15.19. Stages in annular conjunctival autografting: A. a larger graft from the superior bulbar conjunctiva is partially divided lengthwise to obtain an elongated strip of conjunctiva; B. the elongated strip of conjunctiva is wrapped around the limbal defect and sutured in place. (*Cornea* 1997; 16.3:365–368, permission from Lippincott/Williams & Wilkins.)

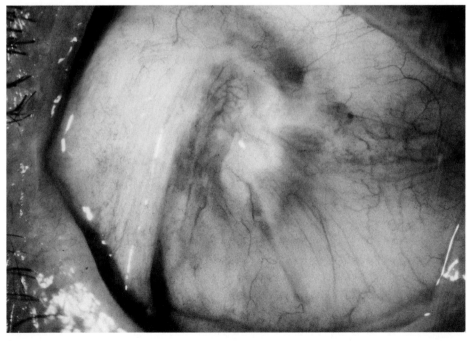

A

Figure 15.20. Annular conjunctival graft in advanced subtotal primary pterygium: A. preoperative state—advanced primary pterygium.

(*Figure continues on the next page.*)

Figure 15.20. (*Continued*) B. 7 days after surgery—the elongated strip is in place around the limbus; C. successful annular conjunctival autografting 6 months after surgery—no recurrence noted; D. 2 years after penetrating keratoplasty: no pterygium recurrence has occurred. Visual acuity correctable to 20/30. (*Cornea* 1997; 16.3:365–368, with permission from Lippincott/Williams & Wilkins.)

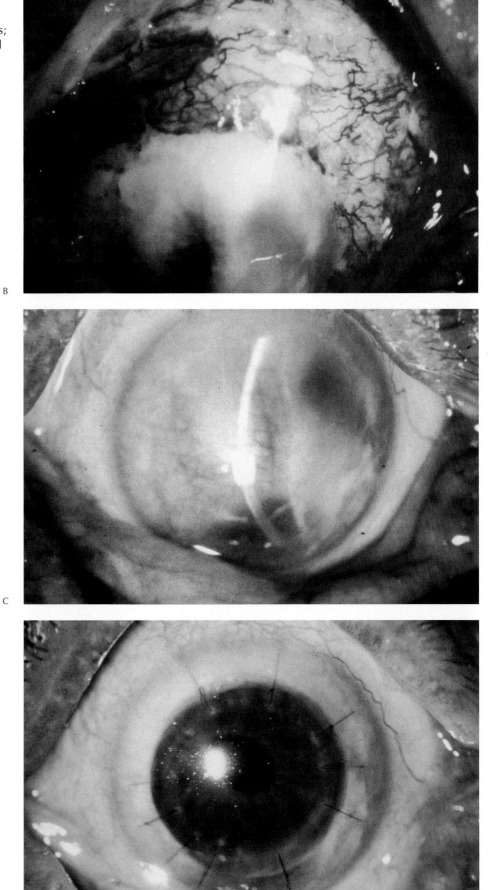

B

C

D

References

1. Thoft RA. Conjunctival transplantation. *Archives of Ophthalmology* 1977; 95:1425–1427.

2. Gómez-Márquez J. New operative procedure for pterygium. *Arch de oftal hispano-am* 1931; 31:87.

3. Kenyon KR, Wagoner MD, Hettinger ME. Conjunctival autograft transplantation for advanced and recurrent pterygium. *Ophthalmology* 1985; 92.11;1461–1470.

4. Tan DTH, Chee SP, Dear KBG, Lim ASM. Effect of pterygium morphology on pterygium recurrence in a controlled trial comparing conjunctival autografting with bare sclera excision. *Archives of Ophthalmology* 1997; 115:1235–1240.

5. Ti SE, Chee SP, Dear KBG, Tan DTH. Analysis of variation in success rates in conjunctival autografting for primary and recurrent pterygium. *Br J Ophthalmol* 2000; 84:385–389.

6. Chen PP, Ariyasu RG, Kaza V, LaBree LD, McDonald PJ. A randomized trial comparing mitomycin and conjunctival autograft after excision of primary pterygium. *American Journal of Ophthalmology* 1995; 120.2:151–160.

7. Singh G, Wilson MR, Foster CS. Long-term follow-up study of mitomycin eye drops as adjunctive treatment for pterygia and its comparison with conjunctival autograft transplantation. *Cornea* 1990; 9.4:331–334.

8. Lewallen S. A randomized trial of conjunctival autografting for pterygium in the tropics. *Ophthalmology* 1989; 96.11:1612–1614.

9. Prabhasawat P, Barton K, Burkett G, Tseng SCG. Comparison of conjunctival autografts, amniotic membrane grafts, and primary closure for pterygium excision. *Ophthalmology* 1997; 104.6:974–985.

10. Starck T, Kenyon KR, Serrano F. Conjunctival autograft for primary and recurrent pterygia: Surgical technique and problem management. *Cornea* 1991; 10.3:196–202.

11. Jaros PA, DeLuise VP. Pingueculae and pterygia. *Survey of Ophthalmology* 1988; 33.1:41–49.

12. Sebban A, Hirst LW. Treatment of pterygia in Queensland. *Australian and New Zealand Journal of Ophthalmology* 1991; 19.2:123–127.

13. Wong VA, Law FCH. Use of mitomycin C with conjunctival autograft in pterygium surgery in Asian-Canadians. *Ophthalmology* 1999; 106.8:1512–1515.

14. Mutlu FM, Sobaci G, Tatar T, Yildirim E. A comparative study of recurrent pterygium surgery. *Ophthalmology* 1999; 106.4:817–821.

15. Manning CA, Kloess PM, Diaz MD, Yee RW. Intraoperative mitomycin in primary pterygium excision. *Ophthalmology* 1997; 104.5:844–848.

16. Yanyali AC, Talu H, Alp BN, Karabas L, Ay GM, Caglar Y. Intraoperative mitomycin C in the treatment of pterygium. *Cornea* 2000; 19:471–473.

17. Singh G, Wilson MR, Foster CS. Mitomycin eye drops as treatment for pterygium. *Ophthalmology* 1988; 95:813–821.

18. Hayasaka S, Noda S, Yamamoto Y, Setogawa T. Postoperative instillation of low-dose mitomycin C in the treatment of primary pterygium. *American Journal of Ophthalmology* 1988; 106:715–718.

19. Mahar PS, Nwokora G. Role of mitomycin C in pterygium surgery. *British Journal of Ophthalmology* 1993; 77:433–435.

20. Caliskan S, Orhan M, Irkec M. Intraoperative and postoperative use of mitomycin-C in the treatment of primary pterygium. *Ophthalmic Surgery and Lasers* 1996; 27.7:600–604.

21. Frucht-Pery J, Siganos CS, Ilsar M. Intraoperative application of topical mitomycin C for pterygium surgery. *Ophthalmology* 1996; 103.4:674–677.

22. Mastropasqua L, Carpineto P, Ciancaglini M, Gallenga PE. Long term results of intraoperative mitomycin C in the treatment of recurrent pterygium. *British Journal of Ophthalmology* 1996; 80:288–291.

23. Sánchez-Thorin JC, Rocha G, Yelin JB. Meta-analysis on the recurrence rates after bare sclera resection with and without mitomycin C use and conjunctival autograft placement in surgery for primary pterygium. *British Journal of Ophthalmology* 1998; 82:661–665.

24. Chen JK, Tsai RJF, Lin SS. Fibroblasts isolated from human pterygia exhibit transformed cell characteristics. *In Vitro Cell Dev Biol* 1994; 30A:243–248.

25. Tan DTH, Liu YP, Sun L. Flow cytometry measurements of DNA content in primary and recurrent pterygia. *Investigative Ophthalmology & Visual Science* 2000; 41:(7)1684–1686.

26. Vrabec MP, Weisenthal RW, Elsing SH. Subconjunctival fibrosis after conjunctival autograft. *Cornea* 1993; 12.2:181–183.

27. Oldenburg JB, Garbus J, McDonnell JM, McDonnell PJ. Conjunctival pterygia. *Cornea* 1990; 9.3:200–204.

28. Fong KS, Balakrishnan V, Chee SP, Tan DTH. Refractive change following pterygium surgery. *The CLAO Journal* 1998; 24.2:115–117.

29. Walland MJ, Stevens JD, Steele ADM. The effect of recurrent pterygium on corneal topography. *Cornea* 1994; 13.5:463–464.

30. Stern GA, Lin A. Effect of pterygium excision on induced corneal topographic abnormalities. *Cornea* 1998; 17.1:23–27.

31. Tomidokoro A, Oshika T, Amano S, Eguchi K, Eguchi S. Quantitative analysis of regular and irregular astigmatism induced by pterygium. *Cornea* 1999; 18.4:412–415.

32. Kim S, Yang Y, Kim J. Primary pterygium surgery using the inferior conjunctival transposition flap. *Ophthalmic Surgery and Lasers* 1998; 29.7:608–611.

33. Jap A, Chan C, Lim L, Tan DTH. Conjunctival rotation autograft for pterygium. *Ophthalmology* 1999; 106.1:67–71.

34. Spaeth ED. Rotated island graft operation for pterygium. *American Journal of Ophthalmology* 1926; 9:649–655.

35. Blatt N. Replantation of pterygium as a method of operation for pterygium. *Ztsch für Augenh* 1932; 76:161.

16
Conjunctival Limbal Autograft

Christopher R. Croasdale, Edward J. Holland, and Mark J. Mannis

Indications

A conjunctival limbal autograft (CLAU) is indicated for patients needing epithelial stem cell (SC) transplantation for management of corneal surface disease due to unilateral limbal stem cell deficiency (Table 16.1). Prior chemical or thermal injuries are the most common causes of limbal SC deficiency. Other etiologies include iatrogenic limbal SC deficiency and extensive limbal or conjunctival neoplasias, such as conjunctival intraepithelial neoplasia, squamous cell carcinoma, and sebaceous cell carcinoma. Although these groups account for the majority of cases of unilateral limbal SC deficiency, it is important to recognize that additional cases can occur as a result of any condition where the common underlying pathology is chronic, usually severe, ocular surface inflammation.

Contraindications

In considering a CLAU for unilateral ocular surface disease (OSD), the vital criterion for tissue selection is that the donor eye be free from any condition that may predispose it to later development of limbal SC deficiency, such as long-term contact lens use, multiple prior surgeries, or glaucoma (where the success of potential future filtering surgery could be adversely affected by prior conjunctival surgery). Jenkins et al.[1] reported on conjunctival limbal autografts in five patients with severe epitheliopathy secondary to chronic contact lens wear. Two of the five procedures failed, and one of the donor eyes developed epitheliopathy. These results are likely due to the fact that the donor tissue was obtained from the fellow eyes that were not normal, in that they had also been exposed to chronic contact lens wear. Patients with contact-lens-induced keratopathy may present with unilateral (typically superior) limbal deficiency. Yet with the exception of the rare instance in which the individual has worn a contact lens only in the affected eye, a CLAU from the other eye is ill advised in any bilateral long-term contact lens wearer due to the risk of causing limbal SC deficiency in the donor eye. If any contraindications exist, either a living-related conjunctival allograft or a keratolimbal allograft is advised.

Past, Present and Future of CLAU

The Evolution of CLAU

Procedures designed to restore normal corneal epithelium have evolved over the past several decades. Epithelial transplantation for severe ocular surface disease was first described in 1977 by Thoft,[2] when he described conjunctival transplantation for monocular chemical burns. This conjunctival autograft procedure used several pieces of bulbar conjunctiva from a normal fellow eye as donor tissue. In 3 of 17 eyes, successful re-epithelialization of the cornea was achieved and was accompanied by improved vision and decreased neovascularization. The mean follow-up time of 9 months was relatively short. In 1982 Thoft reported on an additional 17 cases of ocular surface disease that were managed with a conjunctival autograft.[3] Sixteen of these eyes achieved a stable ocular surface with a median follow-up of 36 months and a range of 12 to 60 months. Ten of these eyes had a significant improvement in vision. In 1982, Vastine et al.[4] reported on the use of conjunctival autografts from fellow eyes in 14 patients, 7 with diagnoses consistent with limbal deficiency. They reported that all 7 of these cases developed a stable ocular surface postoperatively with a median follow-up of 16.5 months and a range of 10 to 18 months.

The conjunctival autograft procedure was based on the concept of conjunctival transdifferentiation.[2,4,5,6] Although a conjunctival autograft is useful to re-establish an intact ocular surface in patients with conjunctival scarring, concerns exist whether this procedure truly results in normal corneal epithelium.[7] Tsai et al.[8] com-

Table 16.1. Ocular surface disease secondary to unilateral limbal stem cell deficiency.

Disease	Pathogenesis of unilateral limbal deficiency
Chemical burn	Direct injury to limbal stem cells; prolonged post-injury inflammation
Thermal burn	Direct injury to limbal stem cells; prolonged post-injury inflammation
Iatrogenic limbal stem cell deficiency	Excision and/or mechanical destruction of limbal stem cells or chronic exposure to toxic medications with damage to stem cells
Neoplasia	Replacement of normal limbal stem cells with neoplastic cells
Contact-lens-induced keratopathy	Hypoxia, mechanical trauma, and chemical toxicity damage to limbal stem cells
Severe keratoconjunctivitis	Multiple possible etiologies with common final pathologic pathway of significant and prolonged ocular surface inflammation of the cornea and limbus

pared the results of limbal transplantation to conjunctival transplantation in a rabbit model of OSD. They reported a significant decrease in corneal neovascularization with limbal transplantation, and the resultant corneal epithelia displayed the corneal phenotype. Conjunctival transplantation resulted in corneal epithelia with the phenotype of conjunctiva. The technique of conjunctival autograft remains a valuable procedure for the management of fornix reconstruction and primary and recurrent pterygium, but the success of conjunctival transplantation for the establishment of the corneal surface when a source of limbal stem cells is not available remains to be determined. It is possible that in some of the patients reported above there was only conjunctival or partial limbal deficiency, so that with transfer of healthy, noninflamed conjunctiva the recipient eye improved because of reduced inflammation, allowing the residual healthy limbal tissue to restore the corneal epithelium to its proper state.

Procedures to transplant the limbus have been devised based on the concept of limbal stem cells. Kenyon and Tseng[9] in 1989 described a modification of the conjunctival autograft, which they named limbal autograft transplantation. In this procedure, conjunctiva and limbus from a normal fellow were used to manage diffuse limbal deficiency in unilateral ocular surface disease, or focal limbal deficiency in unilateral or bilateral disease. Their technique used grafts of bulbar conjunctiva that extended approximately 0.5 millimeter onto the clear cornea centrally, thus containing limbal cells. The authors reported data on 21 cases with 6 months or more of follow-up. Preoperative diagnoses included acute and chronic chemical injuries, thermal injury, contact-lens-induced keratopathy, and surface disease secondary to multiple surgeries. The results were impressive with rapid surface healing in 19 cases, stable ocular surface in 20 cases, improved visual acuity in 17 cases, and arrest or regression of corneal neovascularization in 15 cases. No complications developed in the donor eyes. Seven of 7 patients underwent simultaneous or subsequent successful penetrating or lamellar keratoplasty. Based on the nomenclature system of Holland and Schwartz,[5] this procedure is termed conjunctival limbal autograft.

Present and Future Use of CLAU

CLAU has been a major advance in the management of severe unilateral OSD. These procedures are now widely utilized by many corneal surgeons, and numerous patients have benefitted. As indicated earlier, a concern remains of potentially inducing iatrogenic limbal SC deficiency in the donor eye. Fortunately, the risk appears quite low based on several decades of both our clinical experience, and that of others in the literature.[9]

In Chapter 21, Drs. Isseroff and Schwab discuss exciting recent advancements in ex vivo stem cell expansion, which potentially could eliminate the need for harvesting relatively larger amounts of limbal tissue for autologous SC transfer. Such a breakthrough will be readily welcomed, although with the reality of inequitable availability of economic and medical resources around the world, it would not likely eliminate the usefulness and need for the standard CLAU procedure for many years to come.

Preoperative Considerations

Risks and Benefits

The major benefit in using autologous tissue as the donor source in any ocular epithelial transplantation procedure is that the need for systemic immunosuppression is eliminated, since there is no risk for tissue rejection. Additionally, a CLAU is particularly beneficial for patients with conjunctival inflammation because it provides normal, noninflamed, unscarred conjunctiva in addition to healthy limbal stem cells. These benefits can improve the prognosis for a favorable outcome compared to allograft procedures.

A major concern already discussed is the potential risk for the donor fellow eye. One study has demonstrated that partial removal of full-thickness limbal zone will compromise the donor surface.[10] When a large corneal epithelial defect was subsequently introduced in these eyes, a clinical picture consistent with limbal deficiency occurred. In addition, it has been shown that even the removal of partial-thickness limbal epithelium could cause a milder form of limbal deficiency and abnormal corneal epithelial wound healing.[11] We believe the risk of donor epithelial problems is low especially if less than 6 clock hours of limbal tissue and a moderate amount of conjunctiva are removed from the donor eye. We have not seen complications in the donor eyes of our patients, nor did Kenyon and Tseng[9] in one of the largest series of CLAU in the literature.

Management of Coexistent Pathology

Ocular adnexa and anterior segment structures of patients with severe OSD must be carefully examined. Abnormal globe-to-eyelid anatomy can lead to chronic exposure, chronic inflammation, and direct corneal trauma with resultant complications such as recurrent corneal epithelial erosion, secondary microbial keratitis, vascularization, and scarring. Significant abnormal lid positions such as entropion or ectropion should be corrected prior to limbal transplantation. Trichiasis and distichiasis can be treated with cryotherapy, argon laser, surgical excision, or manual epilation. Palpebral conjunctival keratinization and loss of normal forniceal architecture can be treated with mucous membrane or amniotic membrane grafting.

An assessment of aqueous tear production should be performed. Patients with a low Schirmer test, a scant tear lake, and rose bengal or fluorescein staining consistent with aqueous tear deficiency usually require permanent punctal occlusion. Additional medical management of dry eye from either aqueous or lipid tear deficiency is covered in Chapter 4. Blepharitis should also be treated maximally and is covered in Chapter 3. If lagophthalmos or poor lid closure exists, lateral tarsorrhaphy at the time of surgery will improve chances for success by narrowing the palpebral fissure and improving ocular surface wetting through reduced surface area exposure and tear evaporation.

It is crucial to ask about any past history of glaucoma, and to look for evidence of this condition during the physical examination. Patients with severe OSD are at increased risk for developing secondary glaucoma. Prolonged anterior segment inflammation after chemical and thermal injuries can cause scarring and decreased functioning of the trabecular meshwork and normal aqueous outflow pathways. Chronic topical corticosteroid adds additional risk. Patients with iatrogenic limbal SC deficiency from multiple prior surgical procedures may have poorly controlled intraocular pressures if there is significant scarring of the peripheral angle of the anterior chamber. Glaucoma should be managed aggressively to ensure the best prognosis for visual rehabilitation. Poorly controlled chronic glaucoma is a major risk factor for long-term poor visual outcome in patients who otherwise undergo successful limbal SC grafting.

Surgical Technique

This procedure involves transfer of limbal stem cells from the healthy fellow eye to the diseased eye primarily utilizing conjunctiva as a carrier.

Anesthesia

The procedure involves both eyes. If the patient is healthy and can safely tolerate general anesthesia, this is often our preferred method because it eliminates time constraints of local anesthesia and reduces patient anxiety over a bilateral procedure. Alternatively, local anesthesia can be employed with a peri- or retrobulbar block with or without a VIIth cranial nerve block (O'Brien) for the recipient eye, and topical/subconjunctival anesthesia for the donor eye.

Preparation of the Recipient Eye

Any speculum providing adequate exposure is used. A lateral canthotomy is sometimes necessary to increase exposure. If symblepharon formation has occurred and limits exposure of the ocular surface, it can be released at the limbus.

A 360° limbal peritomy is performed, and conjunctiva is resected posteriorly 2 to 3 mm from the limbus with Westcott scissors. It is important to remove this tissue from the limbus because the new source of epithelium must repopulate the ocular surface prior to reinvasion by the fibrovascular tissue of the conjunctiva. Extensive bleeding can occur due to neovascularization of the injured eye's surface. If this interferes with visualization, one can operate on a single quadrant at a time to control bleeding. Topical epinephrine (1:10,000 dilution) and thrombin applied with surgical spears are useful adjuncts to wet-field cautery. Once the limbal conjunctival tissue is excised, the recipient CLAU sites are prepared. The grafts will be centered at the 12 o'clock and 6 o'clock meridians and will measure approximately 8 mm horizontally by 5–8 mm vertically (no more than 3 clock hours each). If the limbal peritomy and conjunctival recession do not accommodate these dimensions, additional resection is done at the recipient sites as necessary (Figure 16.1A).

Next, abnormal corneal epithelium and fibrovascular pannus are removed by superficial dissection. Various approaches can be useful. Blunt dissection with a cellulose sponge may work. If a dissection plane is established, forceps can sometimes be used to peel off the abnormal tissue in a sheet. However, sharp dissection is often needed in areas to find an adequate tissue plane to create a smooth ocular surface. A No. 64 Beaver or equivalent crescent blade can be used for this maneuver. Care is taken to avoid cutting deep into stroma because of the risk of corneal perforation and postoperative optical distortion from surface irregularity. Bleeding is often encountered with the corneal surface

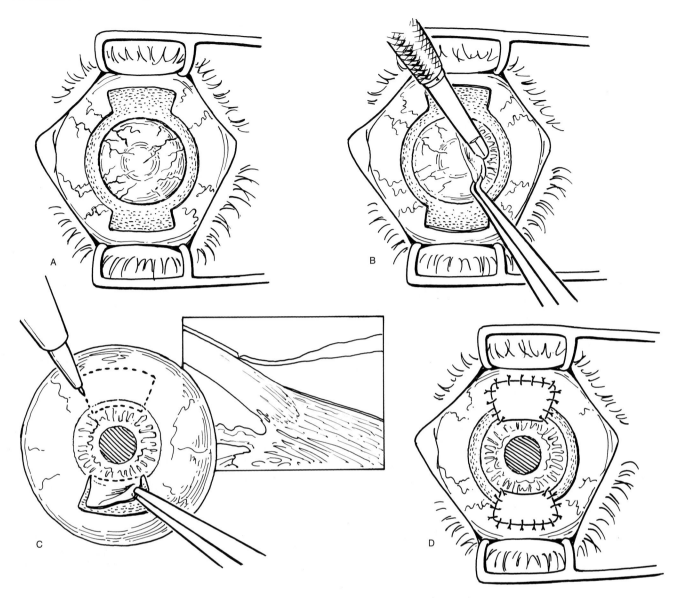

Figure 16.1. Technique for conjunctival limbal autograft (CLAU). (A) Recipient eye preparation. A 360° limbal peritomy is performed with removal of 2–3 mm of bulbar conjunctiva and additional resection at the 12 and 6 o'clock meridians; (B) Abnormal corneal epithelium and fibrovascular pannus are removed by superficial dissection using necessary techniques (peeling, blunt dissection, sharp dissection); (C) Donor tissue harvesting. Conjunctival dimensions of the grafts are marked with a gentian violet marking pen. Inset—Dissection of limbus is carried onto peripheral cornea beyond the vascular arcades. Harvesting begins with the bulbar conjunctival portion and proceeds anteriorly. (D) The conjunctival limbal grafts are transferred to their corresponding anatomic positions on the recipient eye and secured with multiple interrupted 10.0 nylon sutures.

pannus removal, and topical epinephrine and thrombin can be used on this tissue as well (Fig. 16.1B).

When hemostasis is achieved, the surface is moistened, the speculum removed, and the eyelids are closed while the autografts are being harvested from the other eye.

Harvesting the Donor Tissue

The speculum is placed in the fellow eye. The two conjunctival limbal autografts are taken from the corresponding 12 o'clock and 6 o'clock positions. A gentian violet surgical marking pen is used to mark the conjunctival portions of the grafts with the same dimensions as the recipient beds. Light cautery can be used to mark the conjunctival dimensions, although drawbacks include tissue damage and potential fusion of the conjunctiva to the underlying Tenon's capsule. The conjunctiva can be elevated from Tenon's layer with use of a subconjunctival injection of balanced salt solution or anesthetic without epinephrine. The needle entry point into the conjunctiva should be outside of the graft portion to minimize unnecessary defects. Dissection of the graft begins by incising with Westcott scissors along the lateral borders. If possible, the tissue should be completely undermined between the lateral edges before cutting along the posterior edge. This sequence helps keep the tissue on stretch. Once the posterior edge is cut, the thin conjunctival tissue folds and scrolls easily upon itself, making inadvertent damage such as buttonholes somewhat more likely. Non-toothed forceps are recommended to help avoid tearing the tissue. When the graft is completely free it is possible to become confused as to proper orientation. For this reason

it is helpful to include the gentian violet markings within the graft to delineate which side is the epithelial surface (Figure 16.1C).

Once the lateral and posterior edges are free, the conjunctiva is reflected anteriorly over the cornea and blunt dissection is continued anteriorly. When the point of conjunctival insertion at the limbus is reached, further blunt dissection should be performed with a dull scarifier (e.g., Tooke blade) into the peripheral cornea approximately 1 mm beyond the peripheral corneal vascular arcades. Some surgeons may prefer to complete the epitheliectomy with a sharp crescent blade, or even Vannas scissors. The desired corneal epithelial extent of

Figure 16.2. Conjunctival limbal autograft. A. Preoperative photograph of patient with unilateral chemical injury. Note the pannus and central epithelial defect. B. 6 months postoperative showing normal corneal epithelium.

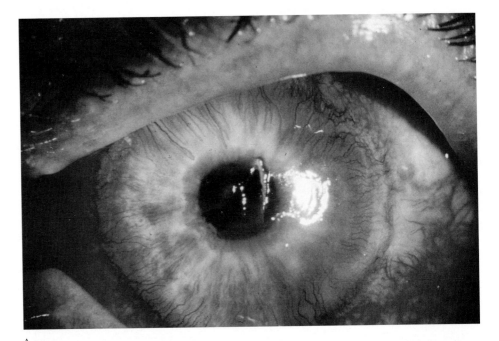

A

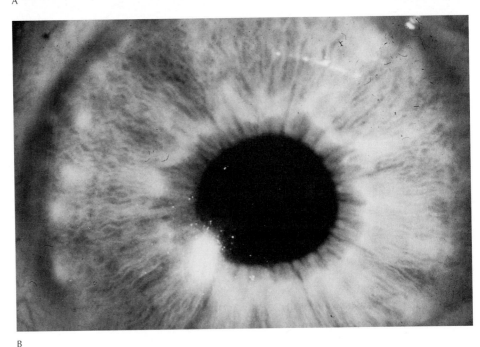

B

the dissection should be lightly marked with any type of blade from the corneal side. It is important to emphasize that this maneuver is essentially a superficial epithelial keratectomy of peripheral limbus and cornea and not a lamellar dissection into stroma or sclera. It is also extremely important to carry the dissection onto the peripheral cornea and to avoid prematurely excising the piece of tissue without the SCs.

Once the tissue is free, it is transferred epithelial-side-upward to a Petri dish and covered with corneal storage media (or balanced salt solution if the former is unavailable). The same procedure is completed at the 6 o'clock position. The donor sites are left open to

heal. The lid speculum is removed and the surface moistened before closing the lids and returning to the recipient eye.

Placement of the Donor Tissue

The recipient eye of the patient is reopened with placement of a speculum. One autograft is sutured at a time into its anatomically correct position (limbus to limbus) with multiple interrupted sutures. We recommend 10-0 nylon over polyglactin (Vicryl) because it causes less postoperative inflammation. Some surgeons use a combination, with 10-0 nylon for the anterior corneal sutures

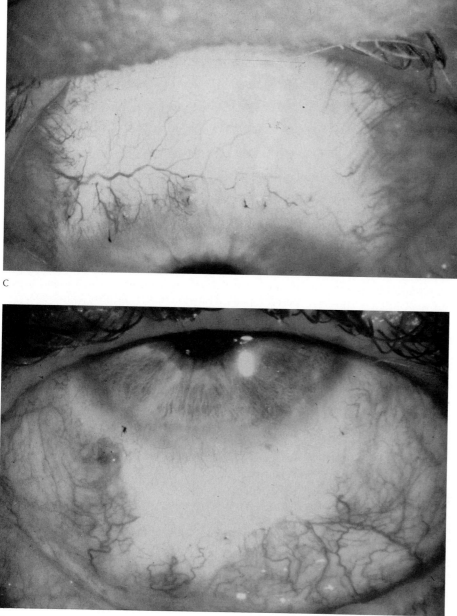

C

D

Figure 16.2. (*Continued*) C. and D. Site of conjunctival limbal autograft in recipient eye. Note the normal appearance of the conjunctival autografts and the chronic injection of the unoperated conjunctiva.

and 9-0 Vicryl for the conjunctival sutures. The corners are secured first, and additional sutures are placed along the conjunctival portions to prevent postoperative dehiscence. The sutures are placed first through the conjunctival graft, then through the recipient episcleral tissue, and finally through the recipient conjunctiva. We cut nylon sutures on the knot and leave short tails with Vicryl sutures. Knots can be left unburied because the bites are short, and attempts to bury them often result in the sutures either breaking or being pulled out accidentally. During suturing, the autograft epithelium should be protected from desiccation and trauma with balanced salt solution and a viscoelastic (Figure 16.1D). Figure 16.2 demonstrates a series of clinical photographs of a patient with a conjunctival limbal autograft.

At the conclusion of the operation, an antibiotic-steroid ointment can be placed on the recipient eye and a drop of antibiotic-steroid solution placed on the donor eye. A patch and protective shield is placed over the recipient eye until the patient is seen the next day.

Adjunctive Use of Amniotic Membrane

There are insufficient data to determine whether the adjunctive use of amniotic membrane with CLAU increases the success of the procedure. Details on the applications of amniotic membrane are covered in Chapter 19.

Proposed advantages include reduced inflammation postoperatively and faster epithelization of conjunctival and corneal surfaces with their appropriate respective epithelial phenotypes. The end result of these processes should be a reduction in postoperative vascularization and scarring. In partial limbal SC deficiency, amniotic membrane may work by providing a more hospitable substrate environment for the healthy remaining limbal SC, thereby facilitating expansion and re-epithelization with normal corneal epithelium.[12]

Disadvantages to the use of amniotic membrane primarily include high cost and relative unavailability. Most surgeons need the tissue only infrequently and lack the resources and facilities to prepare it on their own.

If adjunctive amniotic membrane is available, it can be applied in several ways. On the donor eye it can be placed over the donor graft sites to facilitate faster epithelization with reduced inflammation and scarring. On the recipient eye it can be placed either over the areas of recessed conjunctiva alone, or as a single sheet over both the cornea and exposed sclera. When used only on the exposed sclera and not the cornea, its role is to act as a barrier against conjunctivalization of the cornea. When applied additionally over the cornea, it may facilitate improved epithelization, although in patients with better preoperative visual acuity, it can be expected that vision will be affected until the amniotic membrane absorbs over the first several months.

Postoperative Care

The donor eye is treated with the antibiotic-steroid drops 3 to 4 times daily until epithelization is complete (usually 1 to 2 weeks) and inflammation has subsided. A rare complication is the occurrence of a pyogenic granuloma at a graft donor site.

The recipient eye is treated with a low-toxicity antibiotic several times daily as prophylaxis during epithelization. In addition, nonpreserved artificial tears are used frequently while the patient is awake. Topical steroids are used 3 or 4 times daily for inflammation. It is important to avoid excessive use of preserved topical medications because preservative toxicity can damage the fragile new epithelium. If significant inflammation occurs in the immediate postoperative period, oral steroids should be considered.

Nylon sutures can be left in place for many months. Those that become loose or cause irritation should be removed, preferably after at least several weeks of healing. Vicryl sutures usually loosen over 3 to 4 weeks and require removal if they do not fall out on their own.

References

1. Jenkins C, Tuft S, Liu C, et al. Limbal transplantation in the management of chronic contact-lens-associated epitheliopathy. *Eye* 1993; 7:629–633.
2. Thoft RA. Conjunctival transplantation. *Arch Ophthalmol* 1977; 95:1425–1427.
3. Thoft RA. Indications for conjunctival transplantation. *Ophthalmology* 1982; 89:335–339.
4. Vastine DW, Stewart WB, Schwab IR. Reconstruction of the periocular mucous membrane by autologous conjunctival transplantation. *Ophthalmology* 1982; 89:1072–1081.
5. Holland EJ, Schwartz GS. The evolution of epithelial transplantation for severe ocular surface disease and a proposed classification system. *Cornea* 1996; 15:549–556.
6. Kwitko S, Marinho D, Barcaro S, et al. Allograft conjunctival transplantation for bilateral ocular surface disorders. *Ophthalmology* 1995; 102:1020–1025.
7. Kruse FE, Chen JJY, Tsai RJF, et al. Conjunctival transdifferentiation is due to incomplete removal of limbal basal epithelium. *Invest Ophthalmol Vis Sci* 1990; 31:1903–1913.
8. Tsai RJ-F, Sun T-T, Tseng SCG. Comparison of limbal and conjunctival autograft transplantation in corneal surface reconstruction in rabbits. *Ophthalmology* 1990; 97:446–55.
9. Kenyon KR, Tseng SCG. Limbal autograft transplantation for ocular surface disorders. *Ophthalmology* 1989; 96:709–723.
10. Chen JJY, Tseng SCG. Corneal epithelial wound healing in partial limbal deficiency. *Invest Ophthalmol Vis Sci* 1990; 31:1301–1314.
11. Chen JJY, Tseng SCG. Abnormal corneal epithelial wound healing in partial thickness removal of limbal epithelium. *Invest Ophthalmol Vis Sci* 1991; 32:2219–2233.
12. Tseng SCG, Prabhasawat P, Barton K, et al. Amniotic membrane transplantation with or without limbal allografts for corneal surface reconstruction in patients with limbal stem cell deficiency. *Arch Ophthalmol* 1998; 116:431–441.

17

Living-Related Conjunctival Limbal Allograft

Sheraz M. Daya, Edward J. Holland, and Mark J. Mannis

Indications

The value of a normal limbus in maintaining a normal ocular surface has been well documented on the basis of anatomical and experimental evidence.[1-7] The objectives of epithelial stem cell transplantation are to restore phenotypic corneal epithelium to the corneal surface, to promote the barrier function of the limbus, and to improve surface lubrication, thus providing an improved milieu for maintenance of corneal clarity. Depending on the cause, as outlined in earlier chapters, stem cell deficiency may be bilateral and may also involve the conjunctiva with varying severity ranging from subconjunctival scarring, to keratinization, cicatrization, symblepharon formation, and secondary lid abnormalities. In bilateral disease, the only option for stem cell restoration is the use of allogeneic sources.[8-10] Procedures available include a cadaveric keratolimbal allograft (KLAL), living-related conjunctival limbal allograft (lrCLAL), and more recently, ex vivo stem cell allograft expansion.

Keratolimbal allograft transplantation has the advantage of providing a complete limbus for transplantation and thus a larger load of stem cells with restoration of a barrier to the whole limbus. The practical disadvantage is that it is almost impossible to obtain immune histocompatibility and, with such highly antigenic tissue transplanted into a highly vascularized recipient bed, there is the potential increase risk of graft rejection.[11,12] This risk of rejection may account for the reduced long-term survival of nonmatched keratolimbal allografts. Tsubota reported long-term survival of only 51%,[13] and Ilari reported 50%.[14] Furthermore, depending on cadaver and storage time, there may be a degree of stem cell death, thus reducing the volume of cells transplanted. While there may be limitations on the amount of tissue that can be transplanted in a lrCLAL, there is the advantage of providing some degree of immune histocompatibility,[15,16] thereby reducing the dependency on and dosage of systemic immunosuppressive agents. Additionally, cell death is theoretically limited because of the rapidity of transplantation from donor to recipient and the rapid revascularization of grafted material.

Ocular surface reconstruction can be divided into two components, structural reconstruction and surface restoration. Structural reconstruction involves reduction of ankyloblepharon and symblepharon and treatment of lid abnormalities, whereas surface restoration includes establishment of the barrier function at the limbus and epithelialization of the cornea with phenotypic corneal epithelium. Cadaveric KLAL transplantation alone or in combination with amniotic transplantation may accomplish both successful structural reconstruction as well as surface restoration. On a long-term basis, KLAL may fail to maintain phenotypic corneal epithelium even if structural reconstruction is usually maintained without recurrence of symblepharon.[10,13,17,18]

Since lrCLAL requires a procedure on an individual other than the patient, it is best reserved for eyes in which there is a minimal risk of failure. Eyes that require surface restoration alone are best suited for lrCLAL. Eyes requiring both reconstruction as well as restoration are unsuitable for lrCLAL and are best initially treated by KLAL with amniotic membrane transplant as a first stage, followed by lrCLAL in the event of epithelial failure.

Contraindications and Preoperative Considerations

Contraindications to lrCLAL include:

1. Any ocular surface requiring structural reconstruction.
2. Severe keratinization of the palpebral conjunctiva.
3. Inadequate lid closure.

4. Dry eye.

5. Severe inflammation.

In severe cases of bilateral disease, such as those following chemical injuries and Stevens–Johnson syndrome, severe cicatrization may be associated with lid abnormalities including keratinization, trichiasis, and entropion. Lid reconstructive and corrective procedures are best performed well in advance of epithelial transplantation. The goal of these procedures is to ensure adequate and atraumatic coverage of the ocular surface. Inadequate lid closure and severe keratinization of palpebral conjunctiva are incompatible with successful epithelial transplantation and are an absolute contraindication to lrCLAL. An ocular surface requiring reconstruction has been discussed above and is also a relative contraindication to lrCLAL.

Surface lubrication is crucial for survival of epithelium. Bilateral stem cell deficiency can be associated with severe dryness as a result of cicatrization of the main and accessory lacrimal ducts. The tear function index (TFI)[19] is a method of evaluating status of lubrication, and methods to improve the TFI such as punctal occlusion are best carried out prior to surgery. Epithelial transplant procedures are contraindicated in instances in which there is absolute dryness with no tear function and where improvement is unlikely in the future.[19]

Severe inflammation is a poor prognostic factor, and its presence is also a contraindication to lrCLAL.[16] Treatment during the acute phase of an illness, for instance, soon after a chemical injury, is contraindicated. The goal in this instance would be to stabilize the eye and reduce inflammation. Other procedures, such as amniotic membrane transplantation with or without KLAL, are best utilized to promote epithelialization and downregulation of inflammation.[20–23] Underlying causes of stem cell deficiency, such as ocular cicatricial pemphigoid, must also be adequately controlled prior to surgery. Inflammation, where present, can be controlled by topical and systemic steroids. Furthermore, it is best to have a period of 3 to 6 months free of inflammation prior to surgery.

Since many affected corneas are not transparent, some surgeons might consider performing a simultaneous visually rehabilitative procedure such as a penetrating keratoplasty. One report[16] demonstrated a reduction in corneal opacification with improvement in visual outcome in 70% of eyes following lrCLAL alone, obviating the need for a penetrating or lamellar keratoplasty. In most cases, therefore, it is best to perform a lrCLAL alone and wait for at least 6 to 12 months before considering corneal graft.[24] This allows the cornea to clear and also provides an opportunity for the ocular surface to improve, thereby optimizing graft survival, should it be required.

Surgical Techniques

Donor Selection

Since immune histocompatibility is one of the main reasons for embarking on this course of management, the best HLA-matched relative is the ideal donor. Human leukocyte antigen (HLA) typing is performed on all possible donors. If only parents are available, then HLA matching is not necessary, since the recipient will be a haplotype. Since expression of blood-group antigens has been demonstrated on epithelial cells,[25] ABO matching is also advisable when there are several potential donors available.

Both eyes of the donor are evaluated to ensure there is no underlying ocular history that may preclude donation. A history of glaucoma, for example, would be a relative contraindication because of the possible need for a trabeculectomy in the future. Additionally, chronic use of topical medications and prior contact lens wear with Thimerosal-containing preservatives suggest potential stem cell depletion that could be exacerbated by removal of limbal conjunctiva. A prior surgical history would also be a relative contraindication because of the possibility of iatrogenic stem cell deficiency.[26] One should measure tear breakup time, Schirmer test, and employ rose bengal staining to ensure there is no underlying abnormality.

Following identification of the best-matched living relative, screening for the possibility of blood-borne diseases is necessary. The standard serologic tests required by the Eye Bank Association of America are advised; these include screening for human immunodeficiency virus 1 and 2 and hepatitis B and C.

Anesthesia

Topical retro- or peribulbar anaesthesia can be used for harvesting donor tissue. However, based on cultural and practical considerations, general anesthesia can be employed. The recipient's eye can be similarly anesthetized using retro- or peribulbar anesthesia or, if necessary, general anesthesia.

Harvesting Tissue From the Relative

The nondominant eye of the donor is selected for the conjunctival limbal allograft, if it has not been used for tissue donation before. Since it is customary for surgeons to operate out of one operating room, removal of the donor tissue needs to be accomplished first. The procedure includes standard sterile preparation and draping of the eye. The sites for donation are marked on the donor eye (Figure 17.1A). Methods include a marking pen on the conjunctival surface or a 12-blade radial keratot-omy marker with a gentian violet marking pad. The

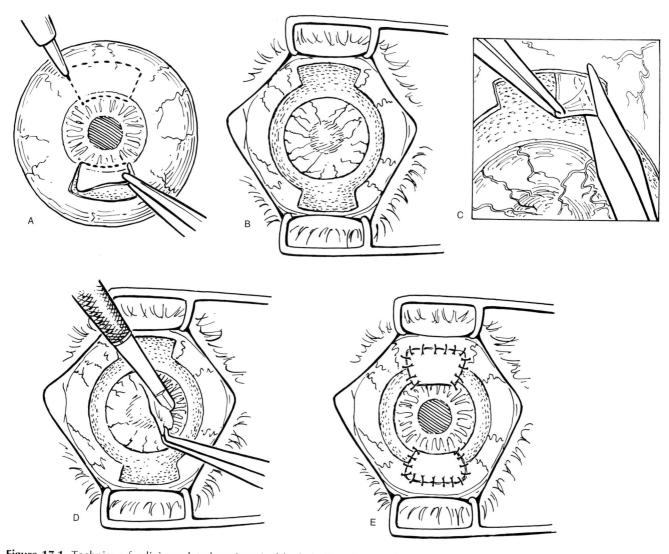

Figure 17.1. Technique for living-related conjunctival limbal allograft transplantation. (A) Harvesting of tissue from the donor eye. Conjunctival dimensions are marked using a gentian violet pen. Harvesting begins in the conjunctiva and proceeds anteriorly. (B) Preparation of the recipient. A 360-degree limbal conjunctival peritomy is performed and conjunctiva allowed to recess. Recipient beds of 3 clock hours are created at the 12 and 6 o'clock meridian. (C) Subconjunctival fibrous tissue is resected. (D) Abnormal corneal epithelium and fibrovascular pannus are removed using necessary techniques (peeling, blunt and sharp dissection). (E) Conjunctival allografts are transferred to corresponding anatomic positions on the recipients and secured with 10-0 suture. (Adapted from Brightbill: *Corneal Surgery. Theory, Technique and Tissue*, 3rd ed., p. 493, by permission of Mosby.)

cornea and conjunctiva are marked. It is best to incorporate the gentian violet markings within the donor tissue. These marks safeguard against inverting the donor tissue on the recipient eye.

Two pieces of tissue, each between 2 and 3 clock hours at the limbus, are resected from the 12 o'clock and 6 o'clock areas, and 5 mm posterior to the limbus (Figure 17.1B). Some surgeons elevate the site with a subconjunctival injection of balanced salt solution. Radial incisions are made at the lateral borders and dissection is performed, undermining the tissue as much as possible. Blunt forceps are used in order to prevent tearing the tis-

sue. The posterior edge is then cut 5 mm posterior to the limbus, and the tissue is reflected anteriorly on to the corneal surface (Figure 17.2). Dissection is continued into the peripheral cornea 1 mm anterior to the vascular arcade. A blunt scarifier (e.g., Tooke knife) is useful in accomplishing this dissection. This does not involve a lamellar dissection into the corneal stroma. Since stem cells are in the basal layer of the epithelium, only a superficial keratectomy is necessary. The author finds Vannas scissors useful in cutting the anterior portion of the tissue once adequate blunt dissection has been performed. The lower blade is placed under the tissue and

Figure 17.2. Donor conjunctival limbal allograft tissue reflected onto corneal surface and dissection carried anteriorly without involving corneal stroma.

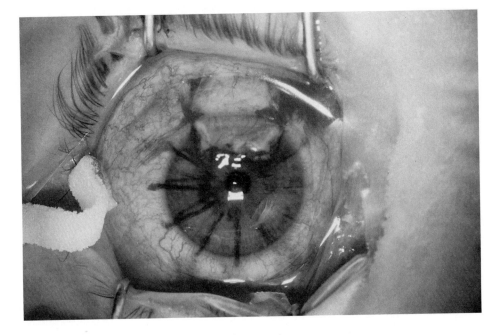

directed anteriorly and flat on the ocular surface. The scissors are advanced after small cuts are made with the mid-shaft of the blade until the tissue is completely resected. The tissue is allowed to float on balanced salt solution or is immersed into corneal storage media if available. Some surgeons leave the donor site alone and proceed to harvest tissue from the second site. Others prefer to advance the posterior conjunctiva to 2 mm posterior to the limbus and to suture the conjunctiva to the episclera using 8-0 polyglactin (Vicryl™, Ethicon) suture. Advancement of conjunctiva minimizes postoperative discomfort and inflammation on the donor eye. Tissue is harvested from the second site in a similar fashion. An antibiotic steroid ointment is placed in the eye, and the eye is patched until the patient is seen the following day.

Preparation of the Recipient Eye and Placement of Donor Tissue

The eye is sterilized and draped in a similar fashion to the donor eye. A speculum is inserted to ensure adequate exposure. Symblepharon, if present, can be lysed in the inferior fornix to enable insertion and expansion of the lid speculum. A 360-degree limbal conjunctival peritomy is performed. The conjunctiva is undermined and allowed to recess 2 to 3 mm from the limbus. Areas of conjunctiva failing to recede adequately are excised along with the limbal skirt of tissue. The recession of conjunctiva is enhanced by excision of subconjunctival scar tissue and thickened Tenon's capsule. This recession is necessary to enable the new source of limbal epithelium to repopulate the corneal surface and to prevent conjunctival tissue from crossing the limbus. Since the area is highly vascularized, there may be excessive

bleeding that can interfere with visualization. Wet-field cautery, topical adrenergics such as viscous phenylephrine 10%, and thrombin can be used to arrest bleeding. Alternatively, simply waiting a short period prior to operating further permits normal clotting mechanisms to achieve hemostasis. The surgeon then prepares the recipient beds for the limbal tissue. This includes removal of recipient conjunctival tissue 3 clock hours at the 6 and 12 o'clock areas and to 5 mm behind the limbus. The abnormal corneal epithelium is then removed. This is usually a vascularized pannus varying in adherence to the underlying stroma. A surgical spear or a lamellar dissector is often most effective in removing the epithelium without removing the stroma. The cornea is frequently thinner as a result of prior inflammation and fibrosis so that the surgeon must avoid removal of deeper layers, which can lead to optical irregularity, further thinning, or even perforation. The harvested tissue is then sutured in the same anatomical orientation with the limbal edge at the recipient limbus. The tissue can be sutured with 10-0 nylon or polyglactin, although some surgeons prefer the former because it is less likely to produce inflammation than absorbable suture. The author's preference is to use 2 clock hours of donor tissue and to stretch this to occupy 3 clock hours of limbus, suturing the tissue with absorbable material. Sutures are tied but not buried to prevent trauma and possible cheese wiring of donor tissue. During the operation, it is essential to protect the tissue from trauma and desiccation by balanced salt solution and viscoelastic material. Once concluded, a steroid-antibiotic ointment is instilled and the eye is patched until the patient is seen the following day. Figure 17.3 demonstrates a living related conjunctival limbal allograft.

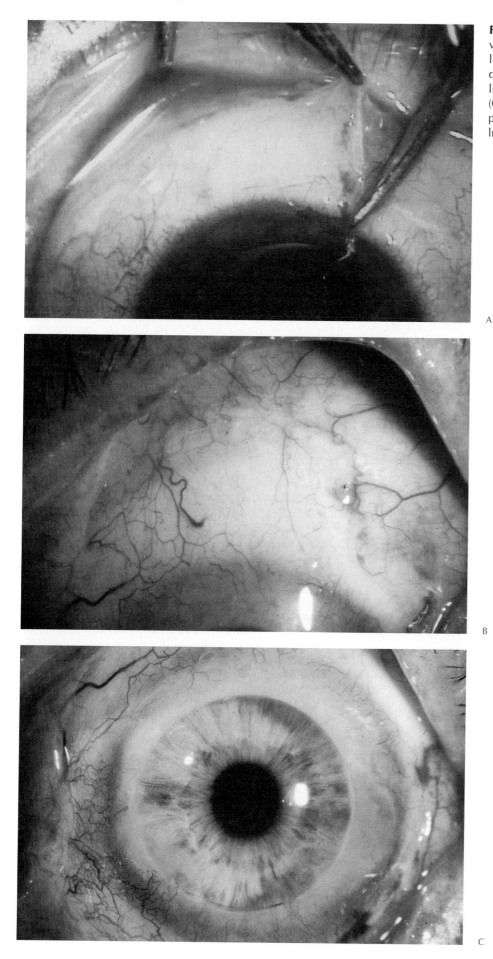

Figure 17.3. Living-related conjunctival limbal allograft. (A) Conjunctival limbal allograft being removed from donor eye. (B) Superior conjunctival limbal allograft in recipient eye. (C) Clear penetrating keratoplasty performed 4 months after lr-CLAL.

A

B

C

Postoperative Management

The goal of postoperative management is to minimize inflammation and promote epithelization in both the donor and host. In the donor, a combination of steroid and antibiotic is used in the donor until epithelization is complete, usually within a few days, and steroids can be gradually tapered over a period of 2 to 3 weeks. In the recipient, vascularization of the grafts is important to ensure survival of stem cells. It is, therefore, essential that the grafts do not move as a result of lid action against the graft site. Keeping the eye patched between eyedrops for at least the first week keeps the grafts in contact with the globe and minimizes the risk of dislodgement. A contact lens can also serve as a bandage preventing the grafts from rubbing against the lid. Preservative-free steroids and antibiotics are instilled 4 times daily. Some also advocate the use of autologous plasma or serum[16,27,28] to provide growth factors for the epithelium. When there is an underlying reduction in tear production, preservative-free tear supplements should be started early. Evidence of slow epithelial healing is best managed by an early tarsorrhaphy.

Immunosuppression

The role of immunosuppression has been debated. Kwitko[15] and Rao[29] in their series did not use systemic cyclosporin A. Daya and Ilari used cyclosporin A indefinitely in all recipients and reported 100% survival at a mean of 26.2 months.[16] Since rejection is the major cause of allograft failure, systemic immunosuppression is advisable, assuming that there is no contraindication. Systemic immunosuppression is commenced on the day of surgery, using a combination of systemic steroids and cyclosporin A (CsA). Steroid regimens vary. The author commences intravenous methyl prednisolone 2mg/kg on the day of surgery followed by 1 mg/kg intravenously for three additional days. Oral prednisolone is then started, the dose varying depending on the degree of inflammation present. Systemic CsA is started at a dose of between 3 and 5 mg/kg/day as a single dose or in two divided doses. A serum trough level is obtained on the fourth day, and the daily dose is adjusted accordingly. A repeat trough level is obtained again on a weekly basis until stable and then 1 to 2 monthly thereafter. Desired therapeutic levels vary between institutions, although they are typically between 150 and 200 ng/ml. The duration of immunosuppression is also variable with some surgeons discontinuing treatment at 12 to 18 months and others maintaining this indefinitely. While on treatment, periodic evaluation of creatinine and blood pressure is essential. In addition, some authors advocate the use of a third oral immunosuppressive, azathioprine, which allows for reduced doses of CsA.[10]

The conjunctival grafts are revascularized within 4 to 7 days and in the following 2 weeks often become swollen with engorged vessels. This phenomenon has been observed in conjunctival autografts and probably represents reactive hyperemia. In some instances, a subconjunctival hemorrhage occurs in the graft. There is no reason for concern, since the grafts do eventually thin.

Living-related conjunctival limbal allograft provides an opportunity to restore the ocular surface in cases of bilateral ocular surface disease. Although this technique permits a degree of histocompatibility matching, there is still the potential for rejection and ocular morbidity. Hence, systemic immunosuppression is recommended. Careful patient preparation is necessary to optimize outcomes. Corneal grafting for visual rehabilitation may not be necessary and is best performed 6 to 12 months following lrCLAL. As with all allograft procedures, close and regular follow-up care is essential to ensure long-term survival.

References

1. Davanger M, Evensen A. Role of the pericorneal papillary structure in renewal of corneal epithelium. *Nature* 1971; 229:560–561.
2. Townsend WM. The limbal palisades of Vogt. *Trans Am Ophthalmol Soc* 1991; 89:721–756.
3. Schermer A, Galvin S, Sun TT. Differentiation-related expression of a major 64K corneal keratin in vivo and in culture suggests limbal location of corneal epithelial stem cells. *J Cell Biol* 1986; 103:49–62.
4. Cotsarelis G, Cheng SZ, Dong G, Sun TT, Lavker RM. Existence of slow-cycling limbal epithelial basal cells that can be preferentially stimulated to proliferate: implications on epithelial stem cells. *Cell* 1989; 57:201–209.
5. Ebato B, Friend J, Thoft RA. Comparison of central and peripheral human corneal epithelium in tissue culture. *Invest Ophthalmol Vis Sci* 1987; 28:1450–1456.
6. Ebato B, Friend J, Thoft RA. Comparison of limbal and peripheral human corneal epithelium in tissue culture. *Invest Ophthalmol Vis Sci* 1988; 29:1533–1537.
7. Chen JJ, Tseng SC. Abnormal corneal epithelial wound healing in partial-thickness removal of limbal epithelium. *Invest Ophthalmol Vis Sci* 1991; 32:2219–2233.
8. Tseng SC. Classification of conjunctival surgeries for corneal diseases based on stem cell concept. *Ophthalmol Clin North Am* 1990; 3:595–610.
9. Holland EJ. Epithelial transplantation for the management of severe ocular surface disease. *Trans Am Ophthalmol Soc* 1996; 94:677–743.
10. Holland EJ, Schwartz GS. The evolution of epithelial transplantation for severe ocular surface disease and a proposed classification system. *Cornea* 1996; 15:549–556.
11. Tsubota K, Toda I, Saito H, Shinozaki N, Shimazaki J. Reconstruction of the corneal epithelium by limbal allograft transplantation for severe ocular surface disorders. *Ophthalmology* 1995; 102:1486–1496.

12. Williams KA, Coster DJ. The role of the limbus in corneal allograft rejection. *Eye* 1989; 3:158–166.

13. Tsubota K, Satake Y, Kaido M, et al. Treatment of severe ocular-surface disorders with corneal epithelial stem-cell transplantation [see comments]. *N Engl J Med* 1999; 340: 1697–1703.

14. Ilari L, Moshegov C, Wee TL, Wiffen SJ, Daya SM. Long term follow up of keratolimbal allografts (KLAL) for the treatment of stem cell deficiency. 103rd Annual Meeting of the American Academy of Ophthalmology, Orlando, FL, 1999.

15. Kwitko S, Marinho D, Barcaro S, et al. Allograft conjunctival transplantation for bilateral ocular surface disorders. *Ophthalmology* 1995; 102:1020–1025.

16. Daya SM, Ilari L. Living related conjunctival limbal allograft for the treatment of stem cell deficiency. *Ophthalmology* (accepted for publication).

17. Daya SM, Bell RW, Habib NE, Powell-Richards A, Dua HS. Clinical and pathologic findings in human keratolimbal allograft rejection [In Process Citation]. *Cornea* 2000; 19:443–450.

18. Tsubota K, Satake Y, Ohyama M, et al. Surgical reconstruction of the ocular surface in advanced ocular cicatricial pemphigoid and Stevens–Johnson syndrome [see comments]. *Am J Ophthalmol* 1996; 122:38–52.

19. Tseng SC, Tsubota K. Important concepts for treating ocular surface and tear disorders. *Am J Ophthalmol* 1997; 124:825–835.

20. Tseng SC, Prabhasawat P, Barton K, Gray T, Meller D. Amniotic membrane transplantation with or without limbal allografts for corneal surface reconstruction in patients with limbal stem cell deficiency. *Arch Ophthalmol* 1998; 116:431–441.

21. Azuara-Blanco A, Pillai CT, Dua HS. Amniotic membrane transplantation for ocular surface reconstruction [see comments]. *Br J Ophthalmol* 1999; 83:399–402.

22. Shimazaki J, Shinozaki N, Tsubota K. Transplantation of amniotic membrane and limbal autograft for patients with recurrent pterygium associated with symblepharon. *Br J Ophthalmol* 1998; 82:235–240.

23. Kim JC, Tseng SC. Transplantation of preserved human amniotic membrane for surface reconstruction in severely damaged rabbit corneas. *Cornea* 1995; 14:473–484.

24. Holland EJ, Schwartz GS. Epithelial stem-cell transplantation for severe ocular-surface disease [editorial; comment]. *N Engl J Med* 1999; 340:1752–1753.

25. Dua HS, Chan J, Gomes JA, Azuara-Blanco A. Adverse effect of blood group ABO mismatching on corneal epithelial cells [letter]. *Lancet* 1998; 352:1667–1668.

26. Holland EJ, Schwartz GS. Iatrogenic limbal stem cell deficiency. *Trans Am Ophthalmol Soc* 1997; 95:95–107.

27. Tsubota K, Goto E, Shimmura S, Shimazaki J. Treatment of persistent corneal epithelial defect by autologous serum application. *Ophthalmology* 1999; 106:1984–1989.

28. Tsubota K. Ocular surface management in corneal transplantation, a review. *Jpn J Ophthalmol* 1999; 43:502–508.

29. Rao SK, Rajagopal R, Sitalakshmi G, Padmanabhan P. Limbal allografting from related live donors for corneal surface reconstruction [see comments]. *Ophthalmology* 1999; 106:822–828.

18
Keratolimbal Allograft

Gary S. Schwartz, Kazuo Tsubota, Scheffer C. G. Tseng, Mark J. Mannis, and Edward J. Holland

Evolution of Keratolimbal Allograft

Keratolimbal allograft (KLAL) is a technique in which allogeneic cadaveric limbal stem cells are transplanted to a recipient eye with severe ocular surface disease (OSD) using peripheral cornea as a carrier.[1,2] The surgical technique has evolved considerably since its inception.

In 1984, Thoft described a technique he termed keratoepithelioplasty (KEP). This technique was the first allograft procedure for the management of severe OSD.[3] "Lenticules" of peripheral cornea were harvested from a cadaveric whole globe, placed evenly around the corneoscleral limbus, and sutured to the sclera. Although Thoft did not describe obtaining limbus with his KEP procedure, since there was not a good understanding of the stem cell theory at that time, it is possible that stem cells were harvested along with the peripheral corneal lenticules. In 1990, Thoft and co-workers modified the original KEP procedure to include limbal tissue with the peripheral cornea and thus described the first true keratolimbal allograft.[4]

A modification of Thoft's KEP technique was described by Tsai and Tseng in 1994.[5] A continuous annular ring of limbal tissue was harvested from a whole globe utilizing a suction trephine. The resultant keratolimbal ring was then subdivided and transferred to the recipient eye.

Tsubota and co-workers, in 1995, reported the use of stored corneoscleral rims for limbal stem cell transplantation.[6] By using stored tissue, they afforded patients several days to coordinate surgery after acquisition of suitable donor tissue.

Holland and Schwartz modified Tsubota's technique by using the stem cells from two stored corneoscleral rims instead of one. In this way, the potential number of transplanted limbal stem cells was doubled.[2,7] Another advantage of the latter procedure was that a contiguous ring of keratolimbal crescents was placed around the recipient limbus, acting as a barrier for potentially invading conjunctival tissue.

In 1996, Sundmacher, Reinhard, and co-workers presented their results of an alternative procedure, which they termed homologous penetrating central limbokeratoplasty (HPCLK).[8,9] In this procedure, a stored corneoscleral rim intentionally trephined off-center to create a 7.7–10 mm penetrating keratoplasty button. The donor graft is created in such a way, so that approximately 30–40% of the circumference of the graft contains limbal tissue. Patients undergoing this procedure benefit from receiving a clear penetrating keratoplasty graft along with limbal stem cells in a single operation.

Indications

Keratolimbal allograft surgery is performed in order to treat severe bilateral ocular surface disorders secondary to limbal stem cell deficiency. It is also a surgical alternative for patients with unilateral disease who fear damage to the healthy fellow eye if used as a source of limbal stem cells. Keratolimbal allograft surgery may be the only choice for obtaining allogeneic tissue if there is no available or willing living relative.

A keratolimbal allograft procedure is ideally suited for disease entities that primarily affect the limbus with minimal or no involvement of the conjunctiva. Aniridia exemplifies the disease process that is probably best suited for KLAL.[10] For similar reasons, KLAL is the optimal procedure in most cases of iatrogenic limbal stem cell deficiency.[11] Most cases of iatrogenic deficiency, whether they involve only sectoral or total limbal involvement, typically have reasonably normal conjunctiva. Patients with total limbal deficiency will require a 360-degree KLAL, while those with sectoral limbal deficiency may require only sectoral KLAL.

Keratolimbal allograft may also be beneficial for patients with limbal stem cell deficiency with mild to moderate conjunctival involvement. Patients with chemical injuries may benefit from this procedure. However, they fare best if the eye is allowed to quiet prior to surgery. Patients with mild Stevens–Johnson syndrome (SJS) or ocular cicatricial pemphigoid (OCP) may also benefit from KLAL, and the chances of graft survival are highest if the inflammation can be controlled prior to surgery.

The success rate with KLAL decreases with increasing conjunctival inflammation. The most severe forms of OSD involve total limbal stem cell deficiency with active conjunctival inflammation (e.g., severe SJS, OCP, and recent chemical injuries). In these cases, total limbal stem cell deficiency is complicated by conjunctival inflammation and scarring, decreased mucin and aqueous tear deficiency, and the potential for keratinization of the ocular surface. Because KLAL does not provide healthy conjunctiva, one might consider living-related conjunctival limbal allograft (lr-CLAL) if a living donor is available.

Preoperative Considerations

One major threat to the success of any ocular surface reconstruction procedure, including KLAL, is the lack of a healthy and stable tear film.[12] If a proper tear film layer is not present on the ocular surface, it must be restored by correcting lid abnormalities, neurotrophic exposure, and severe aqueous tear deficiency. This is especially true for those with decreased reflex tearing. Eyelid abnormalities, such as lagophthalmos, misdirected lashes, and malpositioned or keratinized lid margins should be reconstructed either prior to, or at the conclusion of, KLAL. Great care must be taken when performing KLAL in patients with abnormal or absent blink, since persistent epithelial defects may develop with risk of subsequent scarring and infection.

Severe aqueous tear deficiency with decreased reflex tearing is another relative contraindication to KLAL. In addition to the absence of the nutritive component and mechanical lubrication of the normal tear film, these patients lack essential tear components such as vitamin A and epidermal growth factor (EGF).[13–16] If KLAL is undertaken in such patients, successful surface rehabilitation will be maximized if autologous serum is applied regularly following KLAL.

The success of KLAL is decreased in eyes with significant keratinization of the ocular surface.[17] It has been recognized that conjunctival epithelium is derived from a stem cell population[18] that is separate from that of the limbus.[19] Therefore, KLAL alone is not sufficient to correct eyes with diffuse keratinization caused by concomitant loss of both epithelial stem cell populations. It remains to be determined if simultaneous transplantation of both types of epithelial stem cells may ameliorate this difficult situation.

Uncontrolled, severe inflammation is another poor prognostic factor for KLAL. Even for conjunctival limbal autograft (CLAU), severe inflammation limits its success in acute chemical burns in humans,[20,21] and

chronic inflammation adversely affected the initial success in a rabbit model of total limbal deficiency.[22] Although the exact mechanism remains unclear, inflammatory cytokines such as interferon gamma can upregulate Fas or HLA class II antigen and encourage the epithelium to undergo apoptosis in acute chemical burns.[23] Upregulation of HLA class II antigens in the context of inflammation may augment immune sensitization leading to allograft rejection. These data support the notion that the success of keratolimbal allograft is hampered by uncontrolled inflammation and that suppression of inflammation is an important strategy for improving the outcomes.

The fact that suppression of inflammation is beneficial following KLAL is supported by the favorable results observed when amniotic membrane transplantation (AMT) is used in conjunction with KLAL in inflamed eyes.[24] Amniotic membrane transplantation has been shown to suppress inflammation, facilitate epithelization, and prevent cicatricial complications in acute chemical and thermal burns.[25]

Surgical Techniques
General Considerations

The purpose of performing KLAL is to provide healthy limbal SC's to the recipient host limbus. Because the SC's lie in a narrow, fragile portion of the limbus, they must be delivered attached to a more robust carrier tissue. Using peripheral corneoscleral tissue allows for safe transfer and secure attachment of the SC's to the recipient limbus.

For each of the procedures described below, either retrobulbar anesthetic with a VIIth cranial nerve block or general anesthesia is administered.

Corneoscleral Crescent Technique of Holland/Schwartz

Preparation of the Donor Limbal Tissue
In this technique, the source of tissue is a corneoscleral rim preserved in corneal storage media at 4°C. The central cornea of the corneoscleral rim is excised with a 7.5 mm trephine (Figure 18.1). For pediatric donors with smaller corneas, a smaller trephine is employed. An Iowa™ trephine press is used, and the tissue is placed epithelial-side-down in the standard fashion used for cutting a corneal button for routine keratoplasty. In this way, damage to the limbal stem cells is minimized.

The corneoscleral rim is sectioned into equal halves (Figure 18.2). Scissors are used to dissect the excess peripheral scleral tissue, leaving approximately 1 mm of sclera peripheral to the limbus (Figure 18.3). The posterior one-half to two-thirds of each hemisection is re-

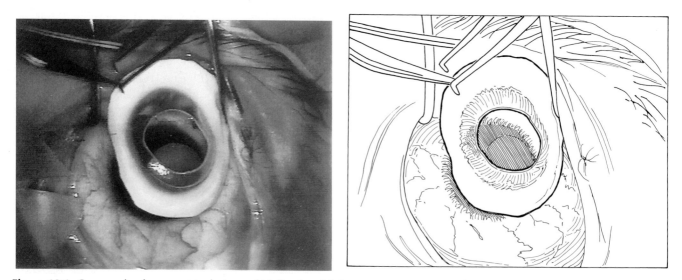

Figure 18.1. Corneoscleral crescent technique of Holland and Schwartz. Donor corneoscleral rim with the central 7.5 mm of cornea removed by trephination.

moved by lamellar dissection using a sharp rounded steel crescent blade (Figures 18.4 and 18.5). These steps are performed under the operating microscope and usually require an assistant to help stabilize the tissue with forceps. The lamellar dissection removes the posterior sclera and posterior stroma, including Descemet's membrane and endothelium. If the graft is too thick, there is greater likelihood that, once transplanted, the friction of the eyelids closing over the surface will impede re-epithelization. If the graft is so thick that a step-off exists between the graft and the cornea, epithelization will be impaired. The posterior tissue is discarded, and the second corneoscleral donor rim is prepared in the same fashion. The four pieces (two from each eye) are then placed epithelial-side-up in storage media solution while awaiting placement later in the operation.

Tissue from two eyes is required in order to have sufficient tissue to place around the recipient limbus without gaps. Previous versions of this technique used tissue from only one eye, with resultant small gaps at the 3 and 9 o'clock limbal positions. Conjunctiva-like tissue often invaded the corneal surface through the gaps in the transplanted tissue using this technique. By transplanting tissue from two eyes (usually three equal pieces representing 100% of the limbus of one eye and 50% of the fellow eye), one and a half times the number of stem cells are transplanted than in those procedures using only one donor eye.

Preparation of the Recipient Eye
Exposure is often difficult in these patients because of superior and inferior symblephara. A speculum is inserted

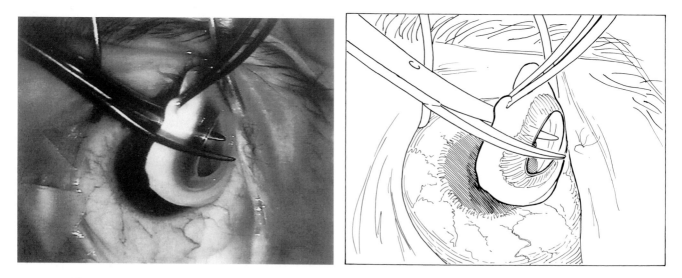

Figure 18.2. Division of the corneoscleral rim to form two hemisection crescents. (Holland and Schwartz)

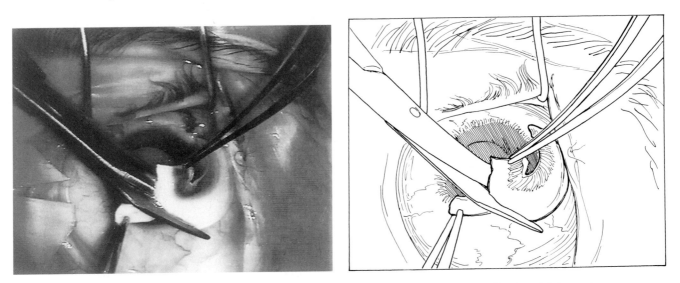

Figure 18.3. Removal of excess peripheral scleral tissue from each crescent. (Holland and Schwartz)

and if needed, a lateral canthotomy is performed. The initial incision is a 360°-limbal peritomy. In most patients with severe OSD, significant bleeding is encountered following the conjunctival incision, and this may necessitate resecting one quadrant at a time. Hemostasis is maintained with topical epinephrine (1:10,000 dilution), thrombin, and wet-field cautery. In areas of symblepharon, conjunctival tissue is first recessed at the limbus and then undermined to allow the conjunctival tissue to fall back: This not only helps create a new fornix, but it also provides more tissue for the palpebral surface. If the initial dissection were made in the fornix and the symblepharon simply excised, there would be a broad area of epithelial defect on the palpebral conjunctival side, leading to further symblepharon formation. Therefore, the symblephara are actually used to help reconstruct the fornix and provide epithelium for the palpebral surface. Care is taken to avoid damaging the superior or inferior rectus muscles in areas of broad symblepharon formation.

The conjunctiva is resected 4 to 5 mm from the limbus to expose an adequately sized bed of denuded sclera on which to position the KLAL tissue. Abnormal fibrovascular pannus and epithelium, which are typically present, are next removed from the surface of the cornea. For superficial keratectomy, blunt dissection with a cellulose sponge is utilized initially, although often semisharp dissection with a rounded steel blade or sharp Westcott scissors is needed to create a smooth surface (Figure 18.6). Care is taken to ensure that the dissection continues in a lamellar fashion, remaining anterior, and that the deep layers of the corneal stroma are not disturbed. It must be borne in mind that the

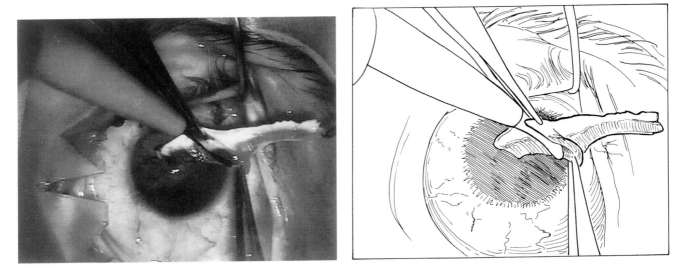

Figure 18.4. Thinning of the KLAL crescent by lamellar dissection; endothelium and posterior two-thirds of stroma are removed. (Holland and Schwartz)

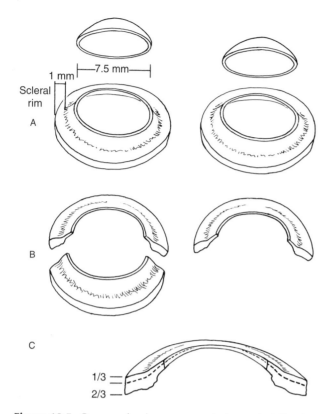

Figure 18.5. Corneoscleral crescent technique of Holland and Schwartz. Schematic diagram of the key steps in preparation of KLAL tissue.

purpose of this dissection is removal of the abnormal fibrovascular conjunctivalized surface that has replaced normal corneal epithelium. Topical epinephrine and thrombin can be utilized to control bleeding during this step also.

Placement of the Donor Tissue

The crescents are placed on the recipient's eye in their proper anatomic orientation with the corneal edges just overlying the recipient limbus (Figure 18.7). The two anterior corners of each crescent are secured at the limbus with interrupted 10-nylon sutures. The corneal edge of the KLAL should lie flush on the recipient cornea. Then the two posterior corners are sutured. An additional suture or two can be placed along the posterior edge if needed for security. Additional crescents are placed end-to-end in the same fashion until the entire circumference of recipient limbus is covered by healthy donor SC tissue (Figure 18.8). To facilitate this close apposition, one of the crescents may be cut into a shorter piece. During the suturing phase of the KLAL, epithelium is protected from both mechanical trauma and desiccation by the use of viscoelastic and balanced-salt solution. If there is a functioning bleb from a prior glaucoma filtering surgery, a gap can be left to preserve the bleb. In situations where a Seton drainage device has been placed, or is anticipated, the limbus can be covered with the new graft tissue without interfering with the success of these glaucoma procedures. The free edges of the recessed recipient host conjunctiva is sutured to the posterior edges of the crescents. At the conclusion of the surgery, the eye is patched and covered with a shield until the patient is seen the next day. Clinical examples of this technique are illustrated in Figures 18.9–18.11.

Corneoscleral Ring Technique of Tsubota

Preparation of the Donor Limbal Tissue

This technique is similar to the one described above except that tissue from one donor corneoscleral rim is used instead of two (Figures 18.12 and 18.13). The donor tis-

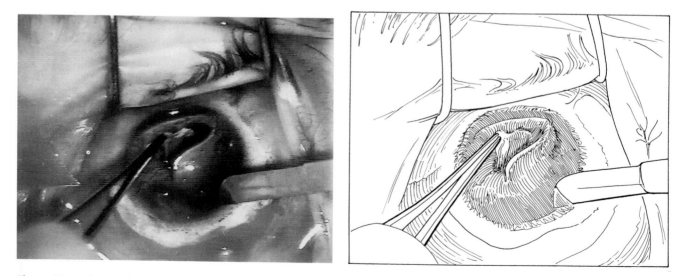

Figure 18.6. Abnormal corneal epithelium and fibrovascular pannus are removed by superficial dissection using blunt and sharp techniques. (Holland and Schwartz)

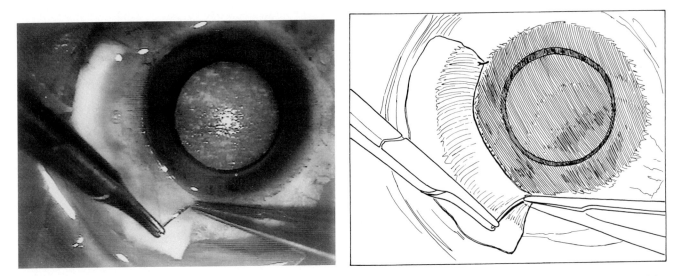

Figure 18.7. Lamellar KLAL crescents are sutured to the recipient eye with proper anatomic orientation. The corneal edges of the KLAL should approximate the recipient limbus. (Holland and Schwartz)

sue is prepared from the conventionally processed corneoscleral button obtained from the eye bank. Theoretically, the potency and capability of the limbal epithelial stem cells should be greater in a young donor. Nonetheless, we noted that the average age of donors was 57.2 years,[26] suggesting that the stem cell reserve may extend to much older donors. Because of the shortage of eye bank corneas in Japan, it would be very difficult to limit the donor source based solely on age.

In addition, a shorter storage time should theoretically be preferable to preserve the viability of the lim-

bal epithelial stem cells. Because of the shortage of donor corneas in Japan, most of the corneas used are imported from an American eye bank. As a result, it regularly takes 6 days after enucleation before the tissue is used for transplantation, explaining the mean tissue-preservation period of 5.9 days that was reported in a previous clinical series.[26] A preliminary study showed that the limbal epithelial stem cells remained viable within such a period of storage time.[27] It is of interest to note that inflammatory cells, such as Langerhans cells, become depleted after several days' storage, suggesting that a theoretical advantage of the longer storage period may, in fact, be beneficial.

The corneal button is preserved in Optisol GS™ (Chiron Technolas, Irvine, CA) as per routine eye bank procedure. It remains to be determined whether this storage medium is ideal for preserving corneal epithelial stem cells. As with Holland and Schwartz's technique, described above, the central cornea of the corneoscleral rim is excised with a 7.5 mm trephine. An Iowa cutting press is used, and the tissue is placed epithelial-side-down in the standard fashion used for cutting a corneal button for routine keratoplasty.

Scissors are used to dissect the excess peripheral scleral tissue, leaving approximately 1 mm of sclera peripheral to the limbus. The posterior one-half to two-thirds of the ring is then removed by lamellar dissection using a sharp rounded steel crescent blade. These steps are performed under the operating microscope and usually require the aid of an assistant. We dissect and remove as much unnecessary tissue as possible leaving thin, ring-shaped limbal tissue containing corneal epithelial stem cells.

In the past, we saved the central corneal button to perform penetrating keratoplasty (PK) simultaneously with KLAL. We do not know whether this may explain the high

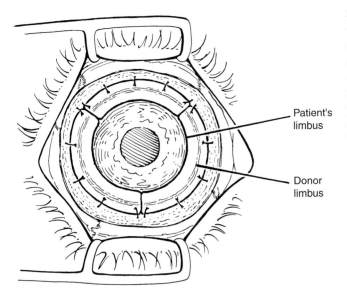

Figure 18.8. Schematic diagram of the recipient eye with three KLAL crescents sutured in place. (Holland and Schwartz)

Patient's limbus

Donor limbus

Figure 18.9. Keratolimbal allograft. (A) Preoperative photograph of an eye after a severe alkali injury. Note the neovascularization, ulceration, and scarring. Visual acuity is hand motions. (B) Photograph taken three months after KLAL. Note the marked regression of the neovascularization and corneal opacification. The patient has a healthy corneal epithelium. (C) Penetrating keratoplasty was performed three months after KLAL. One year postoperatively, visual acuity is 20/30. (Holland and Schwartz)

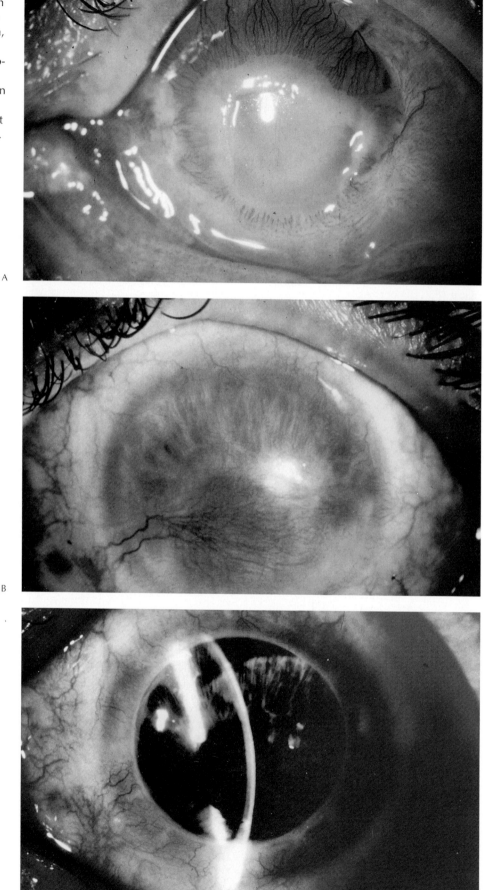

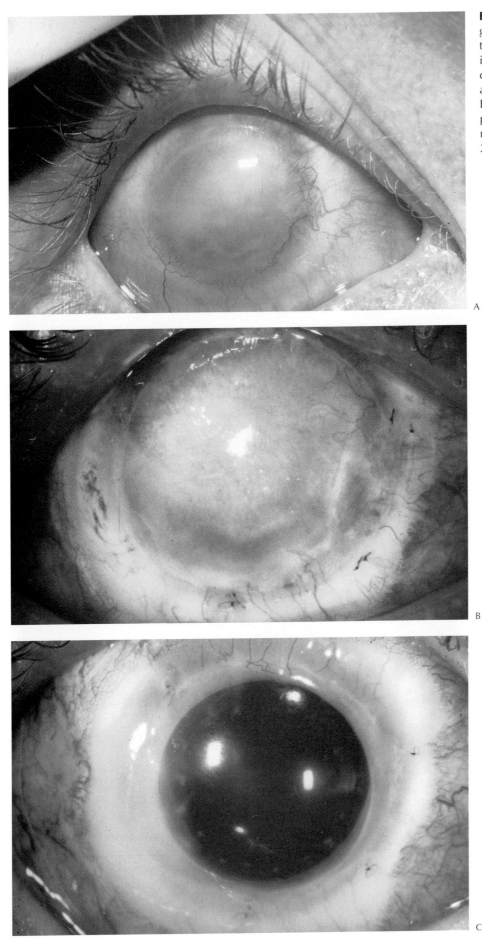

Figure 18.10. Keratolimbal allograft. (A) Severe scarring of a patient's only eye due to a chemical injury. Visual acuity is finger counting. (B) Status post-KLAL with a healthy epithelial surface. (C) Photograph taken one year after penetrating keratoplasty and 15 months after KLAL. Visual acuity is 2/25. (Holland and Schwartz)

Figure 18.11. Keratolimbal allograft in a patient with aniridia.
(A) Status post-penetrating-ker-
atoplasty performed three months
after KLAL. Note healthy epithelial surface. (B) Photograph of
keratolimbal tissue showing
proper anatomic position. (Holland and Schwartz)

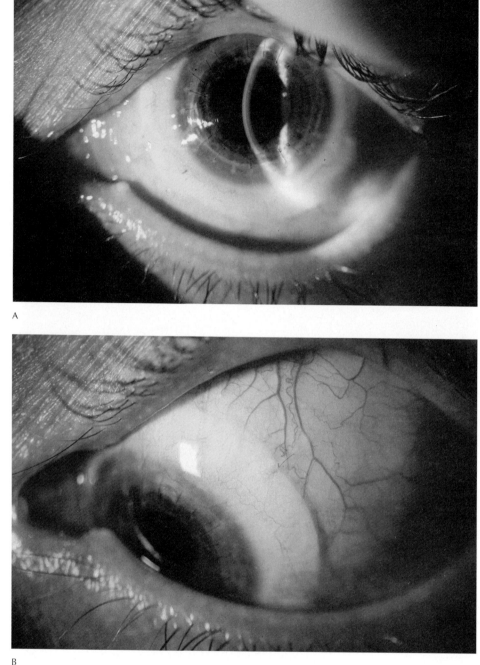

A

B

rejection rate of the corneal graft despite the use of systemic cyclosporin.[24] Holland et al.[10] advocate performing
a PK no sooner than 3 to 4 months following KLAL, and
we try to adhere to this rule if tissue is available.

Preparation of the Recipient Eye
Superficial keratectomy and 360-degree limbal peritomy
are performed, as described in the procedure of Holland
and Schwartz, above. Whenever possible with inflamed
eyes, AMT is performed prior to placement of the KLAL
ring. Amniotic membrane has been used as a substrate

in restoring the ocular surface when the underlying
stroma tissue has been destroyed[27–30] and is described
elsewhere in this text. We noted that amniotic membrane
transplantation, either before or during KLAL, may also
facilitate epithelization and reduce inflammation and
scarring. During limbal transplantation, amniotic membrane is dissected from the chorion and placed on the ocular surface with the epithelial side facing outward. The
membrane is then secured to the eye with eight 9-0 silk
sutures. As much of the ocular surface as possible is covered, with exception of the palpebral conjunctiva.

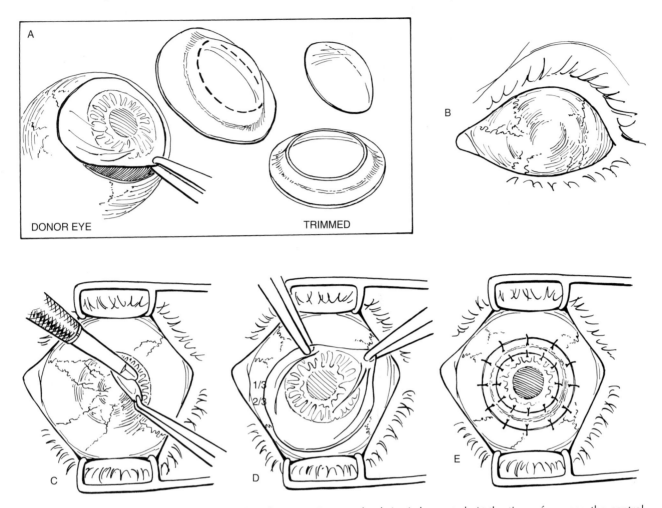

Figure 18.12. Corneoscleral Ring Technique of Tsubota. A. Corneoscleral rim is harvested. At the time of surgery, the central cornea is removed with a 7.5 mm trephine. This creates a central corneal button for a penetrating or lamellar keratoplasty and a corneoscleral ring for the stem cell transplant. B. and C. The recipient eye has the abnormal corneal epithelium removed. A 360° peritomy is performed. D. Amniotic membrane is placed over the cornea and anterior scleral and secured to the sclera. E. The ring-shaped limbal tissue is sutured to the peripheral cornea and limbus. A penetrating or lamellar keratoplasty may be performed.

Placement of the Donor Tissue

The ring-shaped limbal tissue is sutured to the recipient limbal area with interrupted sutures. Four 10-0 nylon sutures are routinely used to secure the central corneal portion. Nine-zero silk or 8-0 Vicryl sutures are used to suture the scleral portion of the limbal graft to the scleral bed. The host conjunctiva is not sutured, but is allowed to adhere to the posterior aspect of the graft of its own accord. At the conclusion of this procedure, a penetrating or lamellar keratoplasty may be performed using tissue from the same corneoscleral button.

Homologous Penetrating Central Limbo-Keratoplasty (HPCLK) Technique of Sundmacher

Preparation of the Donor Limbal Tissue

The source of tissue is a conventionally prepared corneoscleral rim obtained from the eye bank.[8,9] In Sund-

macher's study, transplantation was performed within 24 hours after harvesting and preservation in short-term storage media (Likorol®). The preserved cornea is excised eccentrically, resulting in one-third of the circumference of the button containing limbal tissue (Figure 18.14). Buttons ranging from 7.7 to 10 mm may be cut depending on the diameter of corneal tissue needed for visual rehabilitation in the recipient eye. Unlike the procedures of Holland/Schwartz and Tsubota mentioned previously, the peripheral rim of corneoscleral tissue is discarded.

Preparation of the Recipient Eye

Superficial keratectomy of the central cornea is not necessary, since this tissue will be replaced by the donor button. A trephine is used to remove central corneal tissue as if a standard PK were to be performed. The corneal button that contains limbal stem cells along one-third of its circumference is then secured with suture, much like conventional penetrating keratoplasty in the

Figure 18.13. Patient with
Stevens–Johnson syndrome treated
with a keratolimbal allograft and
amniotic membrane transplant. (A)
Severe ocular surface scarring
with symblepharon formation. (B)
Superficial keratectomy and lysis
of symblepharon. (C) Ocular surface with fibrovascular layer removed. (Tsubota and associates)

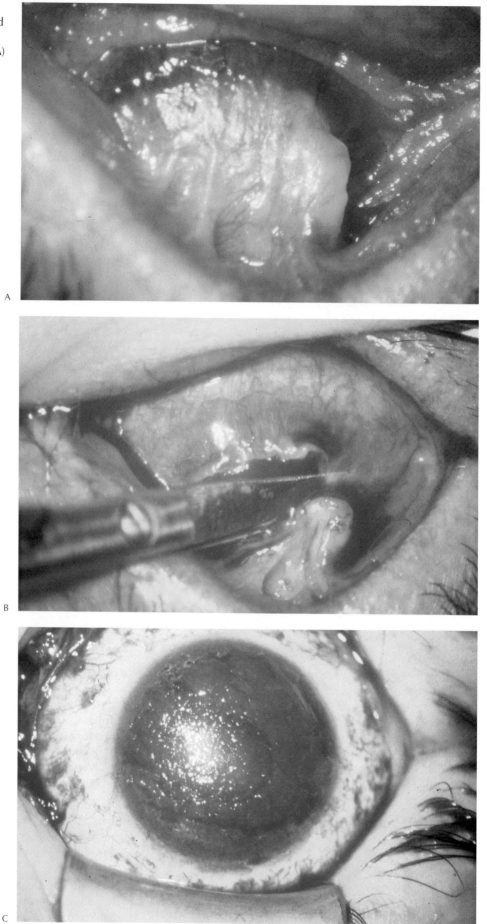

A

B

C

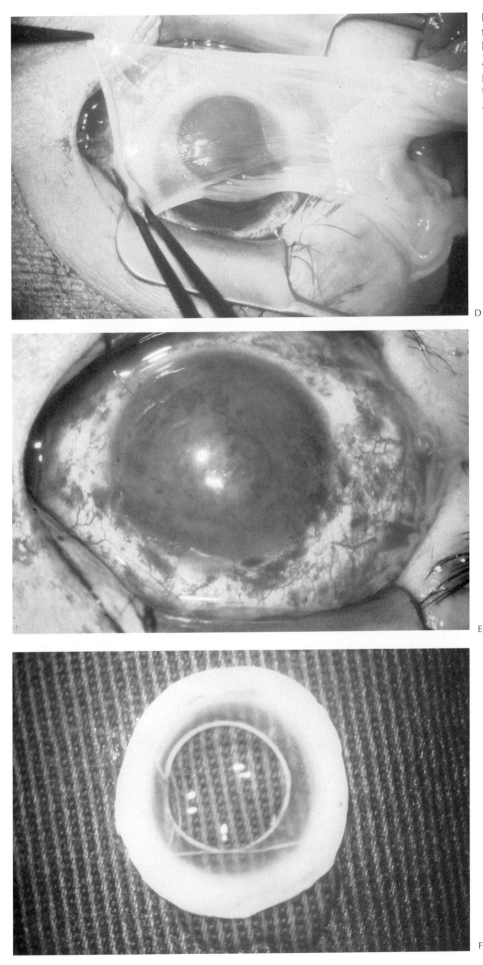

Figure 18.13. (*Continued*) (D) Initial placement of amniotic membrane on the ocular surface. (E) Amniotic membrane sutured into position. (F) Preparation of keratolimbal allograft tissue. (Tsubota and associates)

Figure 18.13. (*Continued*) (G) Completed procedure with amniotic membrane and keratolimbal allograft in place. (Tsubota and associates)

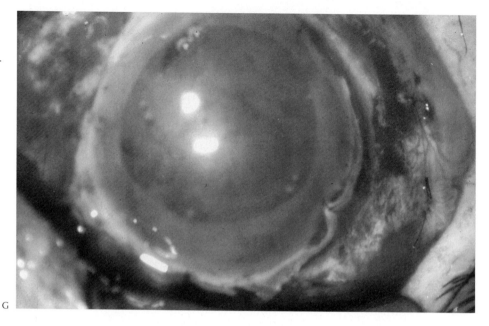

G

central optical axis of the recipient. A patch and a shield are placed over the eye, and the patient is examined the following day.

At the time of Sundmacher's initial report, the mean follow-up time was 9.6 months (range: 1–20 months), and 14 of the 20 grafts (70%) remained clear. The 6 grafts that failed succumbed due to recurrent surface disease in 4 cases, immune reactions in 1 eye, and a combination of surface disease and immune rejection in 1 eye. Ten of the 20 grafts exhibited recurrent surface disease, and in 6 of these there were concurrent immune reactions. In 4 of the grafts (20%), conjunctivalization occurred directly over the transplanted limbal components, and in 7 grafts (35%), conjunctivalization occurred distant from the site of the transplanted stem cells.[1]

The rationale for this approach is the employment of a single allograft for both limbal replacement and optical keratoplasty with protection using systemic cyclosporin A. Nonetheless, 50% of the grafts experienced immune graft reactions despite treatment with the systemic immunosuppressive agent. This may be the result of the transplantation of a larger number of Langerhans cells in these eccentrically trephined donors. The theoretical value of the technique is both relative technical simplicity, the economy of using a single donor for each case, and the immunologic value of a single antigeneic

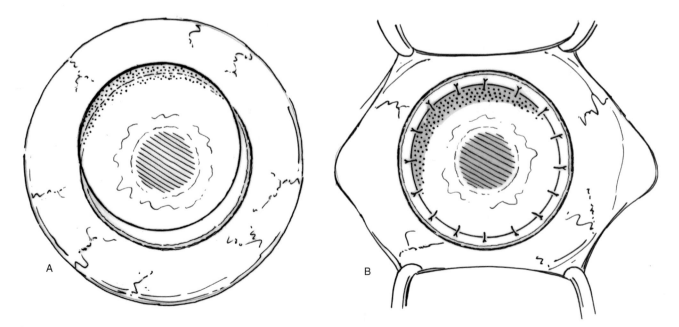

Figure 18.14. Homologous Penetrating Central Limbo-Keratoplasty (HPCLK) Technique of Sundmacher. (A) Eccentrically trephined donor button containing 30-40% limbal stem cells. (B) Donor button placed centrally in recipient corneal bed.

challenge to the recipient. The primary problem, however, remains immune graft rejection that is only partially inhibited by systemic cyclosporin and may theoretically be more frequent due to the larger percentage of Langerhans cells grafted using this technique.

While HPCLK affords the advantage of both a single surgery and a single antigeneic challenge, the results suggest that in the medium and long terms, the success rate as judged by central graft clarity is still less than 30%, largely as a result of immune rejection. The authors plan to investigate the use of alternative immunosuppressive agents and HLA matching in combination with this technique.

Postoperative Care

The key to successful KLAL lies in the postoperative care. Because limbal stem cells are more antigenically active than are central corneal stromal and endothelial cells, the risk of post-operative failure secondary to rejection is much more likely following KLAL than it is following PK. In fact, all patients undergoing KLAL benefit from systemic immunosuppression consisting of corticosteroid, azathioprine and cyclosporin in order to decrease the risk of graft failure secondary to rejection. Systemic immunosuppression following KLAL is discussed more fully in Chapter 22.

In evaluating the success of KLAL, it is important to consider the length of follow-up. When examining a patient with a healthy-appearing ocular surface 3–4 months after PK, it may very well be that one is observing the transplanted adult epithelial cells. In these cases, it may be a year or more before the limbal stem cells are called upon to repopulate the ocular surface. Thus, one cannot pass judgment on the success of KLAL until the patient is at least one year after limbal transplant surgery.

References

1. Tseng S. Concept and application of limbal stem cells. *Eye* 1989; 3:141–157.
2. Holland EJ, Schwartz GS. The evolution of epithelial transplantation for severe ocular surface disease and a proposed classification system. *Cornea* 1996; 15:549–556.
3. Thoft RA. Keratoepithelioplasty. *Am J Ophthalmol* 1984; 97:1–6.
4. Turgeon PW, Nauheim RC, Roat MI, et al. Indications for keratoepithelioplasty. *Arch Ophthalmol* 1990; 108:33–36.
5. Tsai RJF, Tseng SCG. Human allograft limbal transplantation for corneal surface reconstruction. *Cornea* 1994; 13:389–400.
6. Tsubota K, Toda I, Saito H, et al. Reconstruction of the corneal epithelium by limbal allograft transplantation for severe ocular surface disorders. *Ophthalmol* 1995; 102:1486–1495.
7. Croasdale CR, Schwartz GS, Malling JV, Holland EJ. Keratolimbal allograft: recommendations for tissue procurement and preparation by eye banks, and standard surgical technique. *Cornea* 1999; 18:52–58.
8. Sundmacher R, Reinhard T. Central corneolimbal transplantation under systemic cyclosporin A cover for severe stem cell deficiencies. *Graefe's Arch Clin Exp Ophthalmol* 1996; 234:122–125.
9. Reinhard T, Sundmacher R, Spelsberg H, Althaus C. Homologous penetrating central limbo-keratoplasty (HPCLK) in bilateral limbal stem cell deficiency. *Acta Ophthalmologica Scandinavica* 1999; 77:663–667.
10. Holland EJ. Epithelial transplantation for the management of severe ocular surface disease. *Trans Am Ophthalmol Soc* 1996; 19:677–743.
11. Schwartz GS, Holland EJ. Iatrogenic limbal stem cell deficiency. *Cornea* 1998; 17(1):31–37.
12. Shimazaki J, Shimmura S, Fujishima H, et al. Association of preoperative tear function with surgical outcome in severe Stevens–Johnson syndrome. *Ophthalmol* 2000; 107:1518–1523.
13. Tsubota K, Goto E, Shimmura S, et al. Treatment of persistent corneal epithelial defect by autologous serum application. *Ophthalmol* 1999; 106:1984–1989.
14. Tsubota K, Goto E, Fujita H, et al. Treatment of dry eye by autologous serum application in Sjögren's Syndrome. *Br J Ophthalmol* 1999; 83:390–395.
15. Tsubota K. Tear dynamics and dry eye. *Prog Retin Eye Res* 1998; 17:565–596.
16. Tsubota K, Higuchi A. Serum application for the treatment of ocular surface disorders. *Int Ophthalmol Clin* 2000; 40:113–122.
17. Tsubota K, Shimazaki J. Surgical treatment of children blinded by Stevens–Johnson syndrome. *Am J Ophthalmol* 1999; 128:573–581.
18. Wei Z-G, Cotsarelis G, Sun T-T, Lavker RM. Label retaining cells are preferentially located in forniceal epithelium: implications on conjunctival epithelial homeostasis. *Invest Ophthalmol Vis Sci* 1998; 36:236–246.
19. Wei Z-G, Sun T-T, Lavker RM. Rabbit conjunctival corneal epithelial cells belong to two separate lineages. *Invest Ophthalmol Vis Sci* 1996; 37:523–533.
20. Kenyon KR. Limbal autograft transplantation for chemical and thermal burns. *Dev Ophthalmol* 1989; 18:53–58.
21. Kenyon KR, Tseng SCG. Limbal autograft transplantation for ocular surface disorders. *Ophthalmol* 1989; 96:709–723.
22. Tsai RJF, Tseng SCG. Effect of stromal inflammation on the outcome of limbal transplantation for corneal surface reconstruction. *Cornea* 1995; 14:439–449.
23. Tsubota K, Fukagawa K, Fujihara T, et al. Regulation of human leukocyte antigen expression in human conjunctival epithelium. *Invest Ophthalmol Vis Sci* 1999; 40:28–34.
24. Tseng SC, Prabhasawat P, Barton K, et al. Amniotic membrane transplantation with or without limbal allografts for corneal surface reconstruction in patients with limbal stem cell deficiency. *Arch Ophthalmol* 1998; 116:431–441.
25. Meller D, Pires RT, Mack RJ, et al. Amniotic membrane transplantation for acute chemical or thermal burns. *Ophthalmology* 2000; 107:980–989; discussion 990.
26. Kinoshita S, Kiritoshi A, Ohji M, et al. Disappearance of palisades of Vogt in ocular surface diseases. *Jpn J Clin Ophthalmol* 1986; 40:363–366.

27. Tsubota K, Satake Y, Kaido M, et al. Treatment of severe ocular surface disorders with corneal epithelial stem-cell transplantation. *N Engl J Med* 1999; 340:1697–1703.
28. Kim JC, Tseng SC. Transplantation of preserved human amniotic membrane for surface reconstruction in severely damaged rabbit corneas. *Cornea* 1995; 14:473–484.
29. Pires RT, Chokshi A, Tseng SC. Amniotic membrane transplantation or conjunctival limbal autograft for limbal stem cell deficiency induced by 5-fluorouracil in glaucoma surgeries. *Cornea* 2000; 19:284–287.
30. Tsubota K, Satake Y, Ohyama M, et al. Surgical reconstruction of the ocular surface in advanced ocular cicatricial pemphigoid and Stevens–Johnson syndrome. *Am J Ophthalmol* 1996; 122:38–52.

19

Keratolimbal Allograft: Recommendations for Tissue Procurement and Preparation by Eye Banks

Christopher R. Croasdale, Gary S. Schwartz, Jackie V. Malling, and Edward J. Holland

The purpose of this chapter is to facilitate increased usage of keratolimbal allograft (KLAL) transplantation for severe ocular surface disease (OSD) by informing clinicians and eye banks of differences in tissue requirements and preparation for the procedure.

Donor Tissue Selection

In order to obtain appropriate tissue for performing KLAL, the surgeon must both communicate with the eye banks regarding potential availability of tissue and educate the staff of the special requirements of this procedures, which is not commonly performed. If the eye bank is not made aware of specific requirements in tissue selection and preparation, it will be difficult for the surgeon to obtain donor tissue prepared in the desired fashion.

For routine penetrating keratoplasty, most surgeons avoid using tissue from infant donors (usually less than 4 years of age) because of the difficulty of working with the tissue due to its flaccidity as well as its tendency for ectasia postoperatively leading to unpredictable results.[1] Eye banks are aware of this and do not routinely pursue pediatric tissue. Additionally, the incidence of allograft rejection reactions after penetrating keratoplasty was reported to be higher among adults who received pediatric tissue (younger than 6 years of age) compared with adults who received older tissue (donors aged 40 to 70 years).[2] In the KLAL procedures that the authors have performed the pliability of the tissue has not been an issue. We have also not seen any significant differences in rejection episodes based on donor tissue

age. More importantly, we have the clinical impression that tissue from pediatric donors results in more rapid re-epithelization (often 5 to 7 days) of the recipient cornea than tissue from older donors. This observation is not surprising, for it is intuitive that the limbal stem cells (SC) of children would be more active and robust than those of adults. Our preference, therefore, is to use the youngest tissue possible, including neonatal tissue. As an upper age limit, we have avoided using tissue from donors older than 50 years of age. We inform our local eye bank when we have a patient on the waiting list for a KLAL so that they will accept infant tissue that they otherwise would decline or that would be used as research tissue. Additionally, both eyes of the donor should be obtained in order to provide sufficient tissue for the procedure.

Eye Bank Education of Referral Sources

In order to successfully obtain young adult and pediatric donor tissue for performing a KLAL, it is important to educate not only the staff of eye banks, but also referral hospitals and the community. Children's hospitals and neonatal and pediatric intensive care units need to be informed of the need for pediatric donor eyes. From a psychosocial standpoint, offering the option of organ donation to parents and families who are dealing with the loss of a child can aid the grieving process. The knowledge that their child will help provide a gift of sight to another individual can often help bring solace during a difficult time.

Donor Tissue Preparation

General Principles

As with the donor criteria, there are several variations from standard tissue procurement and processing techniques that a prospective eye bank supplier needs to be familiar with. The standard emphasis during tissue procurement for penetrating keratoplasty is avoidance of damage to the corneal endothelium and stroma, with less regard for the epithelium, which normally is regenerated by the recipient host. For tissue to be used for KLAL, it is the donor limbal epithelium that needs to be carefully protected from both trauma and desiccation. Damage to the endothelium or stroma has essentially no bearing on the outcome of KLAL transplants. We prefer that the entire corneal epithelium appear as normal as possible. A grossly normal epithelium indicates that the limbal SC's have probably undergone minimal harm during the procurement.

Whereas most conjunctiva is usually removed during the procurement and processing of tissue to be used for penetrating keratoplasty, we ask for a 3–4 mm peripheral skirt of conjunctiva to remain for KLAL transplantation. Leaving this conjunctival tissue helps minimize damage to the limbal area and allows for some goblet cells to be included along with the transplanted tissue.

If the tissue is to be preserved as a corneoscleral rim, it is preferable to have an increased amount of sclera included in the corneoscleral rim resection from the donor globe, if possible, upward of 4–5 mm. This additional sclera also reduces the likelihood that the limbal stem cells will be damaged during the corneoscleral rim preparation.

Some techniques for KLAL utilize tissue from one donor globe, and, therefore, a single donor can provide tissue for two separate stem cell transplant recipients. However, the authors prefer two corneoscleral rims from the same donor be employed for one recipient. In this way, we provide a greater number of stem cells to the recipient eye than is available from one donor globe. In addition, the remaining keratolimbal donor tissue can be used in the surgical management of symblepharon.

Minnesota Lions Eye Bank Protocol for KLAL Recovery, Processing, and Preservation

The procedure is designed to minimize disturbance and contamination of limbal epithelial stem cells during the recovery of the donor eye and preservation of the corneoscleral button for KLAL transplantation. The technique as performed by the Minnesota Lions Eye Bank (MLEB) meets all current applicable regulatory standards including but not limited to the Eye Bank Association of America (EBAA) standards.[3]

The Minnesota Lions Eye Bank recovers all eye tissue using whole-globe enucleation. The standard enucleation technique is performed with the following changes. The integrity of the epithelial limbal stem cells is carefully maintained by avoiding any contact with the cornea or limbus throughout enucleation. The conjunctiva is cut 360 degrees around the entire globe as far from the limbus as possible (at least 6 mm) using tenotomy scissors.

When the eyes are received at the MLEB, a whole-globe slit-lamp evaluation is performed. The quality of the epithelium, stroma, and endothelium is documented. The tissue is processed and preserved for KLAL for all donor eyes with intact peripheral, and good central, epithelium when the donor is less than 50 years old. Donor and tissue criteria are ultimately determined by the transplanting surgeon. When KLAL tissue is available, the surgeon is informed as soon as possible of the quality of the tissue and the donor history. If the surgeon rejects the tissue, or if the surgeon or patient is unavailable for surgery, then the tissue is distributed for penetrating keratoplasty after meeting all MLEB criteria.

Whole-Globe Technique

If the surgeon prefers to perform KLAL utilizing a whole globe, the tissue is refrigerated at this stage at 2–6°C. The surgeon is contacted at this point because surgery should be scheduled within the next 24 hours. Advantages to the whole-globe technique include relatively fresh tissue that has not been subjected to additional manipulation for storage.

Disadvantages to this technique are numerous. Serological testing must be performed on transplanted tissue to rule out transmittable infectious disease. This testing takes additional time, and in many cases makes it difficult to approve the tissue for surgery in a timely fashion. In addition, with tissue stored as a whole globe, the surgeon, patient, patient's family, and operating room personnel must all be able to commit to the procedure on less than 24 hours' notice. For some patients who live a great distance from a center capable of performing KLAL, use of whole-globe tissue may make surgery for them an impossibility.

Stored Corneoscleral Rim Technique

In 1995, Tsubota and colleagues were the first to report the use of stored corneoscleral rims for stem cell transplantation.[4] They demonstrated that the tissue could be stored up to 5 days using standard eye bank protocol while still maintaining a healthy stem cell and epithelial layer.

The MLEB procedure for processing the corneoscleral rim is as follows. The corneoscleral button excision is performed under a horizontal laminar airflow workbench using sterile technique. The excess conjunctiva (if greater than 6 mm), muscle and fat is bluntly dissected

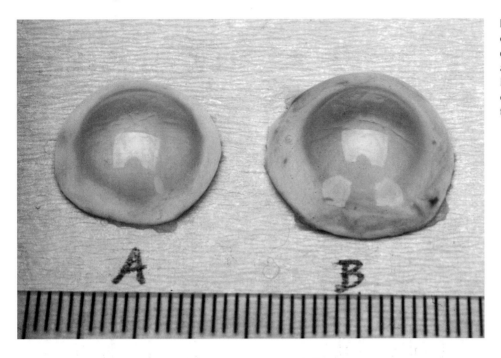

Figure 19.1. Comparison of corneal scleral rim size for standard penetrating keratoplasty (A) and keratolimbal allograft (B). Note the additional scleral and conjunctival tissue for the keratolimbal allograft.

from the posterior sclera (away from the limbus) using iris or tenotomy scissors to aid in decontamination of the globe. The instruments used in this step are isolated from the other items on the sterile field and are used only to remove the conjunctiva from the second eye. The globe is gently placed is a medicine glass of povidone-iodine 1% solution for 3 minutes to allow for decontamination. It is then transferred to a medicine glass of sterile saline (0.9%) using new forceps. The globe soaks in saline until the povidone-iodine is rinsed away, or approximately 1 minute. The entire decontamination process is repeated for the second time.

One globe is then placed on a sterile Petri dish containing two sterile gauze 4 × 4" pads. A small incision is made through the sclera 4–6 mm from and parallel to the limbus using a surgical blade (Figure 19.1). Care is taken to cut through the sclera without rupturing the choroid or deforming the cornea in any way. The scleral incision is extended 360 degrees around the cornea using Castroviejo corneal scissors. The anterior segment is kept intact, and the corneoscleral button should be attached to the choroid only at the scleral spur. The button removal is completed using one pair of fine-toothed forceps to hold the scleral rim of the corneoscleral button stationary while a second pair of fine-toothed forceps is used to gently grasp the choroid underlying the ciliary body just inside the incision. As the ciliary body is pulled down, it will separate and free the corneoscleral rim. The corneoscleral button is placed into a media filled storage chamber endothelial-side-up. The edge of the button is pushed gently down so that media covers the entire button (the cornea is not allowed to float on the surface of the media). The storage-chamber lid is gently tightened without forming air pockets between the lid and the cornea. The pos-

terior chamber of the globe is examined for the presence of the crystalline lens. The second eye is then processed in the same fashion.

There are significant advantages to this technique, for both the patient and the surgeon. The corneoscleral rim tissue can be preserved for 5 days, while whole-globe tissue cannot be utilized after 24 hours. We typically use the tissue within 3 days, but have gone up to our maximum time limit of 5 days in select cases. Because the surgery can be scheduled within 3 to 5 days of procurement of the tissue, the surgeon and patient can take advantage of this extra time and schedule the surgery during routine operating room hours. Performing the surgery in a non-urgent manner also allows the surgeon to do these difficult procedures with the benefit of familiar equipment and operating room staff. The extra time also allows the patient and family more days to prepare for this major surgery.

References

1. Gloor P, Keech RV, Krachmer JK. Factors associated with high postoperative myopia after penetrating keratoplasties in infants. *Ophthalmology* 1992; 99:775–779.
2. Palay DA, Kangas TA, Stulting RD, et al. The effects of donor age on the outcome of penetrating keratoplasty in adults. *Ophthalmology* 1997; 104:1576–1579.
3. Croasdale CR, Schwartz GS, Malling JV, Holland EJ. Keratolimbal allograft: recommendations for tissue procurement by eye banks, and standard surgical technique. *Cornea* 1999; 18(1);52–58.
4. Tsubota K, Toda I, Saito H, et al. Reconstruction of the corneal epithelium by limbal allograft transplantation for severe ocular surface disorders. *Ophthalmology* 1995; 102: 1486–1495.

20
Amniotic Membrane Transplantation for Ocular Surface Reconstruction

Scheffer C. G. Tseng and Kazuo Tsubota

History of Amniotic Membrane Transplantation

Amniotic membrane, or amnion, is the innermost layer of the placenta and consists of a thick basement membrane and an avascular stromal matrix. Amniotic membrane transplantation has been used as a graft or as a dressing (patch) in different surgical subspecialties in early literature.[1] In the English-language literature, a *live* fetal membrane including both amnion and chorion was first used by De Rotth in 1940 as a graft for conjunctival surface reconstruction.[2] Probably due to the inclusion of live cells and the chorion, the success rate was low, i.e., one out of six cases, treating symblepharon and conjunctival defect. In 1940 Brown[3] proposed the use of rabbit peritoneum as a temporary patch to cover the acutely burned ocular surface in order to promote healing and prevent spread of necrosis. Based on this idea, in 1946 and 1947, Sorsby et al.[4,5] used chemically processed "dry" amniotic membrane, termed "amnioplastin," as a temporary patch for treating acute ocular burns. They showed that the earlier the intervention, the shorter the hospitalization. Although a remarkable success was noted, amnioplastin had to be applied repetitively. For reasons still not clear, the use of amniotic membrane disappeared from the literature. As early as 1965, Roper-Hall[6] reviewed the subject of chemical burns and concluded "other materials have been advocated from time to time as temporary grafts with varying enthusiasm."

In 1995 Kim and Tseng[7] reintroduced amniotic membrane for ophthalmic uses. In a rabbit model they showed that 40% of corneas with total limbal deficiency can be reconstructed by replacing the conjunctivalized surface with a preserved human amniotic membrane. As will be described in detail, encouraging results have since been reported by a number of investigators (see Figure 20.1). We attribute such a surge of interest in this new surgical procedure to an improved method of processing and preservation, which has maintained the inherent properties of the amnion.

Mechanisms of Action

The guidelines and operation standards concerning the procurement, processing, and distribution of such a tissue as amniotic membrane, are reported by the Food and Drug Administration, USA (Final Rule: Screening and Testing of Donors of Human Tissue Intended for Transplantation, July 29, 1997), and recently reviewed by Dua.[8] When appropriately processed and preserved (see Figure 20.2), the amniotic membrane can be used for a number of indications, either as a graft to replace the damaged ocular surface stromal matrix, as a patch (dressing) to prevent unwanted inflammatory insults from gaining access to the damaged ocular surface, or a combination of both. Recent reports indicate that potential action mechanisms might include those summarized in Table 20.1.

Compositionally, the basement membrane component of the amniotic membrane resembles that of the conjunctiva.[9] The basement side of the membrane is an ideal substrate for supporting the growth of epithelial progenitor cells by prolonging their life span and maintaining their clonogenicity. This action explains why amniotic membrane transplantation can be used to expand the remaining limbal stem cells and corneal transient amplifying cells during the treatment of partial limbal deficiency[10] and to facilitate epithelization for persistent corneal epithelial defects with stromal ulceration.[11-13] In tissue culture, amniotic membrane supports epithelial cell growth from explant cultures[14-16] or other cultures,[17,18] and maintains their normal epithelial morphology and differentiation.[14,15] The resultant epithelial cells/amniotic membrane can be transplanted back to reconstruct the damaged corneal surface in humans[17,19] and in rabbits.[16,17] The amniotic membrane can also be used to promote nongoblet cell differentiation of the conjunctival epithelium.[15] These data explain

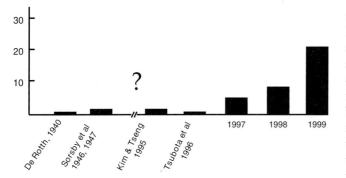

Figure 20.1. History of English-language literature on amniotic membrane transplantation in ophthalmology.

why conjunctival goblet cell density is promoted following amniotic membrane transplantation in vivo.[20]

The stromal side of the membrane contains a unique matrix component that suppresses TGF-β signaling, as well as proliferation and myofibroblast differentiation of normal human corneal and limbal fibroblasts[21] and of normal conjunctival fibroblasts and pterygium body fibroblasts.[22] This action explains why amniotic membrane transplantation reduces scar formation during conjunctival surface reconstruction,[23,24] prevents recurrent scar-

ring after pterygium removal,[25–29] and reduces corneal haze following phototherapeutic keratectomy (PTK) and photorefractive keratectomy (PRK).[30–32] Although such an action is more potent when fibroblasts are in contact with the stromal matrix, a lesser effect is also noted when fibroblasts are separated from the membrane by a distance,[21] suggesting that some diffusible factors might also be involved besides the insoluble matrix components in the membrane. In line with this thinking, several growth factors have been identified in the amniotic membrane.[33] The stromal matrix of the membrane can also exclude inflammatory cells by stimulating them into rapid apoptosis[31,32] and contains various forms of protease inhibitors.[34] This action explains why stromal inflammation is reduced after amniotic membrane transplantation[11,23] and why corneal neovascularization is mitigated,[35] actions important for preparing the stroma for supporting limbal stem cells to be transplanted either at the same time or later.[10,26,36–39]

This action also explains why keratocyte apoptosis can be reduced, and hence why stromal haze is prevented in PRK or PTK by amniotic membrane.[30–32] Future studies are needed to resolve the exact action mechanism.

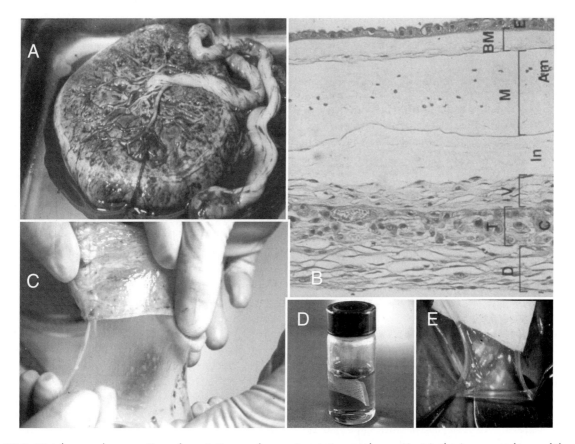

Figure 20.2. Histology and preparation of amniotic membrane. Amniotic membrane (Am) is the innermost layer of the placenta (A) and consists of a thick basement membrane (BM) and an avascular stromal matrix (M), which is apposed to vascularized chorion (C).

Table 20.1. Action mechanisms and observed effects of amniotic membrane transplantation.

Action Mechanisms
- Prolong life span and maintain clonogenicity of epithelial progenitor cells
- Promote non-goblet cell epithelial differentiation
- Promote goblet cell differentiation when combined with conjunctival fibroblasts
- Exclude inflammatory cells with anti-protease activities
- Suppress TGF-β signaling system and myofibroblast differentiation of normal fibroblasts

Observed Clinical Effects
- Facilitate epithelialization
- Maintain normal epithelial phenotype
- Reduce inflammation
- Reduce vascularization
- Reduce scarring

Note: TGF-β: transforming growth factor-β

Table 20.2. Surgical indications for amniotic membrane transplantation.

As a Graft for Conjunctival Diseases
- Pterygium
- Bulbar conjunctival reconstruction after removal of large lesions or scars
- Symblepharon lysis
- Conjunctivochalasis

With or without preserved sclera or pericardium for:
- Bleb leakage or revision
- Scleral melt
- Lid reconstruction
- Orbit reconstruction

As a Graft for Corneal Diseases
- Persistent corneal epithelial defect with or without ulceration
- Partial limbal stem cell deficiency
- Total limbal stem cell deficiency (with limbal transplantation)
- For chemical burns, Stevens–Johnson syndrome
- Painful bullous keratopathy with erosion
- Band keratopathy

As a Patch
- Acute stage of chemical or thermal burns, Stevens–Johnson syndrome
- Preventing scar after PRK or PTK
- Refractory or recalcitrant inflammatory or ulcerative keratitis: HSV, HZO, and vernal

As a Carrier for Expanding Epithelial Stem Cells Ex Vivo
- Limbal stem cell deficiency

Clinical Indications

Based on the action mechanisms and observed clinical effects summarized in Table 20.1, amniotic membrane has been used in the following indications summarized in Table 20.2.

Amniotic Membrane as a Graft for Conjunctival Surface Reconstruction

The action mechanisms summarized in Table 20.1 explain why amniotic membrane transplantation can facilitate epithelialization, maintain normal epithelial phenotype (with goblet cells when performed on conjunctiva),[20] and reduce inflammation, vascularization, and scarring. Based on these therapeutic effects, one can envision that amniotic membrane transplantation can be used for conjunctival surface reconstruction to restore normal stroma and provide a healthy basement membrane for renewed epithelial proliferation and differentiation. The reported literature demonstrates that amniotic membrane transplantation can be used to reconstruct the conjunctival surface as an alternative to conjunctival graft following removal of large conjunctival lesions such as pterygium,[25–29] conjunctival intraepithelial neoplasia and tumors,[23] scars and symblepharon,[23,24,27] and conjunctivochalasis.[40] These results indicate that the reconstructed area can be very large so long as the underlying bed is not ischemic and the bordered conjunctiva has a normal epithelium and subconjunctival stroma. In conjunction with scleral patch graft, amniotic membrane has successfully been used to repair scleral perforation in Marfan's syndrome.[41] As a graft to substitute conjunctival autograft, amniotic membrane can also be used to repair leaking filtration blebs.[42] Amniotic membrane may substitute for conjunctival autograft, and thus may be a better alternative to mucous membrane graft in plastic correction of lid abnormality and orbit reconstruction.

Amniotic Membrane as a Graft for Corneal Surface Reconstruction

Following diagnosis of limbal deficiency, new strategies include the use of amniotic membrane transplantation and limbal stem cell transplantation.[10,36,37] The former is intended to restore the damaged limbal stromal environment, and the latter to restore the limbal stem cell population. Reported clinical experience has demonstrated that this combined approach is effective in treating various degrees of limbal deficiency, depending on (1) the extent of limbal deficiency, (2) the presence or absence of the central corneal transient amplifying cells (TAC), and (3) the depth of central corneal involvement.[10]

One major advance made by amniotic membrane transplantation is that partial limbal deficiency can now be reconstructed by this technique without the use of limbal transplantation.[10] This result, first observed in rabbit experiments at the time when no explanation was available,[7] indicates that patients with partial limbal deficiency can now be treated without long-term use of oral cyclosporin. The second advance is the extremely low incidence of limbal allograft rejection when systemic cyclosporin is concomitantly used and when amniotic membrane transplantation is performed as the first-stage procedure to restore the limbal stromal environment. This effect is presumably attributed to the restoration of a noninflamed limbal stroma. For these reasons, we advise performing a limbal allograft, but not an autograft, as a first attempt to treat unilateral total limbal deficiency or bilateral limbal deficiency with asymmetrical involvement. However, if the limbal allograft fails due to rejection, a limbal autograft can then be used as the last resort. In the latter situation, amniotic membrane is ideal for helping both transplanted limbal stem cells expand on the recipient eye, and the residual stem cells expand in the donor eye. The remaining difficulty remains in those patients who suffer from severe and deep limbal deficiency leading to concomitant transplantation of corneal grafts. We continued to observe a high rate of rejection.[10]

Amniotic membrane can also be applied to treat corneal surface diseases as a graft. When used as a graft or a patch, amniotic membrane can promote healing of persistent corneal ulcers from different causes, including neurotrophic keratopathy caused by various underlying etiologies,[11–13,27] and band keratopathy.[11] This approach is superior to conjunctival flaps or tarsorrhaphy because it preserves a cosmetically more acceptable appearance. A recent multicenter trial shows that amniotic membrane transplantation can be used to treat symptomatic bullous keratopathy caused by aphakia, pseudophakia, or failed corneal grafts.[43] These patients suffered from pain, recurrent erosion, and infection. Although it was advocated for patients without visual potential, it may help eliminate pain in those on the waiting list for corneal transplantation.

Amniotic Membrane as a Patch

Amniotic membrane can also be used as a patch in a temporary or prolonged manner. Experimentally, when used as a patch on a temporary basis this membrane has been shown to reduce corneal haze following PRK or PTK,[30,31] an effect verified in human patients.[27,44] As a temporary patch, amniotic membrane can reduce inflammation, facilitate epithelialization and prevent scarring caused by acute chemical burns in a rabbit model[44] and in human patients.[45] Based on these actions, amniotic membrane as a patch was also used successfully in the acute stage of Stevens–Johnson syndrome,[46] and to suppress refractory inflammation in various ocular surface disorders.[47] Further research in this area may uncover additional applications of using amniotic membrane as a patch.

AM as a Carrier for Supporting and Expanding Limbal Epithelial Stem Cells Ex Vivo for Treating Total Limbal Stem Cell Deficiency

The fact that the amniotic membrane can help preserve and expand limbal epithelial stem cells indicates that it can also be used as a carrier to expand them in in vitro culture. This new approach is applicable to those patients with limited limbal reserve, or who are concerned about having a large part of the healthy limbus removed from the fellow eye or from a living-related donor. In this case, a small limbal biopsy will be performed and the sample placed on the amniotic membrane and appropriately cultured. Within 3 to 4 weeks, such an ex vivo expanded culture, together with the amniotic membrane, can be transplanted to restore the normal corneal surface on limbal deficient corneas. The feasibility of this new approach based on an autologous source has been demonstrated in a short-term rabbit study,[16] and in long-term human patients.[17,19,48] This approach paves the way for using amniotic membrane as a tissue-engineering substrate and may open up new therapeutics by incorporating gene therapies in the future.

Limitations

One should recognize that amniotic membrane transplantation is a substrate transplantation and thus cannot be used to treat ocular surface disorders that are characterized by a total loss of limbal epithelial stem cells or conjunctival epithelial stem cells. Because amniotic membrane transplantation still relies on the host tissue to supply epithelial and mesenchymal cells, it cannot be used to reconstruct the ocular surface that has severe aqueous tear deficiency, diffuse keratinization,[39] absence of blinking in severe neurotrophic state, and stromal ischemia. If not overcome, these conditions present a contraindication for amniotic membrane transplantation.

References

1. Trelford JD, Trelford-Sauder M. The amnion in surgery, past and present. *Am J Obstet Gynecol* 1979; 134:833–845.
2. De Rotth A. Plastic repair of conjunctival defects with fetal membrane. *Arch Ophthalmol* 1940; 23:522–525.
3. Brown AL. Lime burns of the eye: Use of rabbit peritoneum to prevent severe delayed effects. *Arch Ophthalmol* 1941; 26:754–769.
4. Sorsby A, Symons HM. Amniotic membrane grafts in caustic burns of the eye. *Br J Ophthalmol* 1946; 30:337–345.
5. Sorsby A, Haythorne J, Reed H. Further experience with amniotic membrane grafts in caustic burns of the eye. *Br J Ophthalmol* 1947; 31:409–418.
6. Roper-Hall MJ. Thermal and chemical burns. *Trans Ophthalmol Soc UK* 1965; 85:631–640.

7. Kim JC, Tseng SCG. Transplantation of preserved human amniotic membrane for surface reconstruction is severely damaged rabbit corneas. *Cornea* 1995; 14:473–484.

8. Dua HS, Azuara-Blanco A. Amniotic membrane transplantation. *Br J Ophthalmol* 1999; 83:748–752.

9. Fukuda K, Chikama T, Nakamura M, Nishida T. Differential distribution of subchains of the basement membrane components type IV collagen and laminin among the amniotic membrane, cornea, and conjunctiva. *Cornea* 1999; 18:73–79.

10. Tseng SCG, Prabhasawat P, Barton K, et al. Amniotic membrane transplantation with or without limbal allografts for corneal surface reconstruction in patients with limbal stem cell deficiency. *Arch Ophthalmol* 1998; 116:431–441.

11. Lee S-H, Tseng SCG. Amniotic membrane transplantation for persistent epithelial defects with ulceration. *Am J Ophthalmol* 1997; 123:303–312.

12. Kruse FE, Rohrschneider K, Völcker HE. Multilayer amniotic membrane transplantation for reconstruction of deep corneal ulcers. *Ophthalmology* 1999; 106:1504–1511.

13. Chen H-J, Pires RTF, Tseng SCG. Amniotic membrane transplantation for severe neurotrophic corneal ulcers. *Br J Ophthalmol* 2000; 84:826–833.

14. Cho B-J, Djalilian AR, Obritsch WF, et al. Conjunctival epithelial cells cultured on human amniotic membrane fail to transdifferentiate into corneal epithelial-type cells. *Cornea* 1999; 18:216–224.

15. Meller D, Tseng SCG. Conjunctival epithelial cell differentiation on amniotic membrane. *Invest Ophthalmol Vis Sci* 1999; 40:878–886.

16. Koizumi N, Inatomi T, Quantock AJ, et al. Amniotic membrane as a substrate for cultivating limbal corneal epithelial cells for autologous transplantation in rabbits. *Cornea* 2000; 19:65–71.

17. Schwab IR. Cultured corneal epithelia for ocular surface disease. *Trans Am Ophthalmol Soc* 1999; 97:891–986.

18. Koizumi N, Fullwood NJ, Bairaktaris G, et al. Cultivation of corneal epithelial cells on intact and denuded human amniotic membrane. *Invest Ophthalmol Vis Sci* 2000; 41:2506–2513.

19. Tsai RJF, Li L-M, Chen J-K. Reconstruction of damaged corneas by transplantation of autologous limbal epithelial cells. *N Eng J Med* 2000; 343:86–93.

20. Praghasawat P, Tseng SCG. Impression cytology study of epithelial phenotype of ocular surface reconstructed by preserved human amniotic membrane. *Arch Ophthalmol* 1997; 115:1360–1367.

21. Tseng SCG, Li D-Q, Ma X. Suppression of Transforming Growth Factor isoforms, TGF-β receptor II, and myofibroblast differentiation in cultured human corneal and limbal fibroblasts by amniotic membrane matrix. *J Cell Physiol* 1999; 179:325–335.

22. Lee S-B, Li D-Q, Tan DTH, et al. Suppression of TGF-β signaling in both normal conjunctival fibroblasts and pterygial body fibroblasts by amniotic membrane. *Curr Eye Res* 2000; 20:325–334.

23. Tseng SCG, Prabhasawat P, Lee S-H. Amniotic membrane transplantation for conjunctival surface reconstruction. *Am J Ophthalmol* 1997; 124:765–774.

24. Azuara-Blanco A, Pillai CT, Dua HS. Amniotic membrane transplantation for ocular surface reconstruction. *Br J Ophthalmol* 1999; 8339:399–402.

25. Prabhasawat P, Barton K, Burkett G, Tseng SCG. Comparison of conjunctival autografts, amniotic membrane grafts and primary closure for pterygium excision. *Ophthalmology* 1997; 104:974–985.

26. Shimazaki J, Sinozaki N, Tsubota K. Transplantation of amniotic membrane and limbal autograft for patients with recurrent pterygium associated with symblepharon. *Br J Ophthalmol* 1998; 82:235–240.

27. Kim JC, Lee D, Shyn KH. Clinical uses of human amniotic membrane for ocular surface diseases. In: Lass JH, ed. *Advances in Corneal Research.* New York: Plenum Press, 1997; chap. 12.

28. Solomon A, Pires RTF, Tseng SCG. Amniotic membrane transplantation following an extensive removal of primary and recurrent pterygia. *Ophthalmology* 2001; Mar; 108(3): 449–460.

29. Ma DH-K, See L-C, Liau S-B, Tsai RJF. Amniotic membrane graft for primary pterygium: comparison with conjunctival autograft and topical mitomycin C treatment. *Br J Ophthalmol* 2000; 84:973–978.

30. Choi YS, Kim JY, Wee WR, Lee JH. Effect of the application of human amniotic membrane on rabbit corneal wound healing after excimer laser photorefractive keratectomy. *Cornea* 1998; 17:389–395.

31. Wang MX, Gray TB, Park WC, et al. Reduction in corneal haze and apoptosis by amniotic membrane matrix in excimer laser photoablation in rabbits. *J Cat Refract Surg* 2001; Feb; 27(2):310–319.

32. Park WC, Tseng SC. Modulation of acute inflammation and keratocyte death by suturing, blood, amniotic membrane in PRK. *Invest Ophthalmol Vis Sci* 2000; Sep; 41(10): 2906–2914.

33. Koizumi N, Inatomi T, Sotozono C, et al. Growth factor mRNA and protein in preserved human amniotic membrane. *Curr Eye Res* 2000; 20:173–177.

34. Na BK, Hwang JH, Kim JC, et al. Analysis of human amniotic membrane components as proteinase inhibitors for development of therapeutic agent of recalcitrant keratitis. *Trophoblast Res* 1999; 13:459–466.

35. Kim JC, Tseng SCG. The effects on inhibition of corneal neovascularization after human amniotic membrane transplantation in severely damaged rabbit corneas. *Korean J Ophthalmol* 1995; 9:32–46.

36. Tsubota K, Satake Y, Ohyama M, et al. Surgical reconstruction of the ocular surface in advanced ocular cicatricial pemphigoid and Stevens–Johnson syndrome. *Am J Ophthalmol* 1996; 122:38–52.

37. Shimazaki J, Yang H-Y, Tsubota K. Amniotic membrane transplantation for ocular surface reconstruction in patients with chemical and thermal burns. *Ophthalmology* 1997; 104:2068–2076.

38. Tsubota K, Satake Y, Kaido M, et al. Treatment of severe ocular surface disorders with corneal epithelial stem-cell transplantation. *N Eng J Med* 1999; 340:1697–1703.

39. Tsubota K, Shimazaki J. Surgical treatment of children blinded by Stevens–Johnson syndrome. *Am J Ophthalmol* 1999; 128:573–581.

40. Meller D, Maskin SL, Pires RT, Tseng SC. Amniotic membrane transplantation for symptomatic conjunctivochalasis refractory to medical treatments. *Cornea* 2000; Nov; 19(6):796–803.

41. Rodriquez-Ares MT, Tourino R, Capeans C, Sanchez-Salorio M. Repair of scleral perforation with preserved scleral amniotic membrane in Marfan's syndrome. *Ophthalmic Surg Lasers* 1999; 30:485–487.

42. Budenz DL, Barton K, Tseng SC. Amniotic membrane transplantation for repair of leaking glaucoma filtering blebs. *Am J Ophthalmol* 2000; Nov; 130(5):580–588.

43. Pires RTF, Tseng SCG, Prabhasawat P, et al. Amniotic membrane transplantation for symptomatic bullous keratopathy. *Arch Ophthalmol* 1999; 117:1291–1297.

44. Kim JS, Kim JC, Na BK, et al. Amniotic membrane patching promotes healing and inhibits protease activity on wound healing following acute corneal alkali burns. *Exp Eye Res* 1998; 70:329–337.

45. Meller D, Pires RTF, Mack RJS, et al. Amniotic membrane transplantation for acute chemical or thermal burns. *Ophthalmology* 2000; 107:980–990.

46. John T. Transplant successful in Stevens–Johnson syndrome: Human amniotic membrane technique treats acute damage, preserves child's eyesight. *Ophthalmology Times* 1999; 15:10–13.

47. Kim JC. Use of temporary amniotic membrane graft for corneal diseases. Inaugural Scientific Meeting of Asia Pacific Society of Cornea and Refractive Surgery, pp. 49–49. 1998.

48. Schwab IR, Reyes M, Isseroff RR. Successful transplantation of bioengineered tissue replacements in patients with ocular surface disease. *Cornea* 2000; 19:421–426.

21
Ex Vivo Stem Cell Expansion

Ivan R. Schwab and R. Rivkah Isseroff

Introduction

The repair of severe ocular surface disease has been a long-standing challenge and has generated a substantial variety of medical techniques and surgical procedures for repair, with only limited success. There is no "silver bullet" for many of these severe surface problems that bedevil patient and physician alike, including such diseases as Stevens–Johnson syndrome, toxic epidermal necrolysis, ocular pemphigoid, thermal and chemical burns, aniridia, and medication-induced pseudopemphigoid, among others. The pathogenesis of this group of surface diseases seemingly is diverse. Nevertheless, they all have a presumed single common pathway of damage to the corneal epithelial stem cell. These corneal epithelial stem cells are essential to the repair and maintenance of the normal ocular surface. When the stem cells are damaged, they are unable to provide the normal cellular repair mechanisms for the corneal surface. This allows or may even stimulate conjunctiva, or fibrovascular tissue resembling conjunctiva, to overgrow the ocular surface, creating an irregular, scarred, vascularized surface that is insufficient for vision.

The various procedures that have been proposed to correct such problems were doomed to failure until we better understood the role of the corneal epithelial stem cell in the homeostasis of the corneal surface. This understanding has allowed for the autologous or even allogeneic transplantation of such presumed stem cells and their progeny to the damaged ocular surface. Ex vivo expansion of presumed stem cells and bioengineered composite tissues have been viewed as the logical extension of such reparative surgery and may represent the future of ocular surface repair.

The development of corneal epithelial expansion is reviewed in Chapter 12 and will not be addressed in detail here. Understanding of the clinical efforts allows perspective for the impetus of ex vivo stem cell expansion.

Management of Ocular Surface Disease

The management of severe ocular surface disease—including such variable diseases as Stevens–Johnson syndrome, toxic epidermal necrolysis, chemical and thermal burns, congenital abnormalities, cicatrizing conjunctival conditions, and ocular surface tumors—has been a challenging problem. Many different surgical procedures have been tried with varying degrees of success, including mucous membrane grafting from oral or other mucosa, conjunctival flaps, conjunctival free grafts, and lamellar keratoplasty.

Of these procedures, autologous conjunctival transplantation showed the most promise as a tool for restoration of a damaged ocular surface, especially if some normal corneal epithelial stem cells remain in the recipient eye.[1–3] Although these techniques require conjunctival epithelium taken from the normal bulbar surface, the presence of normal corneal epithelial stem cells in the recipient eye will help prevent complete conjunctivalization of the ocular surface from the free conjunctival graft.

The evolution of epithelial transplantation and lamellar keratoplasty took a propitious turn in 1984 when Thoft published his work on keratoepithelioplasty.[4] This remarkable idea included the transplantation of cadaveric corneal tissues to include lenticules of peripheral cornea and limbus with a thin stromal carrier.[4] Thoft advocated this as an alternative to conjunctival transplantation in patients with severe bilateral chemical injuries to the ocular surface.[4] This appeared to be a satisfactory alternative for patients who had little or no normal corneal epithelial surface. However, investigators soon learned that these grafts were difficult to obtain and perform, were readily rejected, and failed to produce convincing results.[5] Human limbal lenticules include the epithelial cells expressing class I human leucocyte antigens (Class I HLA) and are subject to rejection.[5] Nevertheless, this procedure was perhaps the first attempt at the transplantation of corneal epithelial stem cells, although it was not understood as such. Thoft did not have the benefit of our current understanding of the presumed limbal stem cell population. However, he did appreciate the potential of the limbus as an engine for epithelial cellular growth. Later investigators attempted to treat severe chemical burns with large-diameter penetrating keratoplasty and actually did perform the equivalent of an enlarged keratoepithelioplasty.[6,7] Although these procedures probably did transplant limbal corneal epithelial stem cells, many of these patients had problems with eventual epithelial rejection.[6,7] Thoft's work betokened a new age in ocular resurfacing.

With the accumulating evidence of the 1980s and 1990s suggesting that corneal epithelial stem cells resided at the limbus of each cornea, investigators began to consider that complete autologous limbal transplantation could be used to resurface eyes in patients with unilateral surface problems. Armed with this knowledge, surgeons began transplanting autologous limbal tissues to include nearly 180° of the limbus from a healthy eye to a diseased contralateral eye in victims who had only unilateral ocular surface injury or disease.[8–12] This would have been helpful for the recipient eye, but may have been hazardous for the donor eye.[13]

Conjunctival limbal autografts have shown dramatic success in patients with severe and difficult problems.[4–12] Various investigators began using these techniques and obtaining similar results in other forms of stem cell injury or other cases requiring corneal surface reconstruction.[14] Conjunctival limbal autografts were used for acute and chronic chemical injury, thermal burns, contact-lens-induced keratopathy, and ocular surface failure after multiple surgical procedures. Most patients showed consistent visual acuity improvement, rapid surface healing, stable epithelial adhesions, and no recurrent erosion or persistent epithelial defects. Corneal neovascularization stopped or regressed.[4–12] In these studies, some investigators using impression cytology, immunopathology, and light microscopy showed restoration of the corneal epithelial phenotype and regression of the goblet cells from the recipient cornea.[4–12] These grafts showed definite improvement over free conjunctival grafts for conditions requiring the regrowth of corneal epithelium. This simple fact offered further clinical evidence of the authenticity of the limbal stem cell theory. Conjunctival limbal autografts proved to be able to provide corneal epithelial stem cells without the attraction of neovascularization that the conjunctival grafts would often exhibit.

Nonetheless, there are potential problems with this approach. The technique is restricted to unilateral disease, and the donor eye must be completely normal. Failure to notice corneal disease may result in a decrease of vision in the donor eye even if the risk is minimal.[13]

Furthermore, not all patients are willing to risk their uninvolved and healthy eye. In such cases, as well as those with bilateral injuries, it becomes necessary to consider other alternatives, including the use of allografts.

Bilateral severe ocular surface injury or disease, as is usually seen in alkali or thermal burns, is probably more common than unilateral disease. The success achieved with conjunctival limbal autografts led investigators to consider the treatment of bilateral disease with the use of conjunctival limbal allografts, using donor tissue from siblings or other relatives. The success of these allogeneic grafts has led many investigators to advocate such sibling transplants for bilateral injuries.[15] Curiously, the fate of conjunctival limbal allografts in these circumstances is unclear. One would expect the grafts to be rejected, but this does not invariably occur.[16] Allografts may survive in the absence of immunosuppression, although the prognosis improves substantially for patients in whom systemic immunosuppression is utilized.[16] In several well-documented cases, patients who received allografts have improved dramatically with better corneal epithelium.[16,17] This may suggest rejection, yet in each case clinical improvement remained.

Unfortunately for allogeneic transplants, the donor must provide as much as half of his or her limbal tissues. This donation may represent a majority of corneal epithelial stem cells because the advocates of this procedure suggest using the superior and inferior limbus, where we believe the largest number of stem cells are concentrated. This donor location may leave the donor at higher risk of future epithelial surface disease because much of the limbal epithelial stem cell complement may be removed.

The major limitation for conjunctival limbal autografts and allografts, is, therefore, the availability of normal healthy limbal conjunctival epithelium from the contralateral eye or from related donors and the potential threat to the contralateral or donor eye when such limbal cells are removed. Severe burns are difficult to treat with any modality, and it is doubtful that any surface repair consisting of epithelium alone will be sufficient for many of these problems. Extensive damage to the ocular surface causes mucus deficiency and persistent subconjunctival inflammation leading to severe dry eye and fibrosis of the subconjunctival tissue. These are very complicated conditions requiring more complex reconstruction. Some investigators believe that contact with healthy basement membrane is essential and pivotal for the normal epithelialization.[18] If healthy basement membrane is necessary, and that seems likely, transplantation of epithelial cells alone will probably not suffice. Hence, another component to any epithelial graft seemed necessary.

Recently, amniotic membrane has been employed as an organic device to promote the resurfacing of the ocular surface.[19] This remarkable membrane has a single layer of epithelial cells bound to a thick and continuous basement membrane with a full complement of certain subtypes of type IV and V collagen as well as other extracellular factors that are principal basement membrane components.[20,21] Interestingly, certain subtypes of type IV collagen have been recognized histochemically in conjunctival, but not in corneal, epithelial basement membrane.[22] This finding suggests that collagen in the amniotic membrane could serve as a suitable substrate for conjunctival re-epithelization and would be considered substrate for transplantation, especially for corneal epithelial stem cells traditionally found at the limbus. The various laminins known to be present in amniotic membrane could provide signals for hemidesmosomal attachment of epithelium, which could help adherence. Amniotic membrane is known to have a thick basement membrane and has been used successfully for other epithelial cell growth.[23]

Transplanted amniotic membrane seems to promote normal conjunctival re-epithelization while preventing excessive subconjunctival fibrosis. As mentioned above, certain type IV collagen subtypes have been recognized histochemically in conjunctival but not in corneal epithelial basement membrane, and type IV collagen has been recognized in amniotic membrane.[20–22] This finding suggests that the collagen in the amniotic membrane probably serves as a suitable substrate for conjunctival epithelialization and would be suitable for transplantation, as other investigators working with pneumocytes and endometrial cells have suggested.[24,25] Using damaged rabbit corneas as a model, Kim and Tseng demonstrated that the various components of basement membrane mentioned above may well play a role in epithelial healing after de-epithelization, illustrating the role of the extracellular matrix in wound healing.[26]

Cultured corneal epithelial stem cell transplants were considered as early as 1982, when Friend et al. sought to use in vitro epithelial cell cultures on stromal carriers.[27] Unfortunately, this did not meet with much success, possibly because stem cells were not included in the cell cultures. In 1985, Gipson et al. attempted direct transplantation of corneal epithelium to rabbit corneal wounds in vivo.[28] They reported that the adhesion of freshly dissected rabbit corneal basal epithelial cells to denuded basal lamina of corneas can take place within 60–90 minutes in vitro or within 6 hours in vivo.[29] However, these investigators also observed that these epithelial sheets failed to remain adherent to rabbit corneal stroma in vivo after 24 hours.[28] In 1985, Geggel and co-workers applied corneal epithelial cell sheets (obtained by applying dispase grade II to donor rabbit corneas) to a collagen gel (Vitrogen®) and created a safe and nontoxic substrate that allowed for epithelial adherence up to 13 days in vitro.[30] They also discovered that the gel, without the epithelial cells, remained on the rabbit eye and was well tolerated for at least 6 weeks until the end of the animal investigation.[30] Both investigations employed epithelium dissected from the cornea and probably did not include corneal epithelial stem cells.[28–30]

Friend et al. later suggested that adhesion of epithelial sheets obtained from rabbits adhered to stroma in vitro within 24 to 72 hours, and hemidesmosomes formed with host basement membrane at the same time.[31] Additional attempts at in vitro culture and reimplantation continued, but were not successful. Nevertheless, the potential for this work was demonstrated.[22]

Little additional investigation was performed until work by He and McCulley documented that limbal epithelial stem cells could be grown in vitro and would become stratified on type IV collagen-coated collagen shields.[33] These shields could be transferred subsequently to denuded ex vivo human corneal stroma in organ culture. Histologic examination revealed that the epithelial cells had attached tightly to the recipient stromal surface even after the removal of the collagen shield.

Torfi et al. were perhaps the first to report the application of cultured autologous grafts in four patients, with apparent success in three of them.[34] More recently, this procedure has been replicated and reported by a European group.[35] To document the corneal phenotype of the transplanted cells, Pellegrini et al. documented that the cultured epithelia were CK3-positive and represented cells of a corneal lineage.[35] Both groups documented that sufficient corneal epithelial cells to cover the entire corneal-limbal surface can be obtained from a 1 to 2 mm^2 limbal biopsy sample, allowing for minimal stem cell depletion from the healthy eye.[34,35] In both investigations, however, one cannot be absolutely certain of the long-term fate of the transplanted autologous cells or, for that matter, that the transplanted cells were responsible for the improvement in the ocular surface. CK3-positive staining does suggest that these cells were of corneal lineage, but this does not document the source. Do the donated cells persist and proliferate in the recipient eye, or do they stimulate a repair response process and are then gradually replaced by the recipient ocular surface cells?

The evolution of the carrier continued as Tsai presented three cases of autologous stem cell transplantation grown on amniotic membrane.[36] Tsai documented epithelial cell growth by using cytokeratin markers that stained positive with AE5 immunoperoxidase stain to document the multicellular layers of cells on the amniotic membrane, but he did not present a control to document that these cells were not the original amniotic epithelium. Nevertheless, he reported prompt re-epithelialization of the corneal surface in unilateral alkali burns. Tsai et al. later expanded this work to include

6 total patients who received autologous composite grafts consisting of en bloc limbal tissues grown on amniotic membrane.[37] They reported successful re-epithelialization of 4 of these 6 with follow-up of up to 15 months. At the same time, our group reported 10 patients who had received composite bioengineered autologous grafts and 4 patients who received composite bioengineered allogeneic grafts.[38] The donated stem cells for the allogeneic grafts were obtained from living-related donors. Ten of these 14 patients had a successful result, which was defined as restoration or improvement of vision, along with maintenance of corneal re-epithelialization and absence or recurrence of surface disease. Follow-up ranged from 6 to 19 months with a mean of 13 months. Our techniques were slightly different in that our composite graft consisted of the isolation of corneal epithelial cells to be combined with amniotic membrane.[38] This technique may offer the advantage of the elimination of antigenic elements such as allogeneic Langerhans cells, among other elements.

As mentioned previously, investigators have proved that complete autologous limbal transplants have resurfaced eyes with unilateral surface problems.[8–12,14] Unfortunately, this leaves the donor eye at some risk for future surface problems because of the depletion of stem cells from the donor eye. Additionally, this technique does not address bilateral ocular surface injury. The techniques of composite grafting with cultured corneal epithelial (presumed) stem cells and a carrier such as amniotic membrane offer an unrealized potential for successful ocular resurfacing without significant threat to the donor eye.

Current Indications

Corneal and conjunctival epithelial cell injury, degenerations and surface abnormalities are relatively common problems and may become a threat to vision. Ocular surface diseases such as Stevens–Johnson syndrome, toxic epidermal necrolysis, chemical and thermal burns, medication toxicity, recurrent pterygia, certain infectious diseases, ocular tumors, immunologic conditions, radiation injury, inherited and congenital syndromes such as aniridia, among other conditions can severely compromise the ocular surface and cause catastrophic visual loss in otherwise potentially healthy eyes. Treatment is expensive, frustrating, time-consuming, and often unsuccessful. Conjunctival scarring, foreshortening of the fornix, entropion, corneal epithelial keratinization, mucous depletion, and scarring of the ocular surface all contribute to this problem. Ex vivo composite grafting can be considered for all of these conditions, although at this writing the procedure should still be considered investigational. If other procedures offer the patient an improved prognosis, ex vivo composite grafting should probably not be done, reserving this procedure for only those with few other alternatives.

Contraindications

These techniques require a great deal of preparation and laboratory expense and should not be used on patients who have a healthy stem cell population or even a partially healthy stem cell population. Such patients would be well served by simpler techniques. Although it is sometimes not easy to determine if the stem cell population is normal, composite bioengineered conjunctival tissue grafting is in its infancy and should not be considered for patients where other techniques have a satisfactory prognosis. Nevertheless, these ex vivo expanded composite tissue techniques will probably lead us to improved reconstruction techniques for severe ocular surface disease.

Preoperative Considerations

Preoperatively, the donor eye, whether it is autologous or allogeneic, must be biopsied for the necessary complement of stem cells to be expanded in vitro. The donor eye should be healthy without a history or physical signs of injury. While relatively few cells are taken from the donor eye, the remaining complement of cells must be healthy enough to continue the production of normal corneal epithelial cells.

Epithelial cell harvest is done in a similar manner, whether cells are taken from a patient (autologous) or donor sibling (allogeneic). Sterile preparation and draping of the eye is followed by the placement of a lid speculum. Approximately .2 cc of 1% xylocaine is injected beneath the conjunctiva at the superior temporal limbus. A 2 mm² biopsy to include the limbal conjunctiva is harvested and placed in a cellular transport medium for transportation to the laboratory. The limbal conjunctiva is removed as closely to the reflection of the adherent corneal epithelium as possible. Antibiotic ointment is placed, and the eye is covered with a patch for 12 to 24 hours (Figure 21.1).

If the expanded tissue is to be allogeneic, the recipient should be immunosuppressed prior to the transplantation. Immunosuppression may begin a week or two prior to the operation, but the patient's chances probably improve if the immunosuppression precedes the transplantation. Cyclosporin A is the prototype immunosuppressive agent, although suppression levels equivalent to those of renal transplantation may be unnecessary. Nevertheless, the requirements for such grafting are not yet well understood.

Figure 21.1. Biopsy site after limbal tissues removed. Biopsy is improved by removing cells closer to the limbus than is shown in this illustration.

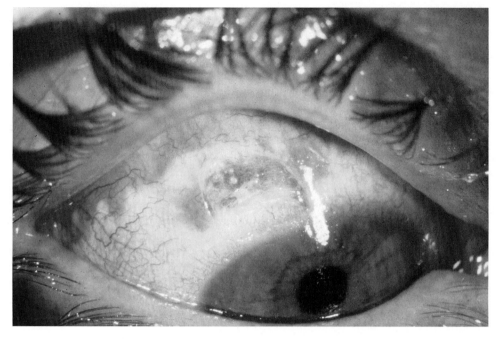

As with any surgical procedure, the patient should be in as good general health as possible, although this procedure is generally done under local anesthesia even when combined with a corneal transplantation. If a corneal transplant is to be combined with the composite graft, and the corneal transplant involves anterior segment reconstruction, then general anesthesia should be considered because of the length of the surgical procedure.

Preparation of the Composite Graft

In our procedure, the 2 mm^2 biopsy was transferred to the laboratory in transport medium. In the laboratory, the epithelium was removed aseptically and transferred to a 60 mm Petri dish. The tissue was washed three times for 5 minutes each with 5 ml of Dulbecco's Phosphate Buffered Saline-Calcium Magnesium Free (DPBS-CMF) (Life Technologies)/5% antibiotic-antimycotic: 10,000u Penicillin-G and 10,000mcg/ml Streptomycin with 25 mcg/mL fungizone (ABAM) (Gemini Bio-Products Inc.), transferring the tissue to a new dish with each wash. The tissue was incubated in a solution of trypsin/edetate disodium (EDTA) solution for 30 minutes at 37°C in a 5% CO$_2$ incubator. The action of the trypsin was inhibited by adding an equal volume of medium that contained 10% fetal bovine serum. The sample was minced with a scalpel blade and centrifuged at 3200 rpm for 5 to 7 minutes. The cells were plated at approximately 1.0×10^6 cells/ml Growth Medium (GM; consisting of Dulbecco's Modified Eagle's Medium, Fetal Calf Serum glutamine,

ABAM, Epidermal Growth Factor, hydrocortisone, and cholera toxin) on two 100 mm dishes with mitomycin-C-treated 3T3 cells. The 3T3 cells had been treated and trypsinized. The dishes containing the corneal cells and the 3T3 feeder cells were placed into a 37° C/5% CO$_2$ incubator. Within 3 days, small colonies of cells formed. At that time, the growth medium was replaced with Keratinocyte Growth Medium (Medium 154 +ABAM and human keratocyte growth supplement, KGM). When the primary dish was at 40–50% confluence, the cells were passed into 4×100 mm dishes (passage #1). These cells were then allowed to reach 40–50% confluence.

Amniotic membrane for human use was obtained from Bio-Tissue™ (Miami, FL) and was stored at −80°C until use. The human amniotic membrane (HAM) from Bio-Tissue™ was thawed in 37°C water bath. The HAM was rolled onto a sterile 100 mm Petri dish containing 15 mL PBS/1%ABAM. The filter paper was removed, keeping the epithelial side up.

The HAM is prepared by removing the amniotic epithelium with trypsinization for 15 minutes followed by gentle scraping. Following removal of the amniotic epithelium, the expanded corneal epithelial cell population for human transplantation is grown onto the amniotic membrane as follows: The HAM is rinsed three times with PBS/1% ABAM. In the fourth rinse bath, the HAM is applied to a circular sterile stainless steel mesh with a 1.5×1.5 cm square cut into the center of the mesh. The center of the membrane is placed over the center of the mesh. Then, the corneal cells, suspended in 0.5 mL GM, are inoculated onto the center of the HAM. The optimal number of corneal cells is

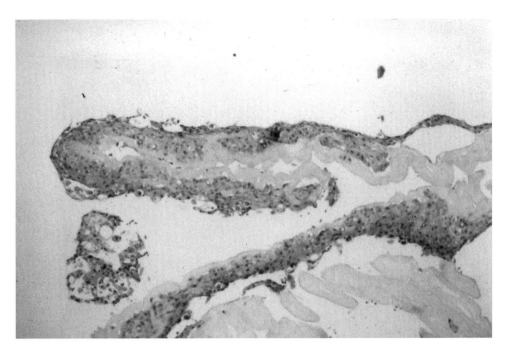

Figure 21.2. In vitro example of corneal epithelial cells growing on denuded amniotic membrane.

1.5–3×10^6 cells. Two mL of GM is added to the dish. The dish with the HAM is then placed into a CO_2 incubator at $37°C$. The HAM is kept covered with GM to prevent drying. More cells are plated if necessary. The medium is changed every two days. One or two days before grafting, the medium is changed to one without ABAM or cholera toxin. The cells are allowed to attach before human transplantation for 10 to 14 days. Before grafting, the medium is aspirated and the graft washed three times with 7 mL PBS, aspirating between washes. After the final wash, 7 mL of unsupplemented DMEM is added to the dish. The dish is placed in an incubation chamber and purged with $95\%O_2/5\%CO_2$. The graft is then ready for transplant (Figures 21.2 and 21.3).

Surgical Techniques

The patients receiving autologous and allogeneic expanded epithelial cell transplants atop amniotic membrane carriers underwent similar procedures. All of the abnormal tissue was removed and the conjunctiva was resected and recessed. The amniotic membrane carrier with expanded corneal epithelial cells was placed atop the defect, and the corneal edge was sewn to the peripheral cornea with 10-0 nylon. The posterior peripheral edge of the amniotic membrane is sewn to the peripheral recessed or resected conjunctiva with 10-0 nylon, and a bandage contact lens was placed to prevent lid trauma. The contact lens was left for approximately 3 months (Figures 21.4 and 21.5). During this

time, the amniotic membrane gradually dissolved, and the peripheral conjunctival sutures were removed. Once the bandage contact lens had been removed, the corneal sutures were also removed.[40] At this writing, we believe that leaving the composite graft intact and not creating a hole is preferable (Figure 21.6).

Postoperative Management

A therapeutic contact lens is placed at the end of the procedure to help ensure that the cells remain in place. Epithelial cell adherence takes weeks, if not months, to complete attachment of the hemidesmosomes. Hence, these cells can be easily removed if not protected during that time. The therapeutic contact lens is left in place for 8 to 12 weeks before consideration of removal to help assist these cells in adhering. The amniotic membrane will dissolve within a matter of weeks, although in some cases fragments may persist for 3 or 4 months, but will completely dissolve leaving only the remaining epithelial cells (Figures 21.7 and 21.8). Systemic immunosuppression should be continued with cyclosporin or a similar agent for at least one year, if it can be tolerated and does not show systemic side effects for those patients receiving allogeneic transplants. Topical treatment with corticosteroids and antibiotics such as a fluoroquinolone is indicated for a period of 3 to 4 weeks. The immunosuppression necessary for allogeneic grafting will also compromise the natural antimicrobial protection inherent to a normal ocular surface. Vigilant observation is essential, since such patients are probably

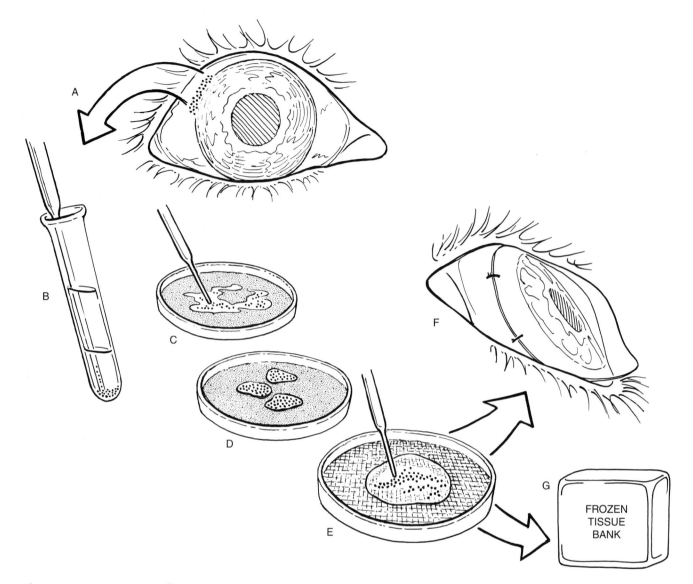

Figure 21.3. Diagrammatic illustration from harvest of cells to surgical procedure. (A) Harvest of donor cells from superior temporal limbus. Approximately 2 mm² tissue is harvested from the limbus. (B) These cells are then transported to the laboratory in a storage medium. (C) The stem cells and epithelial cells are allowed to grow in a culture medium, as mentioned. (D) The stem cells are selected by using only those that form colonies. All other cells, such as Langerhans cells, are removed. (E) Once a pure stem cell/epithelial cell culture has been isolated and grown, it is then transported to amniotic membrane and allowed to grow on this membrane until confluent. (F) The amniotic membrane and stem cells can be transplanted to the ocular surface. This bioengineered tissue can be placed completely across the exposed cornea (beyond the limbus to beyond the limbus), or a central area of clear, corneal stroma can be isolated in a "doughnut" fashion. (G) The remaining cells can be frozen.

at high risk for infectious keratitis. Intraocular pressure should be monitored for steroid response.

Conclusions

Severe ocular surface damage creates frustration for both physician and patient. Often this ocular surface damage covers an otherwise normal eye. Repair of the ocular surface requires an understanding of anatomy and physiology. Ocular surface reconstruction has been evolving as this understanding improves. Recent work suggests that the corneal epithelial stem cell resides at the limbus, and seems to confirm, at least in large part, the "XYZ" hypothesis of Thoft and Friend.[39] Most evidence suggests that corneal epithelial stem cells are necessary to create normal corneal epithelial cells, at least for a prolonged period of time.

This evidence suggests that each stem cell will spawn a limited number of active cells. These transient amplifying (TA) cells will rapidly proliferate for many, but probably not an infinite number of generations of ma-

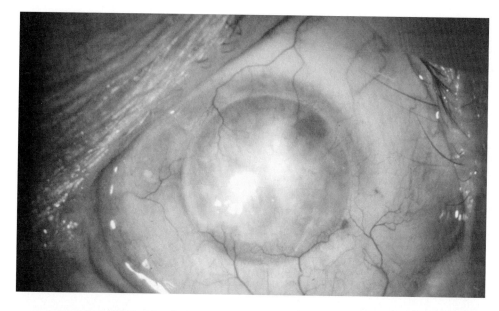

Figure 21.4. Preoperative photograph of patient who had an alkali burn many years previously. He has had multiple attempts at ocular surface repair by corneal transplantation, without success. He continued to have problems with corneal epithelialization.

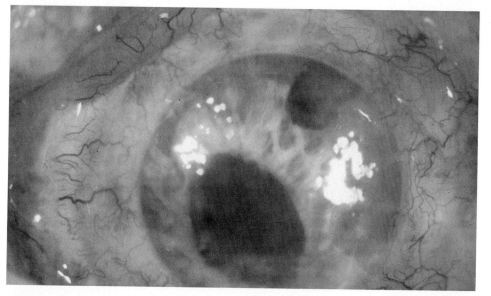

Figure 21.5. Fourteen months postoperative for eye shown in Figure 21.4. The patient had corneal transplant with composite graft overlay. At the time of this writing, the patient remains successful with 14 months follow-up.

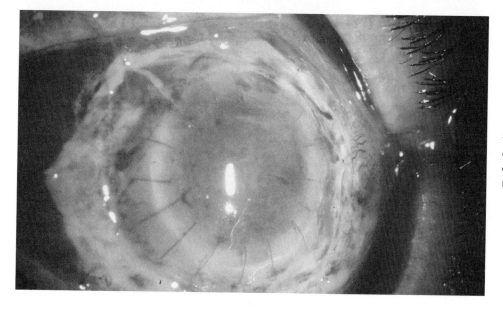

Figure 21.6. An immediate postoperative photograph of an eye that had a severe alkali burn with eventual corneal melt and perforation. He received a corneal transplant and composite bioengineered tissue replacement, and at the time of this writing has a clear and intact ocular surface with 12 months of follow-up, although he has rejected his corneal transplant.

Figure 21.7. Preoperative appearance of an eye that had sustained a thermal and presumed alkali burn with symblephara nasally and superiorly and re-epithelization difficulties.

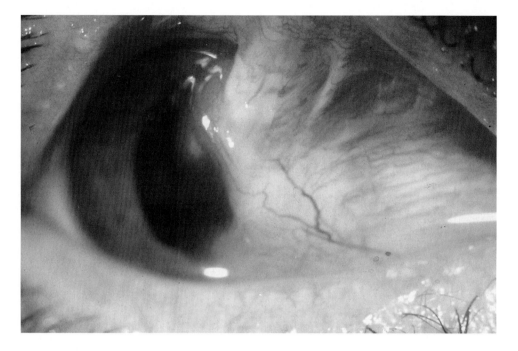

ture corneal epithelial cells. The transient amplifying cells eventually can no longer sustain the metabolic activity, and they themselves stream toward the center of the cornea as fully differentiated cells. The limbal stem cell is then stimulated to create another TA cell and the cycle continues. This differentiation minimizes the demands on the original stem cell. If this model or a similar one for stem cell and corneal epithelial maintainance is true, then corneal epithelial stem cells will be required to re-epithelize a damaged cornea.

The number of corneal epithelial stem cells is clearly finite, and a donor cannot part with all these cells, al-

though it is unclear what percentage of the original stem cell population is necessary to maintain a normal ocular surface. If progress is to be made in the resurfacing of eyes with damaged stem cells, donor stem cells must be used. These can be obtained from autologous tissue, or potentially from allogeneic donors. But there may be danger in acquiring autologous donor stem cells if 80–90% of the complement of stem cells is transferred from one eye to another. Similarly, if living allogeneic donors such as siblings are utilized, there may be a danger to the donor, and this may not be apparent for several years. Hence, for unilateral ocular stem cell dam-

Figure 21.8. Three-month postoperative photograph of the eye seen in Figure 21.6. Some fragments of amniotic membrane remain. The patient continues now with 24 months of follow-up with a clear cornea and no problems with re-epithelization and best corrected 20/70 visual acuity.

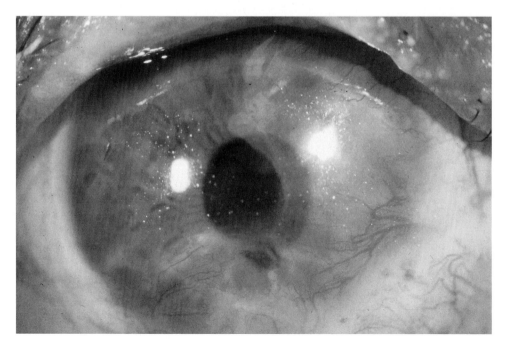

age, and especially bilateral stem cell failure, other techniques must be considered.

Bioengineered skin substitutes have been used in the field of dermatology, and the techniques applied herein are simply extensions of these dermatologic techniques to the eye.[40] In vitro engineering of human skin is already being used for the treatment of burns and chronic nonhealing defects, even if problems remain.[41-43] Cultured ocular surface grafting is a nascent technology that is potentially a powerful tool for ocular surface repair. Such techniques represent a step toward the goal of bionengineered ocular surface transplantation and reconstruction.

References

1. Thoft RA. Indications for conjunctival transplantation. *Ophthalmol* 1982; 89:335–339.
2. Clinch TE, Goins KM, Cobo LM. Treatment of contact lens-related ocular surface disorders with autologous conjunctival transplantation. *Ophthalmol* 1992; 99:634–638.
3. Vastine DW, Stewart WB, Schwab IR. Reconstruction of the periocular mucous membrane by autologous conjunctival transplantation. *Ophthalmol* 1982; 89:1072–1081.
4. Thoft RA. Keratoepithelioplasty. *Am J Ophthalmol* 1984; 97:1–6.
5. Thoft RA, Sugar J. Graft failure in keratoepithelioplasty. *Cornea* 1993; 12:362–365.
6. Kuckelkorn R, Redbrake C, Schrage NF, et al. Keratoplasty with 11–12 mm diameter for management of severely chemically-burned eyes. *Ophthalmologe* 1993; 90:683–687.
7. Redbrake C, Buchal V, Reim M. (Keratoplasty with a scleral rim after most severe eye burns.) *Klin Monatsbl Augenheilkd* 1996; 08:145–151.
8. Kenyon KR, Tseng SCG. Limbal autograft transplantation for ocular surface disorders. *Ophthalmol* 1989; 96:709–723.
9. Coster DJ, Aggarwal RK, Williams KA. Surgical management of ocular surface disorders using conjunctival and stem cell allografts. *Br J Ophthalmol* 1995; 79:977–982.
10. Tsubota K, Satake Y, Ohyamam M, et al. Surgical reconstruction of the ocular surface in advanced ocular cicatricial pemphigoid and Stevens–Johnson syndrome. *Am J Ophthalmol* 1996; 122:38–52.
11. Tsubota K, Toda I, Saito H, et al. Reconstruction of the corneal epithelium by limbal allograft transplantation for severe ocular surface disorders. *Ophthalmol* 1995; 102: 1486–1496.
12. Tan DT, Ficker LA, Buckley RJ. Limbal transplantation. *Ophthalmol* 1996; 103:29–36.
13. Herman WK, Doughman DJ, Lindstrom RL. Conjunctival autograft transplantation for unilateral ocular surface diseases. *Opthalmol* 1983; 90:1121–1126.
14. Shimazaki J, Yang HY, Tsubota K. Limbal autograft transplantation for recurrent and advanced pterygia. *Ophthalmic Surg Lasers* 1996; 27:917–923.
15. Tsai RJF, Tseng SCG. Human allograft limbal transplantation for corneal surface reconstruction. *Cornea* 1994; 13: 389–400.
16. Coster DJ, Aggarwal RK, Williams KA. Surgical management of ocular surface disorders using conjunctival and stem cell allografts. *Br J Ophthalmol* 1995; 79:977–982.
17. Williams KA, Brereton HM, Aggarwal R, et al. Use of DNA polymorphisms and the polymerase chain reaction to examine the survival of a human limbal stem cell allograft. *Am J Ophthalmol* 1995; 120:332–350.
18. Roper-Hall M. Thermal and chemical burns. *Trans Ophthalmol Soc UK* 1965; 85:631–653.
19. Shimazake J, Yang H-Y, Tsubota K. Amniotic membrane transplantation for ocular surface reconstruction in patients with chemical and thermal burns. *Ophthalmol* 1997; 104:2068–2076.
20. Modesti A, Scarpa S, D'Orazi G et al. Localization of type IV and V collagens in the stroma of human amnion. *Prog Clin Biol Res* 1989; 296:459–463.
21. Liotta LA, Lee CW, Morakis DJ. New method for preparing large surfaces of intact human basement membrane for tumor invasion studies. *Cancer Lett* 1980; 11:141–152.
22. Ljubimov AV, Burgeson RE, Butkowski RJ, et al. Human corneal basement membrane heterogeneity: topographical differences in the expression of type IV collagen and laminin isoforms. *Lab Invest* 1995; 72:461–473.
23. Lwebuga-Mukasa JS, Thulin G, Madri JA, et al. An acellular human amniotic membrane model for in-vitro culture of type II pneumocytes: the role of the basement membrane in cell morphology and function. *J Cell Physiol* 1984; 121:215–25.
24. Lwebuga-Mukasa JS, Thulin G, Madri JA, et al. An acellular human amnionic membrane model for *in vitro* culture of type II pneumocytes: the role of the basement membrane in cell morphology and function. *J Cell Physiol* 1984; 121:215–225.
25. Van der Linden PJQ, Erlers JWJ, de Goeij AFPM, et al. Endometrial cell adhesion in an *in vitro* model using intact amniotic membranes. *Fertil Steril* 1996; 65:76–80.
26. Kim JC, Tseng SCG. Transplantation of preserved human amniotic membrane for surface reconstruction in severely damaged rabbit corneas. *Cornea* 1995; 14:473–484.
27. Friend J, Knoshita S, Thoft RA, et al. Corneal epithelial cell cultures on stroma carriers. *Invest Ophthalmol Vis Sci* 1982; 23:41–49.
28. Gipson IK, Friend J, Spurr JJ. Transplant of corneal epithelium to rabbit corneal wound *in vivo*. *Invest Ophthalmol Vis Sci* 1985; 26:901–905.
29. Gipson IK, Grill SM. A technique for obtaining sheets of intact rabbit corneal epithelium. *Invest Ophthalmol Vis Sci* 1982; 23:269–273.
30. Geggel HS, Friend J, Thoft RA. Collagen gel for ocular surface. *Invest Ophthalmol Vis Sci* 1985; 26:901–905.
31. Friend J, Ebato B, Thoft RA. Transplantation of cultured rabbit corneal epithelium *in vitro*. *Invest Ophthalmol Vis Sci* 1987; 28:S53.
32. Roat MI, Thoft RA. Ocular surface epithelial transplantation. *Int Ophthal Clinic* 1988; 28:169–174.
33. He Y-G, McCulley JP. Growing human corneal epithelium on collagen shield and subsequent transfer to denuded cornea *in vitro*. *Current Eye Res* 1991; 10:851–863.
34. Torfi H, Schwab IR, Isseroff R. Transplantation of cultured autologous limbal stem cells for ocular surface disease. *In Vitro* 1996; 32:47A.
35. Pellegrini G, Traverso CE, Franzi AT, et al. Long-term

restoration of damaged corneal surfaces with autologous cultivated corneal epithelium. *Lancet* 1997; 349:990–993.

36. Tsai RJF. Corneal surfaces reconstruction by amniotic membrane with cultivated autologous limbo-corneal epithelium. *Invest Ophthalmol Vis Sci* 1998; 39:S429.

37. Tsai RJF, Li LM, Chen JK. Reconstruction of damaged cornea by transplantation of autologous limbal epithelial cells. NEJM 2000; 343:86–93.

38. Schwab IR, Isseroff RR, Reyes M. Successful transplantation of bioengineered tissue replacements in patients with ocular surface disease. *Cornea* 2000; 343:86–93.

39. Thoft RA, Friend J. The XYZ hypothesis of corneal epithelial maintenance [letter]. *Invest Ophthalmol Vis Sci* 1983; 24:1442–1443.

40. Boyce ST. Cultured skin substitutes: A review. *Tissue Engineering* 1996; 2:255–266.

41. Bell E, Ehrlich HP, Buttle DJ, et al. Living tissue formed *in vitro* and accepted as skin equivalent tissue of full-thickness. *Science* 1981; 211:1052–54.

42. Cuono CB, Langdon RC, McGuire J. Use of cultured epidermal autografts and dermal allografts as skin replacement after burn injury. *Lancet* 1986; 1:1123–1124.

43. Hansbrough JF, Morgan J, Greenleaf G. Advances in wound coverage using cultured cell technology. *Wounds* 1993; 5:174–194.

22
Immunosuppressive Therapy in Ocular Surface Transplantation

Ali R. Djalilian, Robert B. Nussenblatt, and Edward J. Holland

Introduction

Patients with bilateral limbal stem cell deficiency who are not candidates for autologous transplantation generally require allograft tissue to restore the stem cell population.[1] Compared to conventional penetrating keratoplasty, limbal allografts are at significantly higher risk for rejection. This increased susceptibility to rejection is primarily because of the vascularity of the limbal area, which allows greater access for the immune system. It is also due to the greater antigenicity of the limbal tissue, which contains a significant number of Langerhans cells.[2]

Previous studies have demonstrated the importance of immunosuppression in maintaining graft survival following limbal stem cell transplantation.[3–6] Our experience with the keratolimbal allograft (KLAL) procedure in 54 cases further underscored the need for oral immunosuppression.[7] Specifically, among the 28 cases who received oral cyclosporin A (CsA) for 18 months, 24 eyes (87%) achieved a stable ocular surface compared with 16 of 26 cases (62%) who did not get oral CsA (p < 0.05). This and other reports suggest that achieving adequate immunosuppression after KLAL requires oral medications, and that topical therapy alone is insufficient for long-term graft survival. It should be emphasized that immunosuppression is necessary in all patients who receive limbal allografts, even in those who receive HLA-matched living-related tissue.[8]

The use of oral immunosuppressive agents requires careful monitoring and knowledge of the potential side effects. The side effects and adverse reactions due to these medications are the main potential cause of morbidity associated with limbal allograft transplantation. In this chapter, we will review the basic mechanism of rejection and the various topical and oral immunosuppressive regimens available for patients who undergo limbal allograft transplantation.

Mechanism of Rejection

The primary antigens recognized by the immune system include the major histocompatibility antigens (human lymphocyte antigens [HLA]), ABO antigens, and the minor histocompatibility antigens. Class I HLA antigens (HLA-A, -B, and -C) are expressed by all nucleated cells in the body and are found on the corneal epithelium, stromal keratocytes, and endothelial cells, whereas class II antigens (HLA-DR, -DQ and -DP) are present mainly on antigen-presenting cells (APCs) such as macrophages and Langerhans cells.[9] Under the influence of interferon-γ, both corneal epithelial and endothelial cells can also express class II antigens. ABO antigens have been detected primarily on epithelial cells.[10]

During the afferent arm of the immune response, the donor tissue antigens are processed and presented by the APCs of the host for recognition by the T-cells. The donor APCs may also directly present their antigens to T-cells. The main subset of T-lymphocytes that are essential in the sensitization of the host appear to be the CD4+ helper T-(Th-)cells. The HLA class II antigens provide the main antigenic stimulation of these Th-cells. Interleukin-1, which is released by macrophages, helps further to induce the proliferation of Th-cells. Once activated, Th-cells release a number of cytokines including interleukin-2 (IL-2), and interferon-γ. Interleukin-2 stimulates the activation and proliferation of other T- and B-lymphocytes, whereas interferon-γ activates macrophages and induces the expression of class II antigens in the donor tissue. Cytotoxic T-cells (CD8+) directed against class I antigens appear to be the primary effector cells in graft rejection. Antibodies produced by B-cells further contribute to the graft damage by binding to the foreign antigens and attracting other immune cells such as macrophages and natural killer cells. CD4+-cells can also directly participate as cytotoxic effector cells.

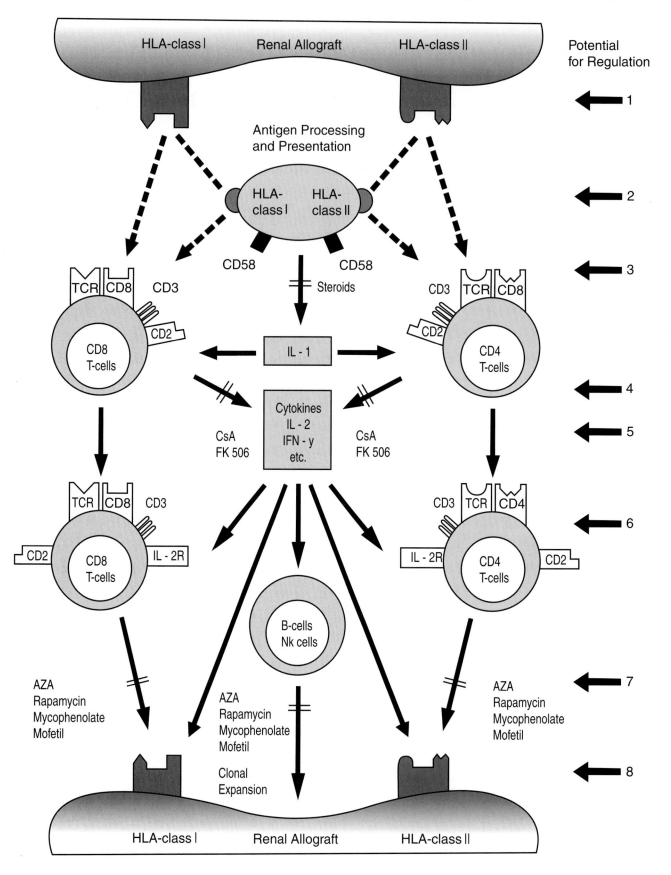

Figure 22.1. Schematic representation of the anti-allograft response showing human lymphocyte antigen (HLA). This antigen is the primary stimulus for the initiation of the anti-allograft response. Also represented are the cell surface proteins participating in antigenic recognition and signal transduction, the contribution of cytokines and cell types to the immune response, and the potential sites for the regulation of the anti-allograft response. Potential sites for regulation are identified on the right. At site 1 histoincompatibility between the recipient and the donor can be minimized (e.g., HLA matching). At site 2 monokine production by antigen-presenting cells can be prevented (e.g., by corticosteroids). Antigen recognition can be blocked (e.g., by OKT3 monoclonal antibodies) at site 3. Site 4 shows where T-cell cytokine production can be inhibited (e.g., by cyclosporin A). At site 5 cytokine activity can be inhibited (e.g., by anti-interleukin-2 antibody). Site 6 shows where cell cycle progression can be inhibited (e.g., by anti-interleukin-2 receptor antibody). Clonal expansion can be inhibited at site 7 (e.g., by azathioprine, rapamycin, mycophenolate mofetil). At site 8 allograft damage can be prevented by masking target antigen molecules (e.g., by antibodies directed at adhesion molecule sites). (Modified from Sharma VJ, et al. *Curr Opin Immunol* 6:784, 1994. Reproduced with permission.)

The anti-allograft response can be manipulated at a number of different levels. The potential sites for regulation of this process are shown in Figure 22.1 and are discussed below (Table 22.1).

Glucocorticosteroids

Corticosteroids are the drugs of choice for both the prevention and treatment of graft rejection. They are currently the most rapid and effective ocular immunosuppressants available. They exert their immunosuppressive effects by nonspecifically inhibiting many aspects of the inflammatory response. They have been shown to block the synthesis of prostaglandins through inhibition of phospholipase A2, decrease cellular and fibrinous exudation, inhibit chemotaxis and phagocytosis, restore capillary permeability, stabilize the lysosomal membranes of polymorphonuclear leukocytes, and when given systemically, reduce the number of circulating T-cells.[11]

Topical Steroids

Topical application of corticosteroids provides good ocular penetration and effective local immunosuppression. Following limbal allograft transplantation, all patients receive topical steroids three to four times a day and are maintained on a tapered dose indefinitely. Overtreatment should be avoided to minimize retardation of epithelial healing. Prolonged use of topical steroids can lead to a number of adverse effects, most importantly glaucoma and cataracts. Many patients with severe ocular surface disease have concomitant glaucoma, which makes them particularly susceptible to steroid-induced elevated intraocular pressure. Most recently we have begun using topical loteprednol (Lotemax) for patients with steroid response.

Loteprednol is a synthetic steroid that is primarily active on the ocular surface and is hydrolyzed by esterases after it enters the aqueous. In a review of 30 patients after penetrating keratoplasty (26 patients) and KLAL (4 patients), there was a 41% mean reduction in IOP (31.1 mmHg to 18.2 mmHg) after switching from 1% prednisolone acetate to 0.5% loteprednol. There were no cases of acute rejection or worsening inflammation during the mean follow-up period of 21.6 weeks.[12] Although not as effective for intraocular inflammation, loteprednol appears to be a reasonable alternative to conventional steroid drops for patients who develop corticosteroid-induced ocular hypertension following corneal or limbal transplantation.

Table 22.1. Immunosuppressive regimen after keratolimbal allograft transplantation.

Agent	Dosage and duration	Monitoring
Corticosteroids		
Topical	qid-qd, indefinitely	IOP, epithelial healing
Oral	1 mg/kg/day, taper over 6 months	BP, serum glucose, weight Gastritis, bone density, lipids
Cyclosporin A		
Topical	2% qid, indefinitely	Epithelial toxicity (vehicle)
Oral	3 mg/kg/day, 12–18 months	Serum level 100–150 ng/dl, Creatinine, BP, lipids, LFTs minerals, urinalysis, CBC
Azathioprine* OR	100 mg/day, 12–18 months	CBC, LFTs
Mycophenolate*	1,000 mg bid, 12–18 months	CBC, chemistries

*Only one of these two agents is used.
IOP—intraocular pressure, BP—blood pressure, LFT—liver function test, CBC—complete blood count.

Systemic Steroids

Systemic steroids are frequently necessary for the management of limbal stem cell transplant patients. Typically, all patients receive prednisone 1 mg/kg/day starting on the day of surgery. Patients are maintained at this dose for 3 weeks and then tapered to 0.5 mg/kg/day by 6 weeks. The prednisone is then slowly tapered (e.g., 25% reduction per month) over 3 to 6 months. Some patients may require a chronic maintenance dose of 5–10 mg/day in order to achieve adequate immunosuppression. Even when used in the short term, systemic steroids can lead to a number of adverse effects. The most notable side effects are osteoporosis, hypertension, hyperglycemia, mood changes, and weight gain. Table 22.2 summarizes all the potential secondary effects associated with corticosteroid therapy.

Before starting patients on systemic steroids, a discussion on the important side effects is prudent and should be documented in the chart. Baseline evaluation should ideally include measuring the blood pressure, serum glucose and electrolytes, as well as a PPD and HIV tests, when applicable. Patients receiving higher doses of systemic steroids should have their blood pressure and serum glucose monitored routinely and treated as indicated until the dose is tapered. Sodium intake may need to be reduced, and potassium supplements may be necessary.

Steroid-induced bone loss is a dose- and duration-dependent process that begins shortly after initiating therapy. It is partly reversible after steroids are discontinued. Currently, it is recommended that all patients should be given supplemental calcium (1000 mg/day) and vitamin D (400 U/day) to retard bone loss. The use of bisphosphonates is recommended for patients at high risk for osteoporosis, including postmenopausal women who are not on estrogen-replacement therapy. Patients on long-term steroids should ideally be monitored with yearly bone scans and treated with bisphosphonates if bone loss is documented.[13]

Patients on systemic steroids, particularly those with a history of peptic ulcer disease or gastroesophageal reflux, would benefit from prophylactic therapy with either an H2 blocker (e.g., ranitidine 150 mg qd-b.i.d.) or a proton pump inhibitor (e.g., omeprazole 20mg/day). The concomitant use of nonsteroidal anti-inflammatory agents can further increase the risk of peptic ulcer disease and should be minimized whenever possible.

Ideally, steroids should be taken as a single dose in the morning. This is not only more physiologic, since the natural peak of adrenal corticosteroid production occurs in the morning, but also allows the patient to sleep better. Splitting the daily dose in two increases the efficacy compared to a single-dose regimen; however, the adverse reactions are likewise increased. Alternate-day dosing has previously been shown to be an effective strategy to reduce the side effects while maintaining the same steroid effect. While this may be a beneficial approach in patients with chronic inflammatory conditions, its role and efficacy in transplant patients has not been studied thoroughly. In general, when tapering steroids the higher doses can be tapered more rapidly, while the lower doses require a slow taper in order to avoid inducing adrenal insufficiency. Patients should also be reminded that corticosteroids are not to be discontinued abruptly, in cases when they are about to run out of medication. Stress doses of steroids should be given at the times of major injuries or surgical procedures.

While corticosteroids are essential for achieving immunosuppression after limbal allograft transplantation, their systemic side effects preclude their use for the long term. Most patients cannot tolerate the high doses necessary to prevent graft rejection if used as a single agent. Therefore, more specific and less toxic agents are used as steroid-sparing medications, allowing the patient to receive lower doses of steroids for shorter durations.

Table 22.2. Secondary effects of systemic corticosteroid therapy.

FLUID, ELECTROLYTES	NEUROLOGIC
Sodium and fluid retention	Headache
Hypertension	Hyperexcitability
Potassium loss	Moodiness
Hypokalemic alkalosis	Psychosis
MUSCULOSKELETAL	**ENDOCRINE**
Muscle weakness and atrophy	Weight gain
Steroid myopathy	Cushingoid state
Osteoporosis	Adrenal suppression
Aseptic necrosis of the femoral	Hirsutism
and humoral heads	Growth suppression in children
Tendon rupture	Diabetes
	Menstrual irregularity
	Hyperlipidemia
GASTROINTESTINAL	
Increased appetite	
Peptic ulcer	**OPHTHALMIC**
Perforation of small and	Posterior Subcapsular Cataracts
large bowels	Glaucoma
Pancreatitis	Central serous retinopathy
DERMATOLOGIC	**OTHER**
Poor wound healing	Increased susceptibility to
Easy bruising	infections
Acne	Thromboembolism
Increased sweating	

Adapted and modified with permission from Nussenblatt RB, Whitcup SM, Palestine AG, *Uveitis, Fundamentals and Clinical Practice*, 2nd ed., Mosby, St. Louis, MO.

Cyclosporin A

Cyclosporin A (CsA) represents a new generation of specific immunosuppressive agents that selectively interfere with immunocompetent cells without causing generalized cytotoxic effects. Structurally, CsA is a hydrophobic, cyclic undecapeptide derived from the fungus *Tolypocladium inflatumgans*. It works mainly on T-cells by binding to an intracellular peptide known as cyclophilin. Cyclophilin is a type of regulatory protein known as immunophilin that seems to control the synthesis of proteins involved in T-cell activation. By inhibiting cyclophilin, CsA blocks the transcription and production of IL-2, thus limiting the activation of CD4+ and CD8+ T-cells. In addition, CsA blocks the production of other lymphokines such as interferon-γ and inhibits the expression of high-affinity IL-2 receptors.[14]

Topical Cyclosporin A

The topical absorption of CsA is hindered by its hydrophobic structure, which cannot penetrate the hydrophilic stroma. To enhance its ocular absorption, a number of vehicles have been used successfully, including olive oil,[15] liposomal encapsulation,[16] and cyclodextrin.[4] Alternatively, the intravenous formulation of CsA can be mixed with artificial tears; however, this requires vigorous shaking of the bottle prior to administration. Most recently, an emulsion formulation has been under investigation in patients with keratitis sicca and may soon be available commercially.[17] Until a commercial preparation becomes available, topical CsA has to be specifically prepared by a pharmacist.

A number of studies have demonstrated topical CsA to be an effective ocular surface immunosuppressant. We have previously reported the use of 2% topical CsA in 43 patients with various anterior-segment inflammatory conditions, including 11 high-risk keratoplasty patients for whom corticosteroid therapy had failed.[15] None of the corneas were rejected during the 7 to 30 months follow-up period. Xu et al. used topical CsA in a rabbit stem cell transplant model and demonstrated that it significantly prolonged graft survival and was comparable to systemic CsA.[6]

Topically, CsA is well tolerated. Patients may experience some discomfort upon instillation and occasionally develop a punctate keratopathy due to the vehicle. Otherwise, no significant ocular side effects have been reported. Studies have also conclusively shown that the systemic absorption of CsA following topical application is minimal.[15] Thus, it is not necessary to monitor blood levels or renal function when only used topically.

Overall, topical CsA is a valuable tool in patients with limbal stem cell transplantation. It provides effective immunosuppression with minimal side effects. Currently, all patients with limbal allografts are placed on topical CsA 3 to 4 times a day and are continued indefinitely. Although it does not eliminate the need for oral CsA in the first 12 to 18 months, it is particularly useful for the long-term management of limbal stem cell patients after oral immunosuppression has been discontinued. The approval of a topical emulsion formulation should make CsA drops more readily available and hopefully eliminate the vehicle-related problems.

Systemic Cyclosporin A

The use of CsA since the early 1980s has had a profound effect on the success of many solid-organ transplants. It is currently the most widely used immunosuppressant in transplant patients, along with steroids. A number of studies have demonstrated its effectiveness in stem cell transplantation.[3–4] As mentioned earlier, we found a statistically significant impact in the surface outcome of patients who were placed on oral CsA following limbal allograft transplantation.[7]

Previously, oral formulations of CsA (i.e., Sandimmune™) had had variable absorption with erratic peak and trough levels. The current microemulsion preparation of CsA (Neoral™) has significantly improved its bioavailability after oral administration. Neoral™ is absorbed more rapidly and predictably, thus making it easier to attain therapeutic drug levels.[18]

In the absence of any contraindications, all of our stem cell transplant patients routinely receive CsA starting at 3 mg/kg/day. Dosages above 150 mg/day are usually given in b.i.d. doses to minimize spikes in the serum levels. Therapeutic drug monitoring for CsA is most commonly done by measuring a predose trough level approximately 12 hours after the last dose. For limbal allograft patients who are concomitantly receiving a CsA-sparing agent (azathioprine or mycophenolate), a trough level between 100 ng/ml and 150 ng/ml is recommended. Higher levels (150–200 ng/ml) may be needed in patients taking CsA as a single agent.

At the start of therapy, serum trough levels are checked frequently (every 2 to 3 weeks) until stabilized, then every 1 to 2 months thereafter. Although monitoring serum trough levels remains the standard, there is increasing evidence that a 2 hour post-dose level is a more accurate predictor of the total effective dose of CsA (area under the curve). Given the more predictable absorption and kinetics of Neoral™, the therapeutic drug monitoring of CsA is likely to change from a pre-dose trough system to a post-dose peak-based strategy.[17]

Monitoring for the side effects of CsA is actually more important than measuring the serum drug levels. A number of dose-related adverse reactions have been associated with systemic CsA. Those most commonly encountered include hypertension, nephrotoxicity, neurotoxicity, hyperlipidemia, and hepatotoxicity. Baseline evaluation for all patients should include blood pressure, serum creatinine, electrolytes, fasting lipids and glucose, liver-function tests, complete blood count, and urinalysis. A history of uncontrolled hypertension, renal insufficiency, and age greater than 60 are considered relative contraindications for the use of CsA.

The blood pressure should be routinely checked at every visit. Nearly half of all patients will experience at least a 10%–15% elevation of blood pressure above their baseline. If the blood pressure remains persistently elevated (systolic > 140 or diastolic > 90) despite a reduction in the dose, antihypertensive therapy should be started.

Nephrotoxicity occurs in 25% to 75% of patients on systemic CsA. Fortunately, it is dose-related and usually reversible if detected early. The serum creatinine should be followed carefully at all times: every 1 to 2 weeks during the first two months, and every month thereafter. If the serum creatinine rises 30% above the baseline, the dose of CsA should be reduced by 0.5–1 mg/kg/day. If the creatinine remains elevated by 30% or more after the dose reduction, CsA should be discontinued for a month until the creatinine level returns to within 10% of baseline. Measuring the creatinine clearance periodically is actually a more sensitive method for detecting nephrotoxicity due to CsA, although it is less practical and less convenient for the patient.

Periodic laboratory evaluation (every 2 to 3 months) should also include liver function tests, serum glucose and electrolytes, calcium, magnesium, fasting lipids, complete blood count, and urinalysis. Mild elevations of the liver enzymes are not uncommon and typically resolve after the dose is lowered. Hyperlipidemia is prevalent (40%) among transplant patients and may warrant treatment if prolonged therapy with CsA is anticipated. Glucose intolerance is seen less frequently with CsA compared with tacrolimus, and occasionally may require treatment.[19–20] Other laboratory abnormalities that can be encountered include hypomagnesemia, hyperkalemia, and thrombocytopenia.

Neurologic toxicity is seen occasionally and may manifest as tremors, paresthesia, headache, and (rarely) seizures. These symptoms usually improve by reducing the dose of CsA. Patients should also be warned about two potentially disfiguring side effects, namely, gingival hyperplasia (9%) and hirsutism (9%). Although usually reversible, gingival hyperplasia may become persistent. Good oral hygiene appears to be effective in preventing the gingival complication. Finally, there are reports of intracranial hypertension (pseudotumor cerebri), cortical blindness, and microangiopathic hemolytic anemia associated with CsA therapy.[21]

The metabolism of CsA is primarily though the cytochrome P450 system and is excreted by the liver. A number of medications have been shown to interfere with the clearance of CsA. The most important drug interactions are those which increase the levels of CsA, thus potentiating its toxicity, and include medications such as acetazolamide, fluconazole, ketaconazole, erythromycin, clarithromycin, diltiazem, and verapamil. In general, any medication that affects the cytochrome P450 system is likely to alter the metabolism of CsA.[22] An interesting interaction is with grapefruit juice, which can increase cyclosporin levels by up to 50%. Patients should also be advised of the potential for such interactions and CsA levels should be monitored more closely when a new medication is added or discontinued.

We typically maintain patients on CsA for at least 12 to 18 months. This is when patients are at the highest risk of rejection. In our experience with 54 cases of limbal allograft transplantation, there was a total of 16 failures, of which 50% (7 cases) occurred during the first 18 months. In patients who develop signs of rejection, oral CsA may be restarted or continued beyond 18 months. Some groups have recommended that patients should remain on oral immunosuppression with CsA (or tacrolimus) indefinitely, given the persistent risk of rejecting the donor stem cells. On the other hand, others advocate a much shorter duration of treatment, and taper off CsA by 3 to 6 months.[4] In the absence of clear evidence supporting the use of lifelong CsA after limbal transplantation, a more conservative approach involving short-term use seems more prudent.

Overall, CsA is invaluable in the management of the stem cell transplant patient. With diligent monitoring, the risk of irreversible toxicity at the recommended doses is quite low. We have treated several hundred patients with various ocular inflammatory conditions with CsA and have not encountered any significant irreversible adverse reactions. The risk of CsA-induced toxicity is even lower when it is used in combination with steroids and a "CsA sparing" agent such as azathioprine or mycophenolate. This allows for lower doses of CsA to be used, thus minimizing its potential risks. Further studies are needed, however, to determine the optimal dose and duration of therapy after limbal allograft transplantation. Nonetheless, CsA remains the cornerstone of immunosuppressive agents for transplantation.

Tacrolimus (FK-506)

Tacrolimus (Porgraf™) is a newer macrolide immunosuppressant derived from the fungus *Streptomyces tsukubaensis*. Its mechanism of action is very similar to CsA. It binds to a different immunophilin, known as FK-506 binding protein. This in turn inhibits the activation T-lymphocytes by blocking the transcription of several lymphokines, most importantly IL-2.

Tacrolimus was first approved in the U.S. in 1994 and is widely used as an alternative to CsA in organ transplantation. Topically, tacrolimus has been shown to be effective in preventing corneal graft rejection in animal models.[23] Like CsA, its topical absorption requires the use of a vehicle such as olive oil. At this time, there are no clinical studies of topical tacrolimus for ocular therapy. Its application in ophthalmology is currently limited to systemic use.

Bioavailability of tracrolimus is variable after oral intake and is best if taken on an empty stomach. The starting dose is 0.15–0.3 mg/kg/day divided in two doses. Therapeutic drug monitoring is required, given its narrow therapeutic index. The target range for tacrolimus trough blood levels is 5–15 ng/ml. Like CsA, it is metabolized by the liver through the cytochrome P450 system, and thus interactions can occur with the same medications mentioned above.

The side effects associated with tacrolimus are similar to those with CsA.[24] Nephrotoxicity is common (40%) and requires monitoring of the kidney function, as outlined above. Likewise, hypertension also occurs frequently with tacrolimus, but it is less common than with CsA. Neurotoxicity is more common compared to CsA and usually presents as headache, tremor, paresthesia, and occasionally seizures. Another important adverse effect that is seen much more frequently compared to CsA is hyperglycemia. The incidence of tacrolimus-induced diabetes may be as high as 20% in transplant patients (compared to 3–4% for CsA). On the other hand, hyperlipidemia occurs less frequently with tacrolimus, while gingival hyperplasia and hirsutism are not seen.[24] Lymphoproliferative disorders including lymphoma have been reported in association with active Epstein–Barr virus infection in patients on tacrolimus.[25]

Tacrolimus is a potent calcineurin-based immunosuppressant quite comparable to CsA. A few studies suggest that it is more effective than CsA in reversing graft rejection, but overall they appear similar for maintaining long-term graft survival.[24] Tacrolimus has been used successfully by other groups to prevent graft rejection after limbal stem cell transplantation.[5] Although neurotoxicity and diabetes are seen more frequently with tacrolimus, the choice between CsA and tacrolimus in stem cell patients is largely a matter of personal experience and preference. With appropriate monitoring, the risk of adverse events can be similarly minimized.

Azathioprine

Azathioprine (Imuran™) is an antimetabolite that blocks the proliferation of dividing cells. After ingestion, it is converted to the active form, 6-mercaptopurine, which competitively inhibits purine synthesis. To effectively block DNA synthesis, it requires the cells to be actively dividing. Thus, azathioprine is most effective if given early in the rejection process in order to inhibit proliferation of B- and T-cells. It is less effective for established graft rejection, since most of the lymphocytes have already proliferated.

Azathioprine has been used extensively in combination with steroids and CsA in organ transplantation. It functions as a steroid and CsA-sparing agent that allows lower doses of these medications to be used. This in turn reduces their associated toxicities. The usual starting dosage is 1–1.5 mg/kg/day. A typical dose for an adult patient is 100 mg/day given as a single or split dose. One important drug interaction is allopurinol, which interferes with the metabolism of 6-mercaptopurine; therefore a lower dose of azathioprine should be used.

Given its nonspecific nature, azathioprine can inhibit the proliferation of other dividing cells. The most common adverse effects seen with azathioprine are leukopenia, thrombocytopenia, and anemia. These myelosuppressive effects are dose-related and typically respond to a dose reduction, or temporary drug discontinuation. Other reported side effects include nausea, diarrhea, alopecia, and rarely hepatotoxicity.

Prior to starting therapy with azathioprine, a complete blood count as well as liver function tests should be performed. The CBC is monitored weekly during the first month, then every two weeks for two months, then monthly thereafter. Liver enzymes should be checked every few months.

Azathioprine remains a useful adjunct for immunosuppressive therapy with an acceptable side effect profile. The introduction of mycophenolate has recently provided an alternative antimetabolite to azathioprine. Although at this time we continue to use azathioprine in our standard three-drug regimen for limbal stem cell patients, mycophenolate mofetil may eventually replace azathioprine if it proves to be more effective, or better tolerated.

Mycophenolate Mofetil

Mycophenolate mofetil (Cellcept™) was approved by the Food and Drug Administration in 1995 for the prevention of acute renal graft rejection. It is a prodrug that is hydrolyzed to mycophenolic acid after oral intake. It selectively inhibits inosine monophosphate dehydrogenase, a crucial enzyme in the *de novo* synthesis of guanosine. In most cells, guanine synthesis can be maintained through an alternate pathway, known as the salvage pathway. However, proliferating lymphocytes require both the *de novo* and the salvage pathways. Thus, mycophenolate specifically inhibits the proliferation of lymphocytes, both B- and T-cells.

Clinically, mycophenolate mofetil has gained wide acceptance as a steroid sparing agent in organ transplantation as an alternative to azathioprine. It is typically used as a part of a triple therapy with steroids and CsA (or tacrolimus). Large clinical trials involving renal transplant patients have shown a lower incidence of acute graft rejection in patients receiving mycophenolate mofetil versus azathioprine (both groups receiving steroids and CsA).[26]

The therapeutic dosage for most patients is 1,000 mg twice a day, although some may benefit from the maximum dose of 3 g/day. It is absorbed rapidly after oral administration. The most commonly reported side effects are the dose-related gastrointestinal problems: abdominal pain, diarrhea, and vomiting (30%–35%).

Leukopenia, anemia and thrombocytopenia are also seen as a result of the myelosuppressive effects of mycophenolate. These side effects usually respond to a reduction in the dosage, or temporary discontinuation of the drug. An increased susceptibility to infections by DNA viruses has also been reported in organ transplant patients taking mycophenolate mofetil.

Currently, mycophenolate blood levels are not used for therapeutic drug monitoring. At the start of therapy, a complete blood count should be obtained and subsequently every month while a patient remains on mycophenolate mofetil. In patients who have been stable on a given dose for more than 6 months, the blood count may be checked every 2 to 3 months.

The clinical experience from solid-organ transplantation appears to support the use of mycophenolate mofetil as an alternative to azathioprine for most patients, particularly those who are intolerant to azathioprine. Currently, we use mycophenolate routinely instead of azathioprine in the management of intractable uveitis. Other groups have reported successful use of mycophenolate for patients with inflammatory eye diseases, as well as high-risk keratoplasty.[27-28] An important consideration is that mycophenolate mofetil is 6 to 7 times more expensive than azathioprine. Although the added benefit of mycophenolate over azathioprine in stem cell transplant patients has not been studied, it is a reasonable choice as an adjunct to steroids and CsA for this group. Perhaps with future studies demonstrating improved outcomes and patient tolerance, mycophenolate may be used routinely in limbal allograft transplantation.

Sirolimus (Rapamycin)

Sirolimus (Rapamune™) is a macrolide immunosuppressant that was approved in 1999 for kidney transplantation. It primarily acts as an antiproliferative agent by blocking the growth-promoting action of cytokines such as IL-2 and IL-4. This antiproliferative action is not limited to T-cells and sirolimus inhibits B-cells, as well as other nonimmune cells such as fibroblasts and smooth-muscle cells. Specifically, it prolongs the cell cycle by inhibiting a protein, mammalian target of rapamycin (mTOR), that regulates the phosphorylation of several cell-cycle-dependent kinases.[29]

Structurally, sirolimus is similar to tacrolimus, and it binds to the same immunophilin, FK-506 binding protein. However, as mentioned earlier, its mechanism of action is different from both CsA and tacrolimus, and sirolimus does not inhibit calcineurin. Clinically, CsA and sirolimus have been shown to act synergistically as immunosuppressants. Tacrolimus and sirolimus appear to competitively inhibit each other in vitro, since they both bind to the same protein. Animal studies, however, suggest that the two may have some additive effects.

Sirolimus is absorbed rapidly after oral administration. Currently, in renal transplant patients it is given as a loading dose of 6 mg on day 1, followed by a maintenance dose of 2 mg once a day. Therapeutic drug monitoring is done by measuring the pre-dose 24-hour trough level. The target range for the trough whole-blood concentration of sirolimus is 5 to 15 mg/ml. Similar to other immunophilins, sirolimus is metabolized by the cytochrome P450 system, and likewise increased levels can be seen with medications such as erythromycin, ketoconazole, and diltiazem. An important interaction is with CsA. In particular, the timing of administration of CsA and sirolimus can significantly affect the sirolimus blood levels. If taken simultaneously, sirolimus appears to have 50% higher levels compared to taking sirolimus 4 hours after CsA (the recommended interval).[30]

Sirolimus is well tolerated. The most commonly reported side effects are hyperlipidemia, thrombocytopenia, and leukopenia. These dose-related problems typically respond to an adjustment in the dosage, while some patients may require lipid lowering agents. Periodic monitoring of the serum lipids and the blood count is recommended. In patients who are also taking CsA, kidney function and CsA levels should be monitored more closely when starting sirolimus.

At this time clinical experience with sirolimus is limited. Based on published reports, it appears to be a good candidate for maintenance immunosuppression as an alternative to azathioprine. By allowing lower doses of CsA to be used, sirolimus can help minimize the potential toxicities with long-term immunosuppression. Moreover, recent studies suggest that sirolimus may actually help induce tolerance. Currently, a rapamycin analog, SDZ-RAD is also in clinical trials. As experience accumulates, sirolimus will likely be an important component of the immunosuppressive armamentarium.

Monoclonal Antibodies

Monoclonal antibodies directed against T-cell antigens have been used extensively to reverse acute graft rejection in solid-organ transplantation. Topical therapy with antibodies is generally ineffective because of poor absorption across the cornea, except in one report wherein liposome-encapsulated anti-CD4 antibodies were used.[16] Local therapy with subconjunctival injection of antibodies to IL-2 receptor was effective in a rat corneal graft model.[31] Similarly, intracameral injection of monoclonal antibodies to CD3 and CD6 were effective in reversing acute corneal graft rejection clinically.[32] However, these modes of delivery are not suitable for repeat administration. Until the development of a suitable form of local delivery, the application of monoclonal antibodies in ocular diseases will be limited to systemic therapy.

Clinically, polyclonal antibodies against T-cells (antilymphocyte globulin, antithymocyte globulin) were first to be used in organ transplantation. In 1981, OKT3 became the first monoclonal antibody approved for transplantation. It is a mouse antibody directed against the T-cell CD3 antigen. Since OKT3 is nonhuman protein, it can elicit an immune response leading to a cytokine-release syndrome manifested as hypotension, bronchospasm, and pulmonary edema.

Recently, two other monoclonal antibodies have been developed that eliminate the cytokine-release problem by being less immunogenic. Daclizumab (HAT [humanized anti-Tac], Zenapax) and basiliximab (Simulect) are both directed against the alpha subunit (Tac/CD25) of the IL-2 receptor of activated T-cells.[33] By blocking the effect of IL-2, they inhibit the proliferation of T-cells. They were studied in the perioperative period and demonstrated to significantly reduce the acute rejection episodes within the first year. Daclizumab was given 24 hours before surgery and every 14 days for a total of 5 doses. Basiliximab was given on day 0 and day 4 only.

We have used Daclizumab to treat patients with intractable uveitis. The results are very promising for this group of patients. It is well tolerated with no significant adverse effects. The main limitation of this treatment modality is that it requires an intravenous infusion. Currently, monoclonal antibodies have not been used in the management of stem cell transplant patients. Perhaps with future studies, it will prove to be a useful adjunct for corneal and limbal transplantation.

Future Therapies

A number of agents have been shown to be effective in cellular and animal studies. One strategy is to prevent transendothelial migration of immune cells using antibodies and antisense oligonucleotides to selectins or adhesion molecules such as ICAM-1 and LFA-1.[34] Another technique is focused on blocking the critical enzymes in the cytokine-signal transduction pathway. Ultimately, the goal in transplantation is to achieve a state of tolerance that would minimize the need for immunosuppression. Oral immunization with donor antigens has been effective in animal models. A promising new approach is to manipulate the costimulatory pathways necessary for T-cell activation. In particular, blocking the B7–CD28 interaction with an immunoglobulin conjugate, CTLA-4Ig, has been shown to induce tolerance in animal models.[35] Eventually, gene therapy will likely provide the ability to specifically manipulate both the graft and the host such that rejection will no longer be a clinical concern.

General Considerations

Patients on immunosuppressive therapy require special attention that may not be routine in most ophthalmology practices. Prior to starting therapy, evaluations should include a medical examination by the primary-care physician, pregnancy status (and plans), PPD and HIV status, as well as the appropriate baseline laboratory tests. A thorough discussion of the potential risks and expected side effects of immunosuppressive therapy is essential. Important considerations for patients on immunosuppression are routine measurement of the vital signs at each visit, a dedicated system to record and follow laboratory results, and communication with the primary-care physician. The treating physician should have a lower threshold for ordering laboratory tests or obtaining consultation when the patient reports a problem. Patients on immunosuppression, particularly steroids, are at increased risk for infections such as Herpes zoster. Appropriate immunizations, including yearly influenza vaccination, are recommended. However, live virus vaccines should be avoided while on therapy, and for 3 months after stopping therapy.

Overall, the safety and efficacy of immunosuppressive therapy has improved tremendously in the past decades. With appropriate monitoring, the risk of irreversible toxicity at the current doses can be acceptably low.

References

1. Holland EJ. Epithelial transplantation for the management of severe ocular surface disease. *Trans Am Ophthalmol Soc* 1996; 94:677–743.
2. Niederkorn JY. Effect of cytokine-induced migration of Langerhans cells on corneal allograft survival. *Eye* 1995; 9(Pt 2):215–218.
3. Shimazaki J, et al. Evidence of long-term survival of donor-derived cells after limbal allograft transplantation. *Invest Ophthalmol Vis Sci* 1999; 40:1664–1668.
4. Tsubota K et al. Treatment of severe ocular-surface disorders with corneal epithelial stem-cell transplantation. *N Engl J Med* 1993; 340:1697–1703.
5. Dua HS, Azuara-Blanco A. Allo-limbal transplantation in patients with limbal stem cell deficiency. *Br J Ophthalmol* 1999; 83:414–419.
6. Xu KP, Wu Y, Zhou J, Zhang X. Survival of limbal stem cell allografts after administration of Cyclosporin A. *Cornea* 1999; 18:159–165.
7. Djalilian AR, Bagheri MM, Swanson PJ, Schwartz GS, Holland EJ. Keratolimbal allograft for the treatment of limbal stem cell deficiency. Oral Presentation, Castroviejo Cornea Society Annual Meeting, October 1999, Orlando, FL.
8. Rao SK, et al. Limbal allografting from related live donors for corneal surface reconstruction. *Ophthalmology* 1999; 106:822–828.
9. Tresesler PA, Foulks GN, Sanfilippo F. Expression of HLA antigens in the human cornea. *Am J Ophthalmol* 1984; 98: 763.
10. Salisbury JD, Gebhardt BM. Blood group antigens on human corneal cells demonstrated by immunoperoxidase staining. *Am J Ophthalmol* 1981; 91:46–50.

11. Duke-Elder S, Ashton N. Action of cortisone on tissue reactions of inflammation and repair with special attention to the eye. *Br J Ophthalmol* 1951; 35:695.

12. Djalilian AR, Sanderson J, Piracha AR, Holland EJ. The use of topical loteprednol etabonate (Lotemax) in corticosteroid induced ocular hypertension following corneal transplantation. Oral Presentation, EBAA annual meeting, October 2000, Dallas, TX.

13. Reid IR. Glucocorticoid osteoporosis—mechanisms and management. *Eur J Endocrinol* 1997; 137:209–217.

14. Belin MW, Bouchard CS, Phillips TM. Update on topical cyclosporin A. Background, immunology, and pharmacology. *Cornea* 1990; 9:184–195.

15. Holland EJ et al. Topical cyclosporin A in the treatment of anterior segment inflammatory disease. *Cornea* 1993;12: 413–419.

16. Milani JK, et al. Prolongation of corneal allograft survival with liposome-encapsulated cyclosporine in the rat eye. *Ophthalmology* 1993; 100:890–896.

17. Stevenson D, Tauber J, Reis BL. Efficacy and safety of cyclosporin A ophthalmic emulsion in the treatment of moderate-to-severe dry eye disease: a dose-ranging, randomized trial. The Cyclosporin A Phase 2 Study Group. *Ophthalmology* 2000; 107:967–974.

18. Keown P, Kahan BD, Johnston A, Levy G, Dunn SP, Cittero F, Grino JM, Hoyer PF, Wolf P, Halloran PF. Optimization of cyclosporine therapy with new therapeutic drug monitoring strategies: report from the International Neoral TDM Advisory Consensus Meeting (Vancouver, November 1997). *Transplant Proc* 1998; 30:1645–1649.

19. Hong JC, Kahan BD. Immunosuppressive agents in organ transplantation: past, present, and future. *Semin Nephrol* 2000; 20:108–125.

20. Keown PA. New immunosuppressive strategies. *Curr Opin Nephrol Hypertens* 1998; 7:659–663.

21. Gijtenbeek JM, van den Bent MJ, Vecht CJ. Cyclosporine neurotoxicity: a review. *J Neurol* 1999; 246:339–346.

22. Campana C, Regazzi MB, Buggia I, Molinaro M. Clinically significant drug interactions with cyclosporin. An update. *Clin Pharmacokinet* 1996; 30:141–179.

23. Kobayashi C, et al. Suppression of corneal graft rejection in rabbits by a new immunosuppressive agent, FK-506. *Transplant Proc* 1989; 21:3156–3158.

24. Vanrenterghem YF. Which calcineurin inhibitor is preferred in renal transplantation: tacrolimus or cyclosporine? *Curr Opin Nephrol Hypertens* 1999; 8:669–674.

25. Cacciarelli TV, Green M, Jaffe R, et al. Management of posttransplant lymphoproliferative disease in pediatric liver transplant recipients receiving primary tacrolimus (FK506) therapy. *Transplantation* 1998; 66:1047–1052.

26. European Mycophenolate Mofetil Cooperative Study Group. Mycophenolate mofetil in renal transplantation: 3-year results from the placebo-controlled trial. *Transplantation* 1999; 68:391–396.

27. Larkin G, Lightman S. Mycophenolate mofetil. A useful immunosuppressive in inflammatory eye disease. *Ophthalmology* 1999; 106:370–374.

28. Reis A, Reinhard T, Voiculescu A et al. Mycophenolate mofetil versus cyclosporin A in high risk keratoplasty. *Br J Ophthalmol* 1999; 83:1268–1271.

29. MacDonald A, Scarola J, Burke JT, Zimmerman JJ. Clinical pharmacokinetics and therapeutic drug monitoring of sirolimus. *Clin Ther* 2000; 22 Suppl B:B101–121.

30. Kaplan B, Meier-Kriesche HU, Napoli KL, Kahan BD. The effects of relative timing of sirolimus and cyclosporine microemulsion formulation coadministration on the pharmacokinetics of each agent. *Clin Pharmacol Ther* 1998; 63:48–53.

31. Hoffman F, et al. Interleukin-2 receptor targeted therapy with monoclonal antibodies in the rate corneal graft. *Cornea* 1994; 13:440.

32. Ippoliti G, Fronterre A. Usefulness of CD3 or CD6 monoclonal antibodies in the treatment of acute corneal graft rejection. *Transplant Proc* 1989; 21:3133.

33. Wiseman LR, Faulds D. Daclizumab: a review of its use in the prevention of acute rejection in renal transplant recipients. *Drugs* 1999; 58:1029–1042.

34. Yamagami S, et al. Suppression of corneal allograft rejection after penetrating keratoplasty by antibodies to ICAM-1 and LFA-1 in mice. *Transplant Proc* 1995; 27:1899.

35. Gerber DA, Bonham CA, Thomson AW. Immunosuppressive agents: recent developments in molecular action and clinical application. *Transplant Proc* 1998; 30:1573–1579.

23
Penetrating Keratoplasty in Ocular Stem Cell Disease

Mark J. Mannis

Introduction

Reconstruction of the ocular surface is often a sequence of procedures that culminates in optical keratoplasty. The surface reconstruction procedures that precede the corneal transplant are designed to optimize conditions for optical function by ensuring a normal interface between the lids and the globe, normal tear function, and, finally, cellular replacement or reconstruction. Despite the fact that roughly 50% of stem cell transplant procedures are followed ultimately by corneal transplantation, there has been relatively little attention in the literature devoted to the special requirements of the corneal graft in the context of stem cell disease. In this brief chapter, we will attempt to provide a logical approach to corneal grafting in the context of the patient who is being treated for a stem cell deficiency.

The overall therapeutic goals in performing a penetrating or lamellar keratoplasty in any patient are (1) to achieve anatomic integration and surface compatibility of the corneal graft; (2) immunobiologic acceptance of the transplanted tissue; and (3) adequate refractive function. In the ophthalmic literature, a great deal of attention has been paid to the phenomenon of graft rejection and its immunomodulation with corticosteroids and other immunosuppressive agents. Likewise there is also a sizable literature that deals with the refractive function of corneal grafts, ranging from studies of regular and irregular astigmatism after keratoplasty, as well as contact-lens fitting and refractive surgical modification of corneal grafts. However, the issue of surface integration has been less extensively covered in the ophthalmic literature, and it is this component that is perhaps most crucial in the patient who has been previously treated, or is currently receiving treatment, for stem cell dysfunction.

In the context of stem cell disease, there are several highly specific factors that become crucial to the survival of the corneal graft. The first is, of course, the degree of severity of the stem deficiency. The extent of a stem cell deficiency is largely dependent on the etiology. As outlined in Chapter 13, the cause of the stem cell deficiency will likely determine whether it is a partial or total deficiency, whether it is associated with inflammation, and whether other components of the ocular surface aside from the stem cells are involved. Determination of these factors is crucial when a corneal transplant is considered as the ultimate rehabilitative step in the process.

The factors that are critical to the survival of a corneal graft include the adequacy of the stem cell reserve, aqueous- or mucin-deficiency dry eye, and anatomic lid abnormalities. In the absence of optimized conditions, the consequence for the corneal graft is that, even with excellent donor material and meticulous surgical technique, the patient may develop persistent nonhealing epithelial defects, secondary ulceration with stromal melting, vascularization and conjunctivalization, and ultimately immune graft rejection. In the context of a noninflamed eye, which has undergone successful stem cell replacement with a procedure such as a conjunctival limbal autograft or keratolimbal allograft, the subsequent placement of a lamellar or penetrating keratoplasty may stress the limits of the available stem cell reserve to produce recurrent ocular surface disease. Therefore, in any patient in which keratoplasty is a component of the therapeutic plan, there must first be an adequate stem cell supply, adequate tear function, and anatomically functional lids.

Review of the Literature

Unfortunately, the existing clinical series that discuss keratoplasty in the context of ocular stem cell disease are, in general, small and have varying degrees of follow-up. This limits our ability to draw any valid conclusions from these studies about which technique is optimal. Nonetheless, there are some general principles of management that can be adduced from these small clinical series. The primary question that has faced ocular surface specialists has been whether stem cell replacement should precede keratoplasty, or whether the best approach is simultaneous surgery. Those who would argue in favor of simultaneous stem cell replacement in penetrating keratoplasty cite the advantages of the need for only a single surgery, the use of a single-donor tissue for both stem cell replacement and keratoplasty, and, therefore, a procedure that presents only a single antigenic challenge. On the other hand, those who advocate sequential procedures suggest that a well-healed, noninflamed eye status post-stem cell transplant is the most favorable condition for a successful corneal graft and will, therefore, be associated with a considerably lower incidence of graft failure.

If one examines the literature over the last decade of the 20th century, there is clearly a division between the advocates of simultaneous combined stem cell transplantation/keratoplasty and those who advocate staged or sequential procedures. In 1989, Kenyon and Tseng[1] presented four cases of conjunctival limbal autograft in 26 consecutive cases in patients who had suffered chemical burns. They recommended that penetrating keratoplasty be performed at least one year after limbal transplantation. In 1997, Theng and Tan published a case report[2] in which a patient received a simultaneous keratolimbal allograft and penetrating keratoplasty with donor tissue from a single donor. The recipient was managed with perioperative immunosuppression and re-epithelized within 24 days. Follow-up of this patient was 21 weeks only, at which time the central cornea remained clear.

Tsubota et al.[3] published a series of 9 patients who underwent combined keratolimbal allograft with penetrating keratoplasty, once again with the donor tissue for the stem cell transplant and the keratoplasty from the same donor tissue. Five of these 9 grafts remained clear after 12.3 months. Although there were 2 episodes of graft rejection and 2 patients required a second limbal graft, visual acuity was improved in all 9 patients. In 1998, Tseng et al.[4] presented a series of 14 eyes that underwent staged procedures, the first stage of which was amniotic membrane transplantation, followed by a combined keratolimbal allograft and penetrating keratoplasty from the same donor. Although staged in a sense, in one group of the patients studied, the penetrating keratoplasties and keratolimbal allografts were performed at the same time, but subsequent to amniotic membrane transplantation. Nine of 14 eyes experienced a penetrating keratoplasty rejection, and 5 of 14 had recurrent surface breakdowns. Three of 14 experienced early keratolimbal allograft rejection. Frucht-Pery et al.[5] presented a small series of three patients with chemical trauma who underwent staged conjunctival limbal autograft, followed by penetrating keratoplasty 3 to 6 months later. Graft epithelialization was complete within 7 to 12 days, and there were no recurrent epithelial defects or graft rejections. In 1999, Tsubota et al.[6] presented a series of 28 eyes with simultaneous penetrating keratoplasty and keratolimbal allograft. The keratolimbal allograft and donor cornea tissue were from the same donor, and cyclosporin A was used systemically, beginning preoperatively and for one month in the postoperative period. Fifteen of 28 (54%) of the penetrating keratoplasties survived, while 13 of 28 rejected. Nine of the 13 had regrafts, and of these, 7 had a second episode of rejection. Four patients underwent a third penetrating keratoplasty.

Croasdale, Schwartz et al.[7] presented a series of 36 cases using staged stem cell transplantation followed by penetrating keratoplasty approximately 3 months later. They employed 2 eyes from the same donor for the keratolimbal tissue and a third donor for the corneal transplant. The patients were treated with topical corticosteroids as well as systemic cyclosporin A for 12 to 18 months. In a subsequent expansion of this series to 54 patients with keratolimbal allograft (personal communication), 35 patients underwent lamellar or penetrating keratoplasty 3 to 4 months post-stem cell graft and were followed for at least one year. Forty of these patients (74%) were stable, and 60% (21 of 35) had successful corneal grafts. Of the 14 failed grafts, 3 succumbed to endothelial graft rejection and 11 to recurrent ocular surface disease.

Rao et al.[8] reported 2 eyes with staged conjunctival limbal allografts, followed by corneal transplantation using limbal tissue from living, related donors. Patients were treated with topical and oral prednisone, and corneal transplantation was performed at 7 and 16 months, respectively, post-stem cell transplant. Both patients developed recurrent epithelial breakdown, although the vision improved to 20/40 in one of these cases.

An alternative approach that has been discussed in greater detail in Chapter 18 is the technique of Sundmacher et al. They employed a single-stage homologous penetrating central limbal keratoplasty using a corneal button harvested eccentrically from the donor eye, so that roughly 40% of the limbus from the donor was transplanted centrally into the recipient.[9] These patients were treated with cyclosporin A, and in 25 eyes of 24 patients, 18 of the transplants failed, either due to recurrent surface breakdown, graft rejection, or a combination of both.

As one can see from this brief summary of several of the major series from the literature that specifically relate to penetrating keratoplasty after stem cell transplant (either keratolimbal allograft or conjunctival limbal autograft), there are three basic approaches. These include (1) simultaneous stem cell graft and penetrating ker-

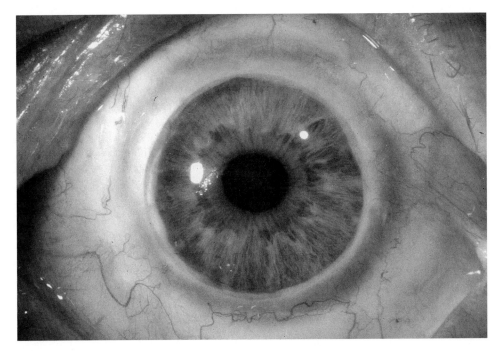

Figure 23.1. Successful penetrating keratoplasty after kerato-limbal allograft. Photograph 10 years postkeratoplasty.

atoplasty using the same donor tissue, (2) the staged approach, which consists of the appropriate stem cell surgery followed by penetrating or lamellar keratoplasty at a later date (Figure 23.1), and (3) a large eccentric donor graft supplying both limbal stem cells and the optimal keratoplasty. Both the simultaneous as well as the sequential approaches have theoretical advantages and disadvantages. The advantage of combined limbal stem cell transplant and penetrating keratoplasty using tissue from the same donor is that this technique (1) uses only a single donor cornea; (2) avoids two separate surgical procedures; and (3) avoids the introduction of additional antigens, thereby potentially diminishing the risk of graft rejection. On the other hand, the simultaneous stem cell/keratoplasty technique is associated with significantly greater technical difficulty. In addition, it is often associated with both increased inflammation at the time of corneal transplant as well as the placement of the graft in a destabilized ocular surface that has not yet had the advantage of stem cell replenishment.

The sequential procedure, on the other hand, also has advantages and disadvantages. Performing the stem cell graft and allowing the eye to heal prior to the keratoplasty affords stabilization of the ocular surface prior to the trauma of the corneal graft, and allows the surgeon to place the corneal transplant at a later date in a relatively noninflamed bed. On the negative side, this approach does require two separate operations, substantially prolongs the rehabilitative process, and, from an immunologic standpoint, presents the recipient with two separate antigenic challenges. As previously stated, the series in the literature to date are generally so lim-

ited in both numbers of patients as well as length of follow-up that no truly definitive conclusions can be drawn as to which procedure is best at this time. Both clearly have theoretical advantages and disadvantages.

Based on the largest series with the longest follow-up, as well as on our own clinical impressions, the authors favor a staged approach, which is more protracted but allows for surface stabilization and resolution of ocular surface inflammation prior to keratoplasty.

Some investigators advocate the use of lamellar keratoplasty instead of penetrating keratoplasty in order to utilize the healthy endothelium of the recipient. This technique eliminates the risk of endothelial rejection and minimizes the hazards associated with intraocular surgery. It is especially useful in cases such as aniridia, in which the final visual outcome will be predictably limited by macular function. Although it has the advantages outlined above, lamellar keratoplasty remains a technically challenging procedure.

Summary

Certain conclusions appear to be clear regardless of the planned surgical approach. The risk of graft rejection and/or recurrent surface disease is higher whenever penetrating keratoplasty is performed in the context of stem cell dysfunction and after a stem cell transplant. In both approaches, the risk of corneal graft rejection is higher than in the keratoplasty population in general. This mandates special considerations in the management of recipient immunosuppression and management of the ocular surface. Finally, larger studies with considerably longer follow-up will be necessary before the ideal surgical and adjunct medical regimens can be determined. It is clear that penetrating keratoplasty plays a significant role in the visual rehabilitative stage of stem cell transplantation. When corneal grafting is necessary after stem cell transplantation, meticulous attention must be paid to nurturing the ocular surface, and to immunosuppression, for the prevention of graft rejection.

References

1. Kenyon KR and Tseng SCG. Limbal autograft transplantation for ocular surface disorders. *Ophthalmol* 1989; 96:709–722.
2. Theng JT and Tan DT. Combined penetrating keratoplasty and limbal allograft transplantation for severe corneal burns. *Ophthalmol Surg Lasers* 1997; 28:765–768.
3. Tsubota K, Toda I, Saito H, Shinozaki N, Shimazaki J. Reconstruction of the corneal epithelium by limbal allograft transplantation for severe ocular surface disorders. *Ophthalmol* 1995; 102:1486–1496.
4. Tseng SCG, Prabhasawat P, Barton K, Gray T, Meller D. Amniotic membrane transplantation with or without limbal allografts for corneal surface reconstructions in patients with limbal stem cell deficiency. *Arch Ophthalmol* 1998; 116:431–441.
5. Frucht-Pery J, Siganos SS. Salomon A, Scheman L, Brautbar C, Zauberman H. Limbal cell autograft transplantation for severe ocular surface disorders. *Graefes Arch Clin Exp Ophthalmol* 1998; 236:582–587.
6. Tsubota K, Satake Y, Kaido M, Shinozaki N, Shimmura S, Bissen-Miyajima H., Shimazaki J. Treatment of severe ocular surface disorders with corneal epithelial stem cell transplantation. *N Engl J Med* 1999; 340:1697–1703.
7. Croasdale CR, Schwartz GS, Malling JV, Holland EJ. Keratolimbal allograft: recommendations for tissue procurement and preparation by eye banks, and standard surgical technique. *Cornea* 1999; 18:52–58.
8. Rao SK, Rajagopal R, Sitalakshmi G, Padmanabhan P. Limbal allografting for related live donors for corneal surface reconstruction. *Ophthalmol* 1999; 106:822–828.
9. Reinhard T, Sundmacher R, Spelsberg H, Althaus C. Homologous penetrating central limbo-keratoplasty (HPCLK) in bilateral limbal stem cell insufficiency. *Arch Ophthalmol Scand* 1999; 77:663–667.

24
Etiology of Limbal Stem Cell Transplantation Failure

Gary S. Schwartz and Edward J. Holland

Introduction

Only a short time ago, patients with severe ocular surface disease (OSD) from limbal stem cell deficiency had a dismal prognosis. The development of limbal stem cell transplantation procedures has dramatically improved our ability to rehabilitate the ocular surface of these patients. Despite these recent advances, there is a significant failure rate both in ocular surface transplantation and subsequent keratoplasty. This chapter will delineate the various causes of limbal stem cell transplantation failure and will discuss potential strategies to improve the success rate.

When evaluating whether a patient has had a successful result, it is imperative to consider the length of follow-up. Evaluation of short-term results (i.e., less than one year) reveals a high success rate with most techniques studied. It must be remembered that penetrating or lamellar keratoplasty in a patient with a total absence of stem cells will do well for the short term. An example of this is the practice of penetrating keratoplasty for patients with aniridia.[1] The aniridic patient with conjunctivalization of the cornea and stromal scarring achieves dramatic improvement in visual acuity immediately after penetrating keratoplasty. However, because aniridic patients have a limbal stem cell deficiency, when the inevitable sloughing of the donor epithelium occurs, it will be replaced by conjunctiva-like tissue. As a result, the ocular surface will fail.

We know from studies of epithelial rejection following keratoplasty that the donor epithelium can survive up to 13 months.[2] Therefore, when stem cell transplantation studies have follow-up of less than a year, it may very well be that the surface appears healthy because of the survival of donor corneal epithelium, rather than from repopulation by the transplanted stem cells.

Other factors important in evaluating success or failure of a particular stem cell transplantation technique is the preoperative diagnosis and severity of disease of the patients enrolled in the study. Patients with total limbal stem cell deficiency will be more difficult to rehabilitate than those with partial limbal stem cell deficiency, and patients with active conjunctival inflammation will have a higher failure rate than those with normal conjunctiva. This concept is discussed in detail in Chapter 13.

Also important are the various factors that one can evaluate in determining success versus failure. Stability of the ocular surface is the fundamental anatomic criterion with which to evaluate stem cell transplantation success. A stable ocular surface has the clinical features of a healthy transparent epithelium and is devoid of neovascularization and inflammation. A stable ocular surface results not only in improvement in visual acuity, but also in resolution of the pain that typically occurs in these patients because of conjunctivalization or persistent epithelial defects.

Another important factor in evaluating success of a limbal stem cell transplantation procedure is visual acuity. This factor is, of course, most important to the patient, and must not be forgotten by the clinician. Unfortunately, many patients with severe OSD have decreased visual acuity secondary to other ocular pathology, such as the aniridic patient with foveal hypoplasia. For this reason, visual acuity cannot be the only measure to evaluate the success of a particular technique.

In the authors' experience, approximately 50% of patients with OSD will require a subsequent penetrating or lamellar keratoplasty for visual rehabilitation. Many of these patients will develop with chronic endothelial rejection with a healthy ocular surface, and therefore graft clarity serves as another determinant of overall success.

The success of ocular surface transplantation has been reported to be between 0–75%.[1,3–5] Rao and co-workers in 1999 reported on their results with living-related conjunctival limbal allograft (lr-CLAL).[3] Donors were HLA-matched, and patients were not given systemic immunosuppression. In all patients, ocular surface went on to fail.

In 1999, Tsubota and co-workers reported their results using a keratolimbal allograft (KLAL) technique.[5] They reported a success rate of 51% (22 of 43 eyes) with a mean of 38 months follow-up (range 1 to 7 years). The authors reported results with KLAL on 25 eyes in 1996.[1] Fifteen of 25 eyes (60%) achieved a stable ocular surface. Follow-up in this study was a median of 20 months with a range of 6–63 months. Kenyon and Rapoza in 1995 reported their results with lr-CLAL.[4] Their patients had a 75% success rate with a mean follow-up of 19.5 months and a range of 10 to 40 months.

Early Stem Cell Transplant Failure

The causes of limbal stem cell transplantation failure can be categorized as early and late. Early failure is defined as occurring less than 12 months from the time of stem cell transplantation. The main causes of early failure include immunologic rejection, inflammation, eyelid abnormalities, and aqueous and mucin deficiency.

Acute rejection typically occurs between 2 and 12 months following transplantation. Review of the literature demonstrates several reports of acute stem cell transplant rejection. In 1993, Thoft and Sugar[6] described patients who had undergone a KLAL procedure that developed epithelial rejection. Clinical findings in these patients included injection, irregular epithelium, epithelial rejection lines, and subsequent epithelial defects. All three cases developed failed ocular surfaces despite aggressive topical anti-inflammatory therapy.

In 1991, Tseng and Tsai[7] reported three cases of rejection of KLAL. Two of the 3 cases were reported to be reversed with oral cyclosporin A. Tan reported 1 case of rejection in five eyes undergoing KLAL.[8] This rejection episode occurred on cessation of oral cyclosporin A 4 months following transplantation. It resulted in local irregularity of the epithelium at the site of rejection, which subsequently resolved.

In 2000, Daya described stem cell rejection as being either acute or low-grade.[9] He described 5 eyes of 4 patients that experienced rejection out of 27 eyes that had undergone KLAL. Four eyes had acute rejection, and one had low-grade rejection. The patients with acute rejection presented at a median of 7.5 months from the time of transplantation (range 2 to 12 months). Patients with acute rejection had symptoms of pain, intense injection at the limbus, edema of the lenticules, punctate epithelial keratopathy, and epithelial defects. Typically, the defects were peripheral and located near the area corresponding to the area of rejection. Three patients had biopsy of the donor tissue that revealed T-lymphocyte infiltration (CD4:CD8, 2:1) with strong HLA-DR (MHC class II) expression. Patients were treated with aggressive oral and topical immunosuppression, and 4 eyes required repeat KLAL for ocular surface rehabilitation.

The authors' clinical experience agrees with what has been described in the literature. Patients note symptoms of pain, redness and photophobia. Clinical examination demonstrates intense injection at the graft-host interface (Figure 24.1), and an epithelial rejection line may be present (Figure 24.2). With timely diagnosis and proper management (see Chapter 22), an acute rejection episode can almost always be resolved. Even though the graft will usually not immediately fail at the time of acute rejection, it has been our clinical experience that

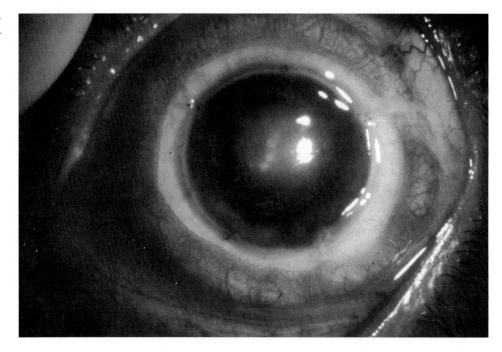

Figure 24.1. Acute stem cell rejection. This patient had a keratolimbal allograft 2 months before. Note the injection at the junction of the recipient conjunctiva and donor limbus.

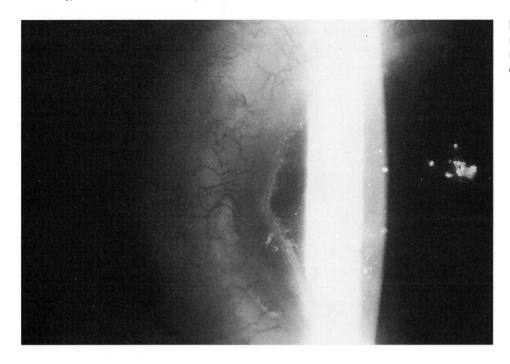

Figure 24.2. Acute stem cell rejection. Note the epithelial rejection line of keratolimbal donor tissue.

patients undergoing immunologic rejection of the stem cell graft do go on to have a higher rate of partial and total ocular surface failure.

Nonimmunologic inflammation is another contributing factor toward transplant failure. Patients with Stevens–Johnson syndrome (SJS), ocular cicatricial pemphigoid (OCP), or severe alkali injuries may have nonspecific inflammation that persists for years. These patients have a higher failure rate with ocular surface transplantation probably due to inflammatory trauma to the delicate transplanted limbal stem cells. In addition, the increased level of inflammation leads to a higher rate of immunologic rejection of the transplanted cells.

Eyelid and adnexal abnormalities can also contribute to limbal stem cell transplantation failure. Entropion, trichiasis and distichiasis can cause failure from chronic, direct trauma to the transplanted stem cell population. Ectropion and lagophthalmos can lead to stem cell failure through exposure and abnormalities in tear film coverage of the ocular surface.

Many patients with limbal stem cell deficiency will also suffer from severe aqueous and mucin deficiency, and keratinization of the ocular surface. In 1996, Holland described keratinization of the conjunctiva as a risk factor for limbal stem cell transplantation failure.[10] Patients with preoperative conjunctival keratinization had a significantly poorer result when compared to those without keratinization. He also described aqueous tear production as another useful parameter to predict outcome. In his study, patients with a Schirmer test of 2 mm or less at 5 minutes without anesthesia had a significantly poorer prognosis.

Late Stem Cell Transplant Failure

Late failure is defined as failure of the ocular surface occurring greater than 12 months after limbal stem cell transplantation. Late causes include sectoral conjunctivalization, low-grade rejection, late acute immunologic rejection, and stem cell transplant exhaustion.

Sectoral conjunctivalization is a process in which a wedge of conjunctiva-like epithelium invades a sector of the cornea (Figure 24.3). Patients present with a slow progression of abnormal, irregular epithelium moving centrally from the limbus. This abnormal epithelium is often accompanied by superficial neovascularization. Impression cytology of this tissue demonstrates goblet cells, and this finding confirms the conjunctival nature of this abnormal tissue. Chronic conjunctivalization will lead to subepithelial scarring; if the central cornea becomes involved, the patient may experience significant visual loss.

Sectoral conjunctivalization is typically seen in gap areas between transplanted areas of stem cell tissue. In the KLAL procedure, it can be seen in areas where a gap has been left at the time of surgery, or areas where there has been contraction during the postoperative healing process. It is not uncommon for conjunctival invasion to occur at the site of prior immunologic rejection.[8] In lr-CLAL procedures, the donor tissue is most often placed in the superior and inferior quadrants, and the nasal and temporal quadrants are left without transplanted stem cell tissue. In these patients, sectoral conjunctivalization will often occur at the nasal and temporal quadrants. This situation is one in which the stem-cell-derived epithelium seems to compete with the abnormal host

Figure 24.3. Conjunctivalization invasion between gaps in keratolimbal allograft donor tissue.

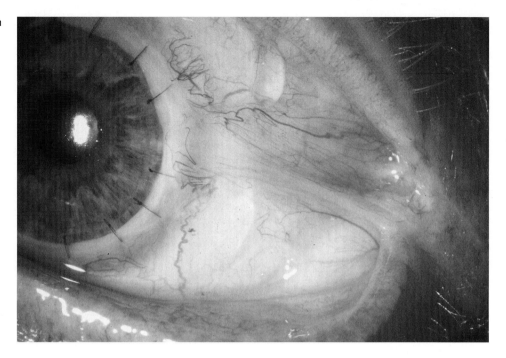

conjunctiva-like epithelium for repopulation of the corneal surface. Fortunately, rapid epithelization by the transplanted tissue usually impedes growth of conjunctiva-like tissue onto the corneal surface.

The treatment of sectoral conjunctivalization is dependent on the size of abnormal epithelium and the amount of inflammation. In cases of quiet eyes with small areas of conjunctival invasion, patients may benefit from sequential conjunctival epitheliectomy as described by Dua[11] (see Chapter 14). Patients with several clock hours or more involvement of the conjunctivalization process may benefit most from a partial repeat stem cell transplant to the involved area. If there is an inflammatory reaction associated with the conjunctivalization process, the clinician must entertain the possibility of chronic immunologic rejection. In these cases, topical and possibly even system immunosuppression may stabilize the ocular surface.

Late failure can also occur because of an episode of acute rejection occurring more than a year after limbal stem cell transplantation. These patients present similarly to those experiencing early failure acute rejection. Patients complain of pain, redness and photophobia. On examination they may have injection at the graft-host interface and may exhibit an epithelial rejection line. As discussed in Chapter 21, the ocular surface of these patients can usually be saved with intense topical and systemic immunosuppressive therapy.

There are also patients who fail late because of chronic, unresolved, low-grade inflammation. This inflammation most likely represents a chronic low-grade form of rejection as described by Daya.[9] These patients will demonstrate mild limbal injection, diffusely or in a sector and they develop conjunctivalization of the cornea in areas corresponding to the conjunctival injection.

The last form of late failure occurs secondary to limbal stem cell exhaustion.[12] In these patients, a slow, quiet conjunctivalization of the corneal surface occurs years after otherwise successful limbal stem cell transplantation (Figure 24.4). It is our clinical impression that this type of failure occurs more commonly following penetrating keratoplasty, or in patients with prior history of acute stem cell rejection. The etiology of stem cell transplant exhaustion are not well understood, and they may, in fact, represent a mild, quiet form of stem cell rejection. We, however, believe it to be secondary to the loss of mitotic activity of the transplanted stem cells over time. Mere transplantation of these delicate cells from one individual may limit their useful life span to 2 to 3 years in many cases. Recipient eyes are often inflamed, and exhibit aqueous tear and mucin deficiency, and these factors may also diminish the lifespan of the transplanted tissue. Subsequent penetrating or lamellar keratoplasty, bringing the added mitotic stress to repopulate the new corneal surface, may transform a marginally functioning transplanted limbal stem population into a case of limbal stem cell exhaustion.

Strategies to Improve Outcomes

Patients with severe OSD disease secondary to limbal SC deficiency provide a significant challenge to the clinician. Long-term success following limbal SC transplantation can be as low as 0% and as high as 75%, depending on the surgical procedure, the preoperative

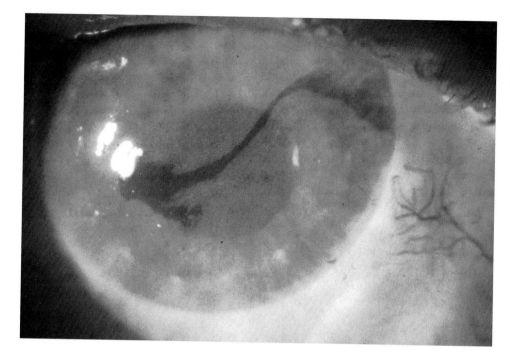

Figure 24.4. Late stem cell failure. Note hazy epithelium and late staining with fluorescein for most of the cornea. A wedge of normal epithelium persists.

diagnoses, and the staging of the patients. Unfortunately, many patients' ocular surfaces may go on to fail despite not only an excellent short-term surgical result, but also diligent postoperative care. Strategies have been developed to improve long-term results following limbal stem cell transplantation. These strategies can be categorized based upon whether they are undertaken preoperatively, intraoperatively, or postoperatively.

Preoperative Strategies

Long-term success following limbal SC transplantation can be maximized by recognizing and correcting certain preoperative risk factors for success. Many patients with limbal SC deficiency with conjunctival inflammation, such as patients with alkali injuries, SJS, or OCP will also have abnormal eyelid architecture. Cicatricial entropion, distichiasis, and trichiasis will often lead to SC transplantation failure from direct trauma. Ectropion and lagophthalmos can lead to failure of the ocular surface from exposure. To maximize outcomes, it is imperative that all eyelid abnormalities be repaired prior to, or concurrently with, the limbal stem cell transplantation procedure.

Patients with severe mucin and aqueous tear deficiencies must also be recognized prior to stem cell transplantation. Patients with severe tear abnormalities should be treated aggressively. We advocate tarsorrhaphy for the majority of patients undergoing SC transplantation. Patients with dry eyes will also benefit from punctal occlusion prior, and nonpreserved artificial tears after, SC transplantation. If a patient has total keratinization of the ocular surface, the surgeon should

consider not performing SC transplantation, since, in our clinical experience, nearly 100% of these patients will go on to eventually fail.

Many patients with severe OSD from limbal SC deficiency will also have significant ocular inflammation. A staging system that includes conjunctival inflammation is discussed in detail in Chapter 13. It is our clinical impression that nonspecific inflammation is a significant risk for limbal SC transplantation failure from both direct trauma to the transplanted cells and an increased likelihood of developing subsequent immunologic rejection. For these reasons, it is imperative that any inflammation be treated aggressively prior to performing limbal SC transplantation. For patients with inflammation from exogenous sources (i.e., alkali, acid or thermal injuries), the eye will often quiet considerably over time. Therefore, it is best to wait months to years after the injury before performing transplantation on these patients. For patients with inflammation from autoimmune sources (i.e., SJS, OCP), the surgeon usually does not have the luxury of the disease quieting down over time. These patients must be treated aggressively with topical and systemic immunosuppression in order to increase the likelihood of SC transplantation success.

Intraoperative Strategies

The most important intraoperative strategies are precise surgical technique, meticulous preparation of the transplanted tissue, and careful selection of the proper surgical procedure. These issues are discussed in detail in other places throughout this text.

Postoperative Strategies

Postoperative strategies exist that are crucial for successful ocular surface rehabilitation following limbal stem cell transplantation. The first of these is the appropriate use of systemic immunosuppression. Systemic and topical immunosuppression are mandatory during the postoperative period to ensure successful transplantation. Many reasons for stem cell transplant failure are related to inflammation. Early failure can be secondary to nonspecific inflammation and may be secondary to acute rejection. Late failure may be secondary to long-term rejection, late acute rejection, chronic low-grade nonspecific inflammation, or stem cell exhaustion (which may have inflammatory causes). Because inflammation is at the root of so many causes of early and late stem cell transplant failure, and because inflammation can normally be treated with aggressive topical and systemic medications, it is imperative to treat patients with failing ocular surface after transplantation with immunosuppression. The overwhelming number of cases of a failing ocular surface can be abated or even reversed with high-dose systemic and topical immunosuppression, and therefore it is our experience that almost all patients with failing surface should be treated with a trial of aggressive immunosuppression.

One other strategy in treating these patients after transplantation is to follow them postoperatively at short time intervals, even while asymptomatic. Early stages of failure such as mild inflammation or conjunctivalization may go unnoticed by the patient. Yet, if the signs and symptoms of these harbingers of surface failure are observed by the clinician, aggressive treatment may be initiated that may prevent subsequent failure of the ocular surface. In the authors' practice we typically examine limbal SC transplant patients at postoperative days 1, 2, and 3, weeks 1, 2, and 4, then monthly for the next 6 months. Obviously, patients may be seen more often as needed.

References

1. Holland EJ, Schwartz GS. The evolution of epithelial transplantation for severe ocular surface disease and a proposed classification system. *Cornea* 1996; 15(6):549–556.
2. Krachmer JH, Alldredge OC. Subepithelial infiltration. A probable sign of corneal transplant rejection. *Arch Ophthalmol* 96:2234–2237, 1978.
3. Rao SK, Rajagopal R, Sitalakshmi G, Padmanabhan P. Limbal allografting from related live donors for corneal surface reconstruction. *Ophthalmology* 1999; 106(4):822–828.
4. Kenyon KR, Rapoza PA. Limbal allograft transplantation for ocular surface disorders. *Ophthalmology* 1995; 102 (suppl):101–102.
5. Tsubota K, Satake Y, Kaido M, et al. Treatment of severe ocular-surface disorders with corneal epithelial stem-cell transplantation. *N Engl J Med* 1999; 340:1697–1703.
6. Thoft RA, Sugar J. Graft failure in keratoepithelioplasty. *Cornea* 1993; 12:362–365.
7. Tseng SCG, Tsai RJF. Limbal transplantation for ocular surface reconstruction: a review. *Fortschr Ophthalmol* 1991; 88:236–242.
8. Tan DTH, Ficker LA, Buckley RJ. Limbal transplantation. *Ophthalmol* 1996; 103:29–36.
9. Daya SM, Dugald Bell RW, Habib NE, et al. Clinical and pathologic findings in human keratolimbal allograft rejection. *Cornea* 2000; 19:443–450.
10. Holland EJ. Epithelial transplantation for the management of severe ocular surface disease. *Trans Am Ophthalmol Soc* 1996; 19:677–743.
11. Dua HS, Azuara-Blanco A: Limbal stem cells of the corneal epithelium. *Surv Ophthalmol* 2000; 44(5):415–425.
12. Holland EJ, Schwartz GS. Epithelial stem-cell transplantation for severe ocular surface disease, editorial. *N Engl J Med* 1999; 340(22):1752–1753.

25
Prosthokeratoplasty in Ocular Surface Disease

Mark J. Mannis

Introduction

The artificial cornea, or keratoprosthesis, is an idea that has fired the imagination and ingenuity of bioengineering ophthalmologists for over two centuries.[1] Over this period of time, investigators have attempted, with varying degrees of success, to produce a truly biocompatible and functional artificial cornea. Several reviews of the history of keratoprosthesis have been published in the ophthalmic literature.[2–8] Keratoprosthesis development cannot be discussed comprehensively in a text of this scope. We will provide only a brief overview of the subject in the specific context of the management of ocular surface disease.

Despite the enthusiasm for the concept of the artificial cornea, most of the clinical attempts at prosthokeratoplasty in both animals and humans have enjoyed only limited success, due to complex issues of materials biocompatibility as well as technical difficulty. Indeed, in the context of severe ocular surface disease, a keratoprosthesis is reserved for the patients in whom surface therapies, reconstructive surgery, and organic transplant are not feasible. It is, in a sense, the last resort.

Prosthokeratoplasty: Current Developments

The modern resurgence of interest in prosthokeratoplasty in the middle of the twentieth century was energized by the observation that slivers of polymethylmethacrylate (PMMA) were well tolerated in the eyes of World War II pilots who had suffered ocular injuries from shattered airplane canopies. This observation led, likewise, to the development of the intraocular lens by Sir Harold Ridley.[9,10] Polymethylmethacrylate became the substance of choice for keratoprosthesis research. It was particularly Stone who engaged in long-term testing of keratoprosthesis made of PMMA.[11,12,13] As the result of these experiments and others, PMMA emerged as the material of choice for the optical portion of the device. During the 1950s and 1960s, considerable efforts were made the world over to find both the best choice of materials as well as an optimal keratoprosthesis design.[14,15,16,17,18]

The last four decades of the 20th century have witnessed a proliferation in keratoprosthesis design (Figure 25.1). Researchers have sought a design that would eliminate the risk of serious complications. The predominant format was the "core and skirt" keratoprosthesis, consisting of an optical cylinder with a mid-stem plate or grid that could be inserted intralamellarly into the surrounding host stroma. Another, less favored, design (the "collar button") consisted of a central stem with anterior and posterior plates or flanges that clamped the cornea like a collar button (Figure 25.2).

Hernando Cardona developed and tested a number of perforating keratoprosthesis models, most of which consisted of a transparent perforating optical cylinder and a skirt to be placed intralamellarly into the surrounding cornea.[19] An early design included a PMMA optic cylinder anchored with an intralamellar fenestrated Teflon plate and covered with sclera or cornea and conjunctiva. The "nut and bolt" keratoprosthesis (1969) was composed of a PMMA shell similar to an external cosmetic contact lens and a 56 diopter polymethylmethacrylate cylinder anchored by both the external plate as well as a retrocorneal nut.[20,21] Experienced surgeons, including DeVoe and Castroviejo, applied Cardona's designs to patients and added their own innovations. These innovations included a through-the-lid implantation technique for end-stage dry-eye patients[21]; a modification that consisted of a through-and-through keratoprosthesis, a pigmented optical cylinder, and a perforated Teflon plate fixed to the cornea. This plate was overlaid with tibial periosteum and conjunctiva.[22] The Cardona device, even though reportedly implanted

Figure 25.1. Various keratoprosthesis types (c. 1960) (Reprinted with permission from W.B. Saunders Company, Philadelphia from Castroviejo, R. *Atlas of Keratectomy and Keratoplasty.* Fig. 13, p. 43. (English Edition), 1966. Originally published as *Atlas de Queratectomias y Queratoplastias*, Salvat Editores, S.A. Barcelona and by permission of Wayenborgh Press, 2001.

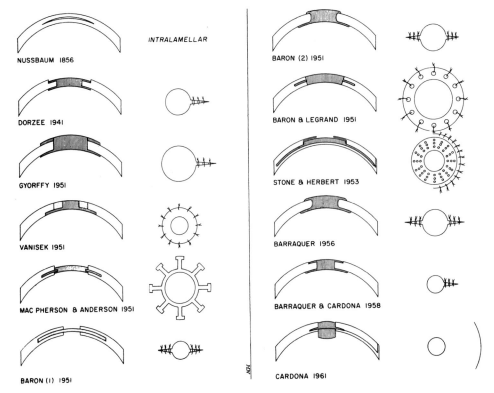

in over 1500 patients, had an extrusion rate of slightly greater than 20%. Buxton reported implantation of 33 Cardona nut and bolt keratoprostheses in 28 eyes with 5 extrusions.[23] Many investigators have published series of varying sizes reporting their outcomes with prosthokeratoplasty.[24–36]

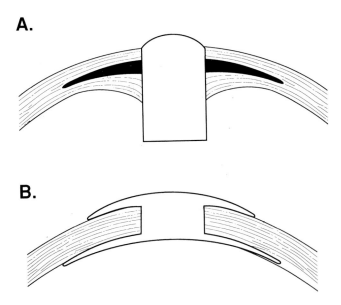

Figure 25.2. The two principal types of keratoprosthesis design employed since 1960. A. "core and skirt" held in place by a plate that is inserted into the surrounding tissue. B. "collar button" type with anterior and posterior plates that clamp the cornea.

The double plated (collar button) type of keratoprosthesis design has been used far less than the "core and skirt" design.[15,37] However, these attempts were largely abandoned in favor of intralamellar fixation models. in the mid-1960s Dohlman and co-workers adopted a collar button design and varied the dimensions as well as the presence or absence of holes and ridges. An additional nub was added for through-the-lid application in the end-stage dry eye.[38,39] (Figure 25.3) Dohlman emphasized the importance of aggressive postoperative management of the keratoprosthesis patient, particularly the management of postoperative inflammation. Approximately 140 patients have had a variation of this type of prosthesis implanted. Lacombe has similarly put a posterior fixation prosthesis to test in a number of patients.[40]

Biomaterials

The two primary technical issues that have emerged in the quest for the development of a successful keratoprosthesis have been (1) the identification of a skirt material that would permit biointegration with the tissue surrounding the cornea and (2) a method of successfully uniting the optical cylinder with the anchoring skirt. A variety of organic and nonorganic biocolonizable materials have been used in an attempt to maximize integration of the keratoprosthesis into the host tissues. Researchers turned to compounds that would permit biointegration with the host corneal tissue. In addition, tissue-derived materials or porous organic and nonor-

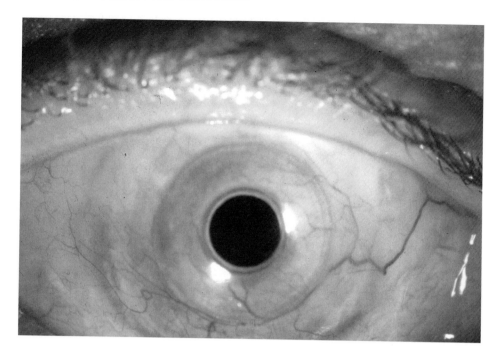

Figure 25.3. Example of a "collar button" keratoprosthesis (Dohlman). Reprinted from Mannis M and Mannis A. *Corneal Transplantation: A History in Profiles*, Wayenborgh Press, 1999; by permission from Wayenborgh Press, Oostende, Belgium.

ganic compounds have been employed. These substances have included cornea, sclera, bone, tooth, and coralline hydroxyapatite,[41] Dacron,[42,43] nylon,[44–46] siliconized Teflon, aluminum oxide ceramic,[33,47,48] proplast (vitreous carbon alloplast),[49,50] Gore-Tex, and Impra.[51–56] The range of polymers employed in prosthokeratoplasty are reviewed in detail elsewhere.[57]

The idea of a fully biointegratable device that might be implanted like a donor cornea has not yet been achieved. This device will require the employment of materials that foster epithelial growth on the anterior exposed surface, and that inhibit the development of retroprosthetic membrane formation and its attendant complications. With the specific goal of biointegration in mind, a variety of skirt materials have been employed, including hydrophilic polymers as described by Caldwell[6] and Chirila,[57,58] among others.

Along with the issue of biocompatibility of the keratoprosthesis with the recipient tissue, the mechanical relationship between the optical cylinder and the prosthesis skirt has emerged as an important technical issue. The problems that develop in the design of keratoprosthetic devices have, in part, related to the mechanical forces exerted on the prosthesis by movements of the eye and lids. Therefore, more recently, researchers have turned to the investigation of flexible keratoprostheses.[6,57]

Notable among these efforts to ensure biointegration and mechanical compatibility has been the work by a group of researchers at the Lions Eye Institute in Western Australia, who are evaluating poly(2-hydroxy ethyl methacrylate) PHEMA for the fabrication of a composite core and skirt (Figure 25.4). Since the optical component as well as the skirt are chemically identical, per-

manently fused, and flexible, the optical core-skirt interface problems that have plagued so many previous keratoprosthesis models may potentially be avoided. The mechanical stress at the skirt/host interface is obviated. In addition, hydrated PHEMA gels have a refractive index similar to human cornea. Copolymers of this type have been used as biomaterials in contact lens technology. The Australian researchers have performed both intrastromal implantations of the material as well as full-thickness implantations in an animal model.[57,58] The clinical viability of this keratoprosthesis design has yet to confront history's test. Still others have looked at buttons of reconstituted collagen in animal models.[59] The clinical efficacy of these newer approaches remains to be demonstrated at the time of this writing.

Prosthokeratoplasty in Ocular Surface Disease

Prosthokeratoplasty has been beset by technical challenges and fraught with complications despite well-documented and very notable successes, some of which have been long term. The primary complications have included dislocation and extrusion of the prosthesis, retroprosthetic membrane formation, secondary glaucoma, endophthalmitis, uveitis, retinal detachment, vitreous hemorrhage, and leakage around the keratoprosthesis with resulting hypotony, among others.

It is clear that, in an eye with severe corneal opacification that is otherwise normal, a keratoprosthesis may provide excellent vision. The question has been for how long—a question even more difficult to answer in the patient with severe ocular surface disease. Although keratoprostheses have now been indwelling for several decades in some patients, the differential survival rates

Figure 25.4. The Chirila keratoprosthesis. (Photograph courtesy
of Traian Chirila and reprinted
from Mannis M and Mannis A.
*Corneal Transplantation: A His-
tory in Profiles*, Wayenborgh
Press, 1999; by permission from
Wayenborgh Press, Oostende,
Belgium.

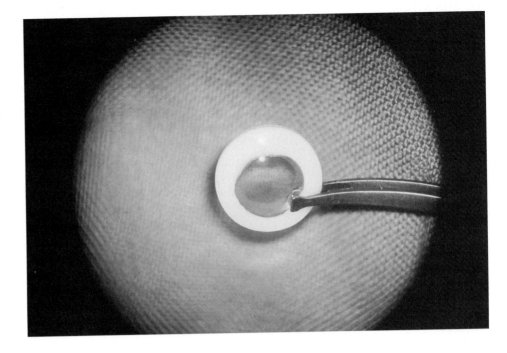

relate, to some extent, to the basic disease entity for which the prosthesis is employed. Patients with severe disturbances of the ocular surface, such as Stevens–Johnson syndrome, have an extremely poor prognosis. Noncicatrizing conditions, on the other hand, may do quite well, while surface diseases such as cicatricial pemphigoid and chemical burns occupy the prognostic midground.[8] As is true in the management of all ocular surface disease, the key factor appears to be the degree of inflammation.

Indications

Implantation of a keratoprosthetic device is generally undertaken when other surface reconstruction efforts for visual rehabilitation have failed, or are deemed unfeasible. As the repertoire of effective stem cell transplant procedures expands, the need for prosthokeratoplasty may diminish. Candidates for prosthokeratoplasty would include patients with severe bilateral chemical or thermal injury and patients with ocular cicatricial pemphigoid or Stevens–Johnson syndrome, in whom organic grafting procedures are not possible.

Complications

The major complications that have hampered prosthokeratoplasty historically and, indeed, to the present day include: (1) necrosis and dissolution of the tissue adjacent to the keratoprosthesis due to the action of proteolytic enzymes (collagenases),[60] which may lead to leakage, hypotony, endophthalmitis, and retinal detachment; (2) glaucoma: the advent of shunt devices in recent years has contributed to the control of this problem in many cases, although cyclodestructive proce-

dures may be necessary to augment pressure control;[61] (3) postoperative uveitis leading to membrane formation, retinal detachment, or macular edema; (4) retroprosthetic membrane formation. This membrane may occur in association with prolonged intraocular inflammation or bleeding in the eye. The YAG laser has been effective in dealing with thinner membranes; however, thicker membranes pose a serious problem.[62] The development of retroprosthetic membranes emphasizes the importance of care peri- and postoperative anti-inflammatory therapy; (5) infection.

No single keratoprosthesis incorporates all the desirable features to date. Progress in the field has been painfully slow, certainly slower than the evolution of tissue transplantation. This slow progress has resulted from the fact that postkeratoprosthesis complications may take years to develop, making it difficult to decide whether a change in a single parameter of design or management may truly make a difference. In addition, the demands of postoperative care in prosthokeratoplasty are considerable in both time and cost, leading to a substantial attrition rate of surgeons interested in the field. Finally, prosthokeratoplasty is technically demanding and is, therefore, practiced by a limited number of surgeons.

The newest generation of keratoprostheses, born of collaboration between ophthalmologists and polymer chemists, may pave the way to successful use of such a device in the patient with severe ocular surface disease. Such a device will allow peripheral tissue ingrowth, provide better optics, allow for the measurement of intraocular pressure, and withstand the pressures and flexures induced by ocular movements. The ultimate success of a keratoprosthesis in the setting of ocular surface disease will depend on its ability to function in the setting of a distinctly abnormal epithelium.

References

1. Mannis MJ and Dohlman CH. The Artifical Cornea: A Brief History. In: Mannis M and Mannis A. (eds.) *Corneal Transplantation: A History in Profiles*. 1999; pp. 321–335. Wayenborgh Press, Oostende, Belgium.

2. Pellier G. *Précis au cours d'operations sur la chirurgie des yeux*. Paris: Didot; 1789.

3. Barnham JJ, Roper-Hall MJ. Keratoprosthesis: a long-term review. *Br J Ophthalmol* 1983; 67:468–474.

4. Abel R. Development of an artificial cornea: I. History and materials. In: Cavanagh HD, ed. *The Cornea: Transactions of the World Congress on the Cornea III*. New York: Raven Press, Ltd.; 1988:225–230.

5. Barber JC. Keratoprosthesis: past and present. *Int Ophthalmol Clin* 1988; 28:103–109.

6. Caldwell DR. The soft keratoprosthesis. *Trans Am Ophthalmol Soc* 1997; XCV:751–802.

7. Leibowitz HM, Vickery T-T, Tsuk AG, Franzblau C. Progress in the development of a synthetic cornea. *Prog Ret and Eye Res* 1994; 13:605–621.

8. Dohlman C. Keratoprosthesis. In: Krachmer J, Mannis M, Holland E, eds. *Cornea*. III vol. St. Louis: Mosby-Yearbook, Inc.; 1997: 1855–1872.

9. Ridley H. Intraocular acrylic lenses after cataract surgery. *Lancet* 1952; I:118–121.

10. Apple DJ, Sims J. Harold Ridley and the invention of the intraocular lens. *Surv Ophthalmol* 1996; 40.

11. Stone WJ, Herbert E. Experimental study of plastic material as replacement for the cornea. *Am J Ophthalmol* 1953; 36:168–173.

12. Stone WJ. Alloplasty in surgery of the eye. *N Eng J Med* 1958; 258:533–540.

13. Stone WJ. Study of patency of openings in corneas anterior to interlamellar plastic artificial discs. *Am J Ophthalmol* 1955; 39:185–186.

14. Cardona H. Plastic keratoprostheses—a description of the plastic material and comparative histologic study of recipient corneas. *Am J Ophthalmol* 1964; 58:247–252.

15. Baron MA. Corneal and lens prostheses in plastic material. *Bull Soc Ophthalmol Fr* 1954; 67:386–390.

16. MacPherson DG, Anderson JM. Keratoplasty with acrylic implant. *Br Med J* 1953; I:330.

17. Sommer G. Neue Versuche zur Alloplastik der Kornea. *Klin Monatsbl für Augenärztliche Fortbildung* 1953; 122:545–554.

18. Chirila TV, Crawford GJ. A controversial episode in the history of artificial cornea: The first use of poly (methyl methacrylate). *Gesnerus* 1996; 53:236–242.

19. Cardona H. Keratoprosthesis: acrylic optical cylinder with supporting intralamellar plate. *Am J Ophhalmol* 1962; 54:284–294.

20. Cardona H. Mushroom transcorneal keratoprosthesis (bolt and nut). *Am J Ophthalmol* 1969; 68:604–612.

21. Cardona H, DeVoe AG. Prosthokeratoplasty. *Trans Am Acad Ophthalmol & Otolaryngol* 1977; 83:271–280.

22. Castroviejo R, Cardona H, DeVoe AG. The present status of prosthokeratoplasty. *Trans Am Ophthalmol Soc* 1969; 67: 207–234.

23. Buxton JN. Personal Experiences. *Trans Am Acad Ophthalmol Otolaryngol* 1977; 83:268–170.

24. Rao GN, Blatt HL, Aquavella JV. Results of keratoprosthesis. *Am J Ophthalmol* 1979; 88:190–196.

25. Aquavella JV, Rao GN, Brown AC, et al. Keratoprosthesis: results, complications, and management. *Ophthalmol* 1982; 89:655–660.

26. Choyce DP. The Choyce 2-piece perforating kerato-prosthesis: 107 cases—1967–1976. *Ophthalmic Surg* 1976; 8:117–126.

27. Choyce DP. Evolution of the Choyce 2-piece multistage perforating keratoprosthesis technique: 1967–1978. *Ann Ophthalmol* 1980; 12:740–743.

28. Sletteberg O, Hovding G, Bertelsen T. Keratoprosthesis II. Results obtained after implantation of 27 dismountable two-piece prostheses. *Acta Ophthalmol* 1990; 68:375.

29. Pushkovskaia NA. Keratoprosthesis as a method of vision in the sequelae of severe corneal lesions (English-language abstract). *Oftalmol ZG* 1985; 3:132.

30. Lund OE. Die Keratoprosthesis. *Der Deutsch Ophthalmol Ges*. Munich: Bergmann; 1977.

31. Moroz ZI. Artificial Cornea. *Microsurgery of the Eye, Main Aspects*. Moscow: Mir; 1987.

32. Worst JGF. Twenty-three years of keratoprosthesis research: present state of the art. *Refract Corn Surg* 1993; 9:188.

33. Polack FM. Clinical results with a ceramic keratoprosthesis. *Cornea* 1983; 2:185–196.

34. Kozarsky AM, Knight SH, Waring GO. Clinical results with a ceramic keratoprosthesis placed through the eyelid. *Ophthalmol* 1987; 94:984.

35. Singh IR. Central and paracentral perforating keratoprosthesis—an experience of 200 cases. *Refract Corn Surg* 1993; 9:191.

36. Yakimenko S. Results of a PMMA/Titanium keratoprosthesis in 502 eyes. *Refract Corn Surg* 1993; 9:197.

37. Barraquer J. Inclusion de protesis opticas corneanas; Corneas acrillicas o queratoprotesis. *Ann Inst Barraquer* 1959; 1:243.

38. Dohlman CH, Schneider HA, Doane MG. Prosthokeratoplasty. *Am J Ophthalmol* 1974; 77:694–700.

39. Doane MG, Bearse G, Dohlman CH. Fabrication of a keratoprosthesis. *Cornea* 1996; 15:179.

40. Lacombe E. Keratoprosthesis by retrocorneal fixation: results in 30 eyes over 3 years. *Refract Corn Surg* 1993; 9:199.

41. Rodan CR, Barraquer-G JI, Barraquer-M JI. Coralline hydroxyapatite keratoprosthesis: K-Pro abstracts: Presented at the Second KPro Study Group Meeting. Rome; 1995.

42. Refojo MF, Kalevar V. Keratoprosthesis with biological interface. *Invest Ophthalmol Vis Sci* 1972; 11:67.

43. Pintucci S, Pintucci F, Cecconi M, et al. New Dacron tissue colonizable keratoprosthesis: clinical experience. *Br J Ophthalmol* 1995; 79:825–829.

44. Girard LJ. Girard keratoprosthesis with flexible skirt: 28 years experience. KPro Abstracts: Proceedings of the first keratoprosthesis study group meeting. *Refract Corneal Surg* 1993; 9:194–195.

45. Girard LJ, Hawkins RS, Nieves R, et al. Keratoprosthesis: a 12-year follow-up. *Trans Am Acad Ophthalmol Otolaryngol* 1977; 83:252–267.

46. Girard LJ. Keratoprosthesis. *Cornea* 1983; 2:207–224.

47. Polack FM. Corneal optical prostheses. *Br J Ophthalmol* 1971; 55:838–843.
48. Polack F, Heimke G. Ceramic keratoprostheses. *Ophthalmol* 1980; 87:693–698.
49. Barber JC, Feaster FT, Priour DJ. Acceptance of a vitreous-carbon alloplastic material, proplast, into the rabbit eye. *Invest Ophthalmol Vis Sci* 1980; 19:182–190.
50. White JH, Gona O. Proplast for keratoprosthesis. *Ophthalmic Surg* 1988; 19:331–333.
51. Legeais J-M, Rossi C, Renard G, et al. A new fluorocarbon for keratoprosthesis. *Cornea* 1992; 11:538–545.
52. Legeais J-M, Renard G, Parel J-M, et al. Keratoprosthesis with biocolonizable microporous fluorocarbon haptic: Preliminary results in a 24-patient study. *Arch Ophthalmol* 1995; 113:757–763.
53. Strampelli B. Osteo-odontocheratoprotesi. *Ann Ottalmol Clin Oculist* 1963; 89:1039–1044.
54. Marchi V, Ricci R, Pecorella I, et al. Osteo-odonto-keratoprosthesis: Description of surgical technique with results in 85 patients. *Cornea* 1994; 13:125–130.
55. Falcinelli G, et al. Osteo-odonto-keratoprosthesis up to date. *Acta XXV Concilium Ophthalmologicum*. Milan: Kugler and Chadini, 1987.
56. Temprano J. Keratoprosthesis with tibial autograft. *Refract Corn Surg* 1993; 9:192.
57. Chirila TV, Hicks CR, Dalton PD, et al. Artificial cornea. *Prog Polym Sci* 1998; 23:447–473.
58. Chirila TV. Modern artificial corneas: the use of porous polymers. *TRIP* 1994; 2:296–300.
59. Devore DP, Kelman CD. Evaluation of collagen-based corneal grafts in the rabbit model. Kpro abstracts: Proceedings of the first Keratoprosthesis Study Group meeting. *Refract Corneal Surg* 1993; 9:208–209.
60. Dohlman CH. Biology of complications following keratoprosthesis. *Cornea* 1983; Volume 2(3)175–176, 1983.
61. Netland PA, Terada H, Dohlman CH. Glaucoma associated with keratoprosthesis. *Ophthalmol* 1998; 105:751.
62. Bath PE, McCork R, Cox KC. Nd:Yag laser discussion of retroprosthetic membrane: A preliminary report. *Cornea* 1983; 2:225.

26

Developing a Logical Paradigm for the Clinical Management of Severe Ocular Surface Disease

Edward J. Holland, Mark J. Mannis, and Gary S. Schwartz

Choosing the appropriate management plan for the patient with severe ocular surface disease, specifically from stem cell deficiency, requires a careful assessment of the nature of the surface pathology as well as its extent. Important factors to consider include laterality of disease, the extent of injury to the limbal stem cells, and the presence and cause of conjunctival inflammation.

The first determination that must be made is whether one or both eyes are involved. Laterality of disease is the most significant prognostic factor for restoration of the ocular surface and for visual prognosis. One of the first decisions is whether to operate on patients with only one involved eye, since they still have good vision in the opposite eye. Factors that influence the decision to operate include the occupational need for binocular vision, the integrity of the injured eye, or the degree of disruption of the patient's life secondary to chronic pain and inflammation in the injured eye. Figure 26.1 is a flow diagram outlining our approach to decision-making in management of the patient with unilateral stem cell deficiency. The discussion that follows will amplify the information in the diagram.

Unilateral Disease

Unilateral Conjunctival Disease

In the patient with unilateral disease, we must decide if the disease is primarily conjunctival, primarily limbal, or a combination of the two. A patient with unilateral disease limited to the conjunctiva does not require a limbal stem cell transplant procedure for surface restoration. A conjunctival autograft from the same eye or from the healthy fellow eye is the appropriate treatment. Indeed, if the disorder is limited to the conjunctiva, it is important not to harvest limbal tissue in order to avoid unnecessary insult to the limbal stem cell population. If autologous donor conjunctiva is not available, amniotic membrane can be used as a conjunctival substitute; the latter, however, is a less effective treatment than conjunctival autograft.

Unilateral Limbal Disease

In the patient with unilateral limbal disease, the appropriate treatment is determined by the extent of the limbal deficiency. For patients with partial limbal disease, especially with less than 50% stem cell involvement, a sequential conjunctival epitheliectomy may be an effective procedure. If this procedure fails, a stem cell replacement procedure should be considered.

Total unilateral limbal deficiency (or partial limbal deficiency that failed conservative treatment) without significant conjunctival disease requires a source of stem cell replacement. The fellow eye is clearly the best source of replacement stem cells, since autologous tissue eliminates the risk of allograft rejection. In these cases, a conjunctival limbal autograft (CLAU) is the most appropriate procedure. An alternative procedure may be an autograft of ex vivo expanded limbal stem cells, although at this writing the procedure is still in developmental stages.

Unilateral Combined Conjunctival and Limbal Disease

In this circumstance, the prognosis is more guarded due to both limbal stem cell disease and conjunctival dysfunction. Sources of stem cell replacement for these patients are similar to those for patients with unilateral limbal disease. However, in these patients amniotic membrane may be used because of the presence of con-

Figure 26.1. Flow diagram for management of the patient with unilateral stem cell deficiency.

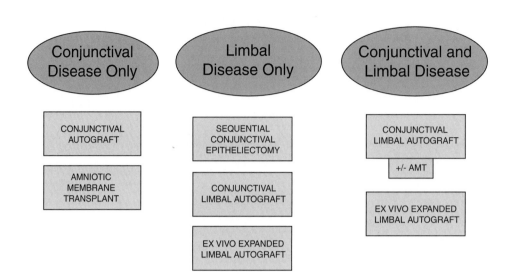

junctival inflammation. In this circumstance, ex vivo stem cell expansion may also be employed.

Bilateral Disease

A far more challenging clinical problem is the patient with severe bilateral surface disease. Figure 26.2 is a flow diagram that outlines our approach to the patient with bilateral stem cell deficiency. The key differentiating point in these patients is the extent and activity of conjunctival inflammation.

Limbal Disease with Normal Conjunctiva

With partial limbal involvement (<50%), sequential conjunctival epitheliectomy may be effective. However, in the vast majority of cases, limbal involvement requires a limbal stem cell transplant procedure. We feel that the procedure of choice in these patients is a keratolimbal allograft (KLAL), since it affords the most abundant source of stem cells and employs (relatively) readily accessible cadaveric donors. Conjunctival replacement is not required in these situations.

Figure 26.2. Flow diagram for management of the patient with bilateral stem cell deficiency.

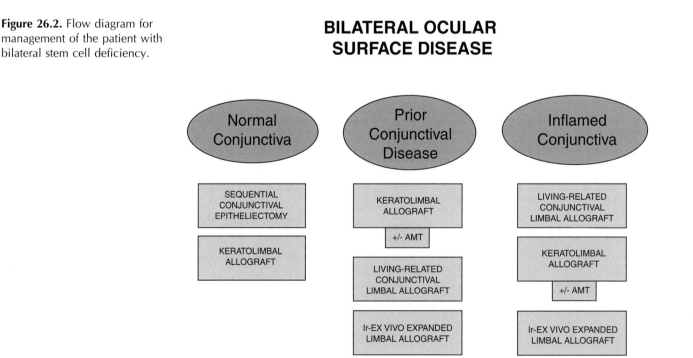

Limbal Disease with Prior Conjunctival Disease

This category includes patients who have suffered past injury or disease of the conjunctiva and have had time to allow for the resolution of inflammation and acute surface injury. In such patients, the decision will be whether to use a KLAL, or a living-related conjunctival limbal allograft (lr-CLAL). If the residual conjunctival damage is minimal, a KLAL may be the procedure of choice. If there are no living relatives available as donors, KLAL may be the only choice. However, if the extent of residual conjunctival injury is significant, the lr-CLAL, which provides conjunctiva as well as limbal tissue, may be a better choice of procedure. Ex-vivo expansion of a living related stem cell donation may be applicable in the future.

The decision to add amniotic membrane to the stem cell transplant procedure will be dictated by the presence of significant conjunctival disease.

Limbal Disease with Inflamed Conjunctiva

Bilateral limbal stem cell deficiency accompanied by conjunctival inflammation represents the worst prognostic category. Prior to any surgical intervention, every effort must be made to mitigate conjunctival inflammation. To this end, we employ both topical and systemic immunosuppression and anti-inflammatory therapy. It may also be extremely important to defer surgical intervention until inflammation has partially subsided, and the surface has stabilized.

The first choice of treatment in this group of patients is a living-related conjunctival allograft (lr-CLAL), since this donor procedure provides conjunctival epithelium and goblet cells in addition to limbal stem cells. Amniotic membrane transplantation is a useful adjunct in such cases because it helps in suppressing conjunctival inflammation.

If a living relative is not available as a source of donor tissue, KLAL is the next option with adjunct amniotic membrane transplantation. Ex vivo stem cell expansion may also be employed in such cases.

Finally, if there is significant preoperative keratinization of the bulbar conjunctiva and cornea and/or no aqueous tear production, stem cell surgery has a very poor prognosis. In such cases, a keratoprosthesis may be the only alternative available to the patient.

Case Presentations

The following clinical examples illustrate management decision-making in severe ocular surface disease:

Case 1: A 42-year-old Caucasian farmer presents with a unilateral nasal pterygium in the left eye and is symptomatic with chronic waxing and waning redness and irritation and, more recently, distortion of vision.

Diagnosis: Pterygium.

Procedure: Conjunctival autograft.

Comment: Conjunctival autograft is the procedure of choice for limited conjunctival pathology, as exemplified by a pterygium. An alternative approach is amniotic membrane transplantation (AMT). However, AMT may be associated with a higher rate of recurrence, and is more costly.

Case 2: An 82-year-old woman has a history of extracapsular cataract extraction, a subsequent trabeculectomy, and a 15-year history of treatment with pilocarpine. From the 11 to 1 o'clock meridians, there is a wedge-shaped area of abnormal epithelium with vascular pannus representing sectoral stem cell deficiency. She complains of redness and blurred vision.

Diagnosis: Sectoral iatrogenic stem cell deficiency.

Procedure: Sequential conjunctival epitheliectomy.

Comment: In the setting of partial limbal deficiency of less than 50% of the limbal tissue, surgical removal of the abnormal epithelium is a possible option. This technique may require several sequential resections. If this procedure fails, then stem cell replacement with a sectoral KLAL should be considered.

Case 3: A 24-year-old construction worker sustained a severe alkali injury to the left eye. There was no involvement of the right eye. After management of the acute disease and a waiting period of 6 to 8 months to allow surface inflammation to subside, surgical treatment was undertaken.

Diagnosis: Severe unilateral alkali injury with conjunctival and limbal deficiency.

Procedure: Conjunctival limbal autograft (CLAU).

Comment: This procedure is well established and remains the preferred treatment for unilateral stem cell and conjunctival deficiency. The risk to the fellow donor eye is minimal in the absence of any previous injury to that eye, and this approach avoids the need for immunosuppression. In the presence of continued conjunctival inflammation, amniotic membrane can be employed.

Case 4: A 38-year-old woman has a history of aniridia and progressive conjunctivalization of the entire cornea. There is significant anterior stromal scarring associated with the epitheliopathy. Visual acuity is 20/400 OU. Her best recorded acuity was 20/80, and in the past foveal hypoplasia was documented. The patient also has unstable intraocular pressure despite the use of multiple topical antiglaucoma medications.

Diagnosis: Limbal stem cell deficiency secondary to aniridia and poorly controlled glaucoma.

Treatment: (1) Glaucoma tube shunt; (2) keratolimbal allograft; (3) lamellar keratoplasty (staged procedures).

Comment: We recommend surgical intervention for glaucoma management if the patient requires more than one topical glaucoma medication. When the glaucoma is controlled, a KLAL should be carried out for rehabilitation of the ocular surface. If significant corneal stromal scarring remains after a successful stem cell transplant procedure, consideration of lamellar or penetrating keratoplasty is reasonable. We chose a lamellar keratoplasty for this patient due to her limited visual potential. Although technically challenging, lamellar keratoplasty avoids the added risk and morbidity of an intraocular procedure in this patient. Additionally, it avoids the risk of endothelial rejection following penetrating keratoplasty.

Case 5: This 56-year-old farmer has a history of injury to both eyes from anhydrous ammonia 25 years prior to this examination. There is total conjunctivalization of both corneas and subconjunctival fibrosis, but no active conjunctival inflammation. There is foreshortening of the inferior fornices bilaterally.

Diagnosis: Old alkali injury without active inflammation.

Treatment: Options for treatment include KLAL or lr-CLAL.

Comment: If there is extensive conjunctival scarring and symblepharon formation, lr-CLAL is the preferred procedure. If conjunctival involvement is less severe and/or a relative is not available, a cadaveric donor for KLAL is a reasonable option. Adjunct amniotic membrane may also be employed.

Case 6: A 48-year-old woman took an oral nonsteroidal anti-inflammatory agent for joint pain and developed severe Stevens–Johnson syndrome one year prior to presentation. Clinical findings include conjunctival injection, symblepharon, total corneal conjunctivalization, and trichiasis of the upper and lower lids.

Diagnosis: (1) Conjunctival and limbal deficiency secondary to Stevens–Johnson syndrome; (2) cicatricial entropion and trichiasis.

Treatment: (1) Repair of the anatomic lid abnormalities prior to stem cell transplantation; (2) living-related conjunctival limbal allograft and amniotic membrane transplantation.

Comments: Living related conjunctival tissue is necessary because of the extensive conjunctival damage. Amniotic membrane is useful because of the active conjunctival inflammation.

Although there is certainly more than one way to manage this spectrum of problems, the ophthalmologist should take into account, as illustrated in the foregoing cases, the laterality and extent of the disease. In addition, any consideration of surgical rehabilitation of the patient with ocular surface disease must first take into account the function of the ocular adnexa, as well as the adequacy of the tear film. Finally, many of these patients have both complex general medical as well as other eye problems requiring close monitoring. The local and systemic immunosuppressive agents required as adjuncts to surgical treatment add yet another layer of complexity to their safe and successful management. Therefore, comprehensive management using a team approach including ophthalmologist, internist, and technical support will best ensure a successful outcome.

Index

NOTE: Page numers in italics refer to illustrations; page numbers followed by the letter *t* refer to tables.